The A-Z Encyclopedia of Food Controversies and the Law

The A-Z
Encyclopedia of
Food Controversies
and the Law

Volume 1

A–P

ELIZABETH M. WILLIAMS
AND
STEPHANIE JANE CARTER

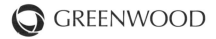 GREENWOOD

AN IMPRINT OF ABC-CLIO, LLC
Santa Barbara, California • Denver, Colorado • Oxford, England

Library of Congress Cataloging-in-Publication Data

Williams, Elizabeth M. (Elizabeth Marie), 1950–
    The A-Z encyclopedia of food controversies and the law / Elizabeth M. Williams and Stephanie J. Carter.
        p. cm.
    Includes bibliographical references and index.
    ISBN 978-0-313-36448-8 (hard copy : alk. paper)—ISBN 978-0-313-36449-5 (ebook) 1. Food law and legislation—United States. I. Carter, Stephanie J. II. Title.
    KF3869.W53   2011
    344.7304'232—dc22   2010039262

ISBN: 978-0-313-36448-8
EISBN: 978-0-313-36449-5

15   14   13   12   11   1   2   3   4   5

This book is also available on the World Wide Web as an eBook.
Visit www.abc-clio.com for details.

Greenwood
An Imprint of ABC-CLIO, LLC

ABC-CLIO, LLC
130 Cremona Drive, P.O. Box 1911
Santa Barbara, California 93116-1911

This book is printed on acid-free paper ∞

Manufactured in the United States of America

Contents

List of Entries

Topical List of Entries

ADVERTISING

Advertising of Alcohol Products
Advertising of Food
Children and Food

AGENCIES AND ORGANIZATIONS

Center for Consumer Freedom
Center for Science in the Public Interest
Centers for Disease Control and
   Prevention
CPR Food Industry Dispute Resolution
   Commitment
Department of Health and Human Services
Environmental Protection Agency
Federal Trade Commission
Food and Drug Administration
National Organic Standards Board
Occupational Safety and Health
   Administration and Slaughterhouses
   Safety
U.S. Department of Agriculture
World Trade Organization

AGRICULTURAL LAW/FARMING AND AGRICULTURE

Agricultural Disaster Assistance Program
Agricultural Personal Property, Taxation,
   and Exemptions
Agricultural Revenue Insurance
Agriculture and Livestock, Urban
Carson, Rachel
Chicken, Organic
Clean Water Act
Cloning
Community-Supported Agriculture
Cooperatives
Cooperatives, Agricultural
Environmental Protection Agency
Ethanol
Family Farm in Bankruptcy,
   Reorganization of
Farm Bill
Farm Labor Laws and Regulations
Farm-to-Table Prices
Farms, Corporate
Farms, Family
Federal Crop Insurance
Fish Farming
Foie Gras, Bans on
Foraged Foods
Free-Range Farming
Genetic Engineering
Growth Hormones
Humane Slaughtering Practices
International Plant Protection
   Convention
Irradiation
Loans and Banking, Agricultural
Packers and Stockyards Act
Perishable Agricultural Commodities Act
Pesticides
Poultry Products Inspection Act
Runoff, Agricultural
Seeds, Genetically Engineered
Soil, Organic
Subsidies
Sustainability
Taxation, Agricultural
Transportation of Agricultural Products,
   Interstate
Treaty on Plant Genetic Resources for
   Food and Agriculture
U.S. Department of Agriculture

LEGAL SYSTEM

LEGISLATION

LITIGATION

MEAT AND POULTRY INDUSTRIES

RESTAURANT LAW AND ISSUES

Americans with Disabilities Act and
   Restaurants
Business Meals, Tax Deductions
Copyright of Recipes and Dishes
Credit Cards and the Restaurant Industry
Equal Employment Opportunity
   Commission and Restaurants
Espionage, Food
Franchises and Restaurants
Hazard Analysis Critical Control Point
Health Regulations, Local Restaurant
Minimum Wage Law and Restaurant
   Workers

Molecular Gastronomy
Pelman, et al. v. McDonald's
   Corporation
Portion Sizes
Restaurant Labeling, Non-Nutritional
Restaurant Leasing
Restaurant Nutritional Labeling
Service Animals in Restaurants and
   Grocery Stores
Sweetened Drinks, Taxes on
Trans Fat
Zoning

SALES

Alcoholic Beverage Control Stores
Alcohol, In-State Distribution of
Alcohol, National Distribution of
Credit Cards and the Restaurant Industry
Distribution of Food
Farm-to-Table Pricing

Foie Gras, Bans on
Forbidden Foods
Internet Sales
Interstate Commerce
Pricing

STATE LAW

Alcohol, In-State Distribution of

State Legal Systems

TAXES AND TAX LAW

Agricultural Personal Property, Taxation,
   and Exemptions
Business Meals, Tax Deductions
Fior D'Italia v. United States
Green Markets and Taxation
Groceries, Taxes on
Internet Sales

Interstate Sales
Prepared Foods, Taxes on
State Law and Federal Law,
   Conflicts between
State Laws, Conflicts between
Sweetened Drinks, Taxes on
Taxation, Agriculture

THREATS AND FOOD

Biological Warfare and Food
Bioterrorism Act of 2002
Espionage, Food

Federal Anti-Tampering Act
Food as a Weapon

TRADE/IMPORT/EXPORT

Appellation d'origine contrôlée
Boycotts
Embargoes

European Union Regulations
Fair Trade
Genetic Engineering

Preface

This encyclopedia, the first devoted to food and the law, offers nearly 200 entries that allow a general reader who is interested in food to understand the legal concepts applicable to food. It covers the way that the powers of the three branches of government—the executive, the legislature, and the judiciary—impact the process of the development of law. In addition, this text lays out issues that the states impact and discusses the role of local governments.

The encyclopedia is designed to address food on a larger scale, as in policies and laws that reflect social trends. In addition to discussing the specific laws, this reference makes it possible to understand how food affects our society and, conversely, how our society affects food. It is aimed at students looking for information on food controversies or interested in food law. It is also aimed at the general public, such as health advocates and parents, who want to know more about the major food issues of our time (organics, genetic engineering, bioterrorism, food safety, and obesity lawsuits) and how the law works. Readers will find a fascinating window into the restaurant business, food business, and food service industries, as well as current farming practices.

The encyclopedia is easily searchable, written in plain English without jargon, and contains the current state of the law of food and drink in the United States and, where applicable, in the world. The underlying legal principles are also summarized; if, for example, one is interested in reading about the obesity lawsuits but does not really understand the court system, one can also read about the court system. It is our hope that this resource gives readers a depth of understanding that is greater than what would be gotten from merely reading about the lawsuits in the popular press.

The introduction presents an overview and sets the philosophical construct of the encyclopedia. A Topical List of Entries lists the broadest topics of food law so that readers can find those of interest quickly.

The encyclopedia is arranged alphabetically by topic. We have tried to provide a wide range of topics so that the reader can not only see the way that food law touches everything and everyone—after all, we all eat—but the reader will also see how intertwined the law is in our lives. Law is influenced by literature, politics, economics, religion, and aesthetics. Thus, the range of entries is vast, from legislation, people, actions, rules and regulations, legal cases, food and beverage industry controls, restaurants, and organizations. It addresses the special concerns of children and those with allergies and disabilities. It encapsulates fast food to organics and sustainability and the environment. Health topics include coverage on alcohol and soda, nutrition, food supplements, labeling, and obesity. There is a strong focus on the business of food in regard to commerce, taxes, trademarks, and even food espionage. There is something for everyone.

Although we did try to give examples of specific cases that were food related, we did not fill each entry with legal citations. Readers should be able to get the complete information within the entry without access to a law library.

The entries contain cross-references to related entries or related appendix material, either within the entry as **bolded** entry names or after entries as "See Also" listings. Most entries also have further reading suggestions—books, articles, laws, and cases, or Web sites—for follow-up and more in-depth research.

If readers wish to discover more cases, books, or articles, a local law library and the Internet should be good places to start. Although many of the cases can be found on the Internet, some of the articles and books are only available in a library. We hope that readers' interests are sufficiently piqued to seek these other sources of information.

The Chronology, a listing of important events in the development of food law, is another supplement to the entries. The development of law is cumulative, based on what has come before; thus, knowing the order in which the law developed is important. In addition, the chronology places each development in history, so that one can see the context in which issues are taken up by Congress and the courts.

The Appendix contains a number of primary documents: court cases; laws, regulations, and regulatory review, and international agreements. The court cases were chosen to illustrate those covered in the entries. Reading the cases will allow the reader to understand legal reasoning of courts, as well as see specific cases that have influenced the law of food. Other documents illustrate what is covered in regulations. Seeing the level of detail given in regulations written about a particular subject allows the reader to see why courts may need to fill in gaps in regulation and how regulations affect the conduct of business. We hope that as you read the cases, perhaps seeing a court's words for the first time, you can see the source of so much of what happens in our lives every day.

Other documents are laws. Reading the general nature of the laws illustrates the need for regulations, which are written in even more detail than legislation. The documents also illustrate international conventions and how they affect the law of food. Although these documents are designed to supplement the entries, if one reads them in the order that they are presented, they unfold into another way to understand and approach law, by gradually revealing how courts apply the law and how legislation supplies it.

The contributors are not all lawyers, but they all work with food law in their work. They are chefs, writers, academics, and lawyers.

We hope that this set becomes a valuable reference tool, but it is not designed to be a substitute for the counsel of an attorney. It contains the law as it relates to food from the soil and water through manufacturing and processing to transportation and distribution to restaurants and grocery stores and farmer's markets. This is the law of food from field to fork.

Elizabeth M. Williams and Stephanie Jane Carter

Introduction

In the 21st century, we have seen an interest in food develop and then explode into a national obsession. Not only are people debating taste—which type of chocolate tastes best, and should it be dark or milk—but they are extending the debate to include many factors that impact the production of food and the morality of eating.

Perhaps there was a time when food was merely fuel for the body, but no more. Today, food is the arena of debate. It is the analog for the entire gamut of moral questions that we face today—trust in government, public health, environmental impact, sustainable practices, humane treatment of animals, responsible treatment of workers, prepared foods and preservatives, and the list goes on and on.

The thing that links us all as human beings is the need to eat and drink. So it seems natural that eating has given rise to this great debate. And as people crystallize their ethical and political positions on various aspects of food and eating, they also tend to want to impose their positions on others. They accomplish this through the law.

Sometimes local law is the vehicle for change, as in the Chicago ban on the sale of foie gras in restaurants in the city in 2006. The Chicago city council enacted the ordinance as a response to activists who convinced the council that the image of the city would be enhanced by this enlightened stand on the forced overfeeding of ducks and geese. Although the ban survived a court challenge, the city council ultimately repealed the law. While the law was in effect, there was clamor on both sides over the rectitude of the ban. People cared.

Humans have regulated and restricted food and food production throughout history. In the United States, some of these restrictions have become adopted by federal, state, or local legislation. Five justifications for regulating food have evolved—the two original and historical justifications and three additional more modern ones:

1. Religion—restrictions on sale and manufacture of certain foods because of religious beliefs
2. Consumer protection—legally imposed limitations put on what may be included in food sold to consumers and the requirement for certain product labeling
3. Health—legally imposed limitations of what may be claimed by food product manufacturers, limitations regarding manufacturing and handling of food to avoid tainted and spoiled food, and limitations in the use of certain "unhealthy" ingredients
4. Power and class—limits on who may have access to food

5. Animal rights—limits on food production methods that are considered cruel
   and unnecessary to the animals to be eaten

Any of these justifications may form the basis for legislation or regulation that controls accessibility to or restriction from particular foods or beverages. However, whatever the motivation for government action may be, not all justifications are morally or constitutionally supportable. To assess the constitutionality of legally imposed regulation, it is necessary to balance rights and dangers rigorously to distinguish the bitter pill of power and control from benign and benevolent protection.

It is the role of the U.S. Constitution to limit government interference with our basic freedoms, the freedom to eat what we choose being inherent in life, liberty, and the pursuit of happiness. Any limitation on the rights of citizens is an inherently serious and important topic. Because everyone eats, these restrictions affect everyone. Restrictions on constitutional rights for whatever reason are serious and should be justified for only the most important reasons. Knowing the justification tells us something about the society and its values. That justification can be either so important that it overrides the protected freedom to eat what we please, or the justification fails to be compelling and is thus unconstitutional.

In applying this analysis a court, ultimately the U.S. Supreme Court—the final arbiter of constitutionality—is figuratively determining where to place a phantom fulcrum on a balance. On the one side rest the reasons to restrict and on the other the reasons to allow. Deciding which rights to protect and how to protect them is a process in constant flux. And today reasonable people can differ as to the need to protect the public from its own actions and the need to protect the right of the public to make personal choices.

In determining which justifications provide a moral or constitutional basis for the restriction of the consumer's access to food stuffs, we should examine each of these justifications separately. As is usual in life, they do not fall neatly into categories, but overlap messily.

Religious Belief and Right-Eating

Today's progressive society and principles of separation of church and state or some other form of secularism require us both to tolerate the religious beliefs of others and to refrain from legally imposing our beliefs on them. Thus, if a person desires not to consume alcohol or caffeine for religious reasons, that person is free to abstain. At the same time, those substances are available to others. For example, in the United States, the religiously observant may refrain from drinking or eating products that contain caffeine, some may refrain from drinking alcohol, and yet others may not eat pork or shell fish, but all of these products are generally available. The religious proscriptions are not secular legal proscriptions, because of the constitutional principle of the separation of church and state established in the First Amendment to the Constitution. The desire of the religious to use the law to limit the choices of those citizens who do not share their beliefs would not be supported by the Constitution.

Although actual religious beliefs have not caused restrictions, sometimes it is the fervor manifested by food zealots of one stripe or another that has become a threat to the pleasures of the table, cultural food customs (known as foodways by anthropologists), and the constitutional rights of nonbelievers. Beliefs about proper eating can rise to the level of pious cult, complete with the need to proselytize and convert others, and to impose beliefs on others by force. These people might justify the use of force—here the force of law—because of their belief that they are morally right and that they are protecting those who do not eat properly from their own ignorance.

Religion as a basis for food restriction is not a constitutionally protected justification. The freedom to practice one's own religion or one's own lack of religion is a highly protected constitutional right, and the legal imposition of the religious beliefs of others on a society is an immoral and unconstitutional use of government power. However, religion is respected, so it is possible to label foods as acceptable according to certain religious laws. There is legislation, such as kosher and halal labeling, that is regulated to ensure that religious laws are actually complied with as a form of consumer protection.

Consumer Protection

Protecting the consumer from adulterated food has a long history. In medieval Europe, guild laws protected the honest craftsman as well as the unwary consumer. As food is processed outside of the sight of the consumer, it gives rise to the need for laws to protect the consumer from the unscrupulous. The more elaborate the processing, transforming the food into a different product, the more important consumer protection laws are. The safety and condition of processed food are not transparent; thus, defects are not observable by simple inspection.

In some instances, consumer protection protects the health of the consumer, for example, by prohibiting the addition of or substitution of unwholesome products. The recent recall of dog food containing adulterants is an example of the problem caused by unseen additives.[1] Other consumer protection laws protect the quality of the product, for example, real maple syrup sold in a bottle labeled maple syrup, instead of maple-flavored syrup.[2] The purpose of the consumer law is to ensure that the consumer gets what is promised.

In other words, consumer protection law is a use of law to keep the consumer safe from the deceptive and immoral acts of others. It has been established that buyers can be protected within constitutional bounds, even though the legislation that protects consumers causes some restriction of the unfettered rights of sellers and manufacturers. Subsets of the consumer protection law are the labeling laws, informing the consumer of nutritional information about processed products. The more information there is about products, the more informed the consumers' choices can be. The two basic controversies over labeling are what information

---

[1]See the various listings on the recall site of the Food and Drug Administration, http://www.fda.gov.

[2]Vermont Statutes Annotated, Title 6, Chapter 32, Sections 481 et seq.

should be disclosed and who should disclose. But no one can force the consumer to use the information in a healthful manner, and the consumer has the right to make poor choices.

Health

Closely related to consumer protection, regulations to protect our health are generally considered to be acceptable limitations on freedom. As with consumer protection arguments, the more processed a food is, the more we need to rely on the government to protect us. As we learn that a particular cookie may contain peanut oil and a child is allergic to it, reading the label that discloses ingredients is a proper use of the law and regulation to protect our health. However, banning peanut oil, because some people are allergic to it, is overreaching.

Public health is protected in other ways—for example, limiting the number of rodent hairs present in our food. But the sense of balance—what is the health risk versus what is the cost of restriction to freedom—is the key to a constitutional justification for restriction. Here, the science of food and nutrition becomes central to finding this balance. In assessing the health risk, we must rely on scientific study, which sometimes must be approached with skepticism. The scientific community cannot always agree on methodology, the number of tests to run, the number of subjects that are representative, and the proper algorithm to use to extrapolate its findings to fit the general population. Without scientific consensus, government restrictions may be ill-founded, premature, and extreme.

For example, with the support of the U.S. government, hydrogenated vegetable oil was developed to substitute for animal fats used in cooking.[3] It was touted as a healthful alternative to lard and butter, and it had a long shelf-life. Advertising campaigns urged people to eschew lard and butter in cooking and substitute hydrogenated oil. As a result, at least one generation has grown up preferring the taste of hydrogenated oil. Now scientific tests have suggested that trans fat, formed by the use of hydrogenated oil can be harmful to our health.[4] The scientifically manipulated, once "healthful" food, is now demonized. There have been attempts to ban foods containing trans fat. The city of New York has imposed such a ban.[5] Of course, we can live without hydrogenated oils. Using the law to protect our health, the government must take the least restrictive path, and the restriction should be based on well-established science. The limitations put on food manufacturers is small, and there are alternatives that will not be noticeable to the consumer.

---

[3]Greg Critser, *Fat Land* (New York: Houghton Mifflin, 2001), 15.

[4]Dariush Mozaffarian, Martijn B. Katan, Alberto Ascherio, Meir J. Stampfer, and Walter C. Willett "Trans Fatty Acids and Cardiovascular Disease," *New England Journal of Medicine* 354 (April 2006): 1601–613.

[5]Title 24, Rules of the City of New York, Article 81 (NY City Health Code), section 81.08, voted December 5, 2006.

Banning through the Courts

Besides bans created by legislation, a trend in the United States has been to use the courts as a means to enforce a ban. A lawsuit against McDonald's (2005), claiming that it had caused a person to become fat, a lawsuit against Kentucky Fried Chicken (2006) because its product contained trans fat, and a threatened lawsuit against Kellogg's (2007) because it markets sugary cereal to children are examples of the use of the courts to advance the agenda of consumers.[6] The existence of these lawsuits shows the degree of fervor of belief held by the health advocates, as well as the interesting position of the corporations re-inventing themselves in the court of public opinion.

Power and Class

Being able to have this discussion about freedom and choices is a lesson in the continued distinction between those who are well off and educated and those who are not. The moral issues that are raised by those who can afford the healthiest food—let us call this the food that is organic, grown using sustainable methods, untainted by hormones and antibiotics—and those who eat the mass-produced food that is less expensive, are myriad. But these are not necessarily constitutional issues. The societal issue is that all have access to food that is wholesome and sustains life.

Too often, it is the poor who are forced to eat and to allow their children to eat the least expensive, fat-laden, and sugar-laden foods. In trying to arbitrate these food choices, it may be precisely because the foods are fat- and sugar-laden that they are affordable. By changing the standard of acceptability, we may be making people unable to afford to eat. As Starbuck's scrambles to eliminate trans fat from its muffins, people who never set foot in a Starbuck's, because the latte there costs more than an entire meal, may not receive any benefits. The efforts to manipulate our food, however well-meaning, may be creating a further divide by class and power and economics.

Animal Rights

A recent, visible achievement of animal rights activists and food is the banning of the sale of foie gras in the city of Chicago, although the ban was subsequently repealed. Foie gras is a luxury item unnecessary for survival. Fighting for the availability of foie gras, then, makes the advocates seem elitist and selfish. In addition, the number of producers of foie gras is small, and they are not an organized lobby. This makes them an ineffective group when lobbying for

---

[6]*Pelman v. McDonald's Corp.* 396 F. 3rd 508, 2005 U.S. App. LEXIS 1229 (2d Cir. NY, 2005);, CSPI press release, June 12, 2006, http://www.cspinet.org/new/200606121.html; Kellogg's press release, June 14, 2007 http://www.kelloggcompany.com/uploadedFiles/KelloggCompany/Home/Press%20Release%20-%20U%20S.pdf; CSPI press release, June 14, 2007, http://www.cspinet.org/new/200706141.html.

themselves. A successful campaign against the foie gras producers can be seen as a blow to the small farms movement, since most foie gras producers are small independent farmers, not large corporate producers. Their vulnerability to animal rights activists merely parallels their overall vulnerability in an ever-encroaching corporate farm atmosphere.

It remains to be seen whether other industries will also be attacked in the same way or whether practices will be required to be improved rather than the product itself banned. Beef and chicken are so basic to the American diet that if humane treatment of animals becomes a true public concern, it is unlikely that it will result in the ban of beef and chicken.

Regulation and Administration

Finally, there are rules and regulations that are not about freedom to choose, but about order and the functioning of the rules themselves. These are rules that require reporting and self-regulation, adherence to inspection schedules, and the payment of fees. These administrative laws represent the governmental function of maintaining order. They are just as important and must be followed just as assiduously as the laws for protection and safety. Paying taxes, creating data bases of information, zoning, and registering businesses are all examples of everyday administration.

Sometimes administration and morality become entangled in the law. The regulation of alcohol sales is an example of this conjoined function. The regulation reflects the concern regarding the morality of alcohol sales and the specifics of the administrative tasks. The differences in the laws from state to state reflect the different attitudes about the morality of alcohol. But even with the occasional confusion of purpose, the administrative laws are all important in making sure that business can operate, trusting that by following the law that contracts will happen, there will be orderly flow of permits and licenses, and that the rules of operation are the same for everyone to create a level playing field.

Economics and Politics

The politics of power is reflected in food law just as it is in all other aspects of life and law. Agribusiness and the subsidies under the various farm bills, anti-trust, and control of groceries and stockyards, and deceptive business practices in packing houses all reflect the power of lobbying, political policy making, and the reaction to unfairness, such as civil rights laws.

The American ideal is to be a nation of laws. The unspoken implication of this maxim is that each person is equal in the eyes of the law. But politics and money have produced laws that have consequences that do not fall equally on all. Food subsidies, special taxes, and the shifting of burdens from government to individuals all have economic and policy consequences that make a knowledge of the applicable law more important today than ever before.

Globalization

The increasing globalization of the economy and culture mean that Americans eat food from all over the world, whether or not we are aware of it. Farmers and food manufacturers ship food from the United States to all parts of the world, both as a part of commerce and as a form of foreign aid. And the global economy means that investments made in the United States may be affected by laws applicable in countries where multinational corporations operate across oceans. All of these factors make an awareness of international law as it affects food important and relevant. It is relevant in developed nations that use the finished product, as well as developing countries that provide raw materials.

Policy

Food law both reflects and influences the way we live and the way we eat. Just as Upton Sinclair exposed practices about stockyards and meatpacking that were not illegal, but which offended and alarmed the country, writer Michael Pollan is affecting the way people want to eat and what they expect in their food. Sometimes it is enough to let the market influence production and choices, as people vote with their wallets. Sometimes the swell of opinion in a certain direction will result in changes in the law. And changes in the law result in changes in behavior and attitude.

This is the unwritten law of chicken and egg, each influencing the other, seamlessly reflecting each other. Does the written law reflect society's values and norms or influence them? The answer is it does both. Knowledge of the law of food allows a person to both recognize what is reflected from society and influence food law by putting pressure on legislative bodies, bringing lawsuits, and informing the public.

Elizabeth M. Williams
New Orleans 2010

Chronology

1202   The Assize of Bread, proclaimed by King John of England, prohibits the adulteration of bread with peas and beans and other substances. Considered the first food safety law in England.

1789   Adoption of the U.S. Constitution, containing the commerce clause, forms the underlying authority for much of U.S. law affecting food and drink.

1862   President Abraham Lincoln appoints Charles M. Wetherill to the Department of Agriculture. He begins the Bureau of Chemistry, which later develops into the Food and Drug Administration.

1883   The Bureau of Chemistry expands its studies in food adulteration, headed by Harvey W. Wiley (chief chemist), also known as the "Father of the Pure Food and Drugs Act."

1898   A Committee on Food Standards is formed by the Association of Official Agricultural Chemists. The food standards are adopted in many states. There is growing interest in establishment of national standards and regulations.

1906   Author and journalist Upton Sinclair publishes *The Jungle*, a novel/exposé of the Chicago meat-packing industry through the human story of the immigrants who worked and lived around the plants.

1906   Meat Inspection Act, which comes directly out of outcry over Upton Sinclair's novel, *The Jungle*, is passed addressing the unsanitary conditions, use of dyes and poisonous substances as preservatives, and banning false claims from the sales of patent medicines.

1906   Pure Food and Drug Act of 1906 requires that all foods and drink in interstate commerce be properly labeled and free from adulterants, considered the beginning of the Food and Drug Administration.

1907   Certified Color Regulations are passed, certifying seven colors that could safely be used in food.

1908   The U.S. Supreme Court in the case of *North American Cold Storage Company v. Chicago* rules that the city of Chicago has the right to seize and destroy food that has been contaminated by vermin in the interests of public health over issues of due process.

1913   The Gould Amendment to the Pure Food and Drug Act of 1906 is the first law to require that food packages be clearly marked by weight or other suitable measure, such as numerical count.

1914   *US v. Lexington Mill and Elevator Company*. In this case the U.S. Supreme Court holds that the use of nitrates in bleached flour could not be prohibited without showing that the presence of nitrates was harmful to health. The presence of the nitrates is not in itself illegal without such a showing.

1920   Eighteenth Amendment to the U.S. Constitution, which bans the manufacture, sale, and transportation of alcohol for human consumption, officially beginning the period popularly known as Prohibition.

1921   The Packers and Stockyards Act is passed in response to the findings of the Federal Trade Commission that there is gross manipulation of the marketplace by meat packers and stockyards resulting in unfair monopolies and fraudulent practices.

1924   *US v. 95 Barrels Alleged Apple Cider Vinegar.* In this case the U.S. Supreme Court affirms that the Food and Drug Act prohibits the use of deceptive, fraudulent, and misleading claims, even if technically true.

1933   The Twenty-first Amendment to the U.S. Constitution repeals the Eighteenth Amendment and ends Prohibition.

1935   The Federal Alcohol Administration Act is passed to allow for the establishing of regulations and control of the alcohol industry after the repeal of Prohibition.

1938   Food, Drug, and Cosmetic Act of 1938 includes standards for quality and fill-of-container in foods, factory inspections, and expansion of remedies for violations. This law greatly expands the role of the Food and Drug Administration (FDA) and includes cosmetics.

1939   The first food standards are promulgated, beginning with tomatoes.

1946   The Administrative Procedures Act is finally enacted after almost 10 years of effort. During this year, 18 new regulatory agencies are established as a part of the New Deal of the administration of Franklin D. Roosevelt. This act lays the foundation for the issuance of government regulations by such agencies as the FDA and the U.S. Department of Agriculture.

1947   The Lanham Act, also known as the Federal Trademark Act, takes effect after passage in 1946. This act establishes the laws of trademark protection in the United States.

1949   The FDA issues what is called the Black Book of industry procedures and practices, officially, *Procedures for the Appraisal of the Toxicity of Chemicals in Food.*

1950   The Oleomargarine Act requires that margarine that is colored yellow be labeled in an obvious way so that consumers are not deceived into thinking that it is butter.

1954   Miller Pesticide Amendment states standards for maximum residue of pesticides in unprocessed agricultural products.

1958   The Food Additives Amendment establishes the requirement that new additives be established as safe.

1958   The FDA publishes the first "generally regarded as safe" list, establishing the principle that using substances from the list is permissible without further establishment of safety.

1960   The Color Additive Amendment requires that colors be established as safe to be used in cosmetics, drugs, and food.

1960   The Delaney Amendment bans the approval of any color additive shown to cause cancer.

1962   Rachel Carson's *Silent Spring* is published by Houghton Mifflin, warning of the environmental problems caused by the pesticide DDT. This is considered the trigger for the environmental movement.

1963   The Food and Agriculture Organization (FAO) of the United Nations establishes the Codex Alimentarius Commission. The Codex Alimentarius is a suggested international code of good food practices, sanitary regulations, and other matters related to food production. The Commission makes recommendations to the FAO and the United Nations.

1964   Food Stamp Act marks the beginning of the modern Food Stamp program.

1965   The Equal Employment Opportunity Commission is established as an independent agency to prosecute the claims of discrimination in employment after the passage of the Civil Rights Act of 1964.

1966   The Fair Packaging and Labeling Act is passed as a consumer protection law that requires informative and accurate labels.

1969   The FDA begins sanitation inspections into many industries—shellfish, milk, roadside travel facilities–in interstate commerce. The obligation had previously been the duty of the Public Health Service.

1970   The Egg Products Inspection Act is adopted by Congress to ensure the safety of egg handling, transportation, and sale.

1970   The Environmental Protection Agency is established to ensure the safety of the water and air in the United States.

1971   The Center for Science in the Public Interest is founded as a nonprofit advocacy and watchdog organization to ensure public awareness of health problems caused by many factors including unhealthy food practices.

1972   The Federal Water Pollution Control Amendments establish the goal of eliminating pollution in the surface waters of the United States.

1973   Outbreaks of botulism cause the FDA to issue standards regarding food processing and canning of low acid foods.

1977   The Saccharin Study and Labeling Act is passed after the artificial sweetener, saccharine, is banned from the "generally regarded as safe" (GRAS) list. Public demand for the sweetener causes the passage of the act, which allowed its use but required prominent labeling.

1977   The Clean Water Act mandating the elimination of discharge of toxins into streams and waterways is passed.

1979   The Department of Health, Education, and Welfare (HEW) is divided and the new Department of Health and Human Services is established, retaining most of the duties of HEW except education.

1982   After the Black Book, the FDA publishes the Red Book, *Toxicological Principles for the Safety Assessment of Direct Food Additives and Color Additives Used in Food.*

1990   The Americans with Disabilities Act is passed, recognizing the rights of those people with disabilities to have access to public accommodations, such as restaurants, and to require employers to make reasonable accommodations for them in the workplace.

1990   The Organic Foods Production Act establishes the infrastructure to write the regulations of the organic food industry and the creation of the National Organic Program and the National Organic Standards Board.

1992   Nutrition Facts are required on consumer packaging of foods, reorganized on a per serving basis and written in an easy-to-read chart.

1993   The European Union is established through the Treaty of Maastricht, creating a framework for laws governing all of the participating nations in Europe.

1994   The FDA approves the first genetically engineered product, a tomato.

1994   Dietary Supplement Health and Education Act exempts vitamins and mineral supplements from the jurisdiction of the FDA.

1996   The Saccharine Notice Repeal Act allows for the repeal of saccharine notice.

1996   The Center for Consumer Freedom is founded by lobbyist Rick Berman to represent the interests of the food industry and to educate the public about pending laws and regulations.

1997   The Food and Drug Administration Modernization Act revises many agency practices and regulates health claims asserted for consumption of foods.

2000   Dietary supplements are limited in the types of statements that can be made for their products.

2001   Eric Schlosser writes *Fast Food Nation: The Dark Side of the All-American Meal*, uncovering the practices of the fast food industry and its effect on American diets.

2002   Scholar Marion Nestle writes *Food Politics: How the Food Industry Influences Nutrition and Health*, exposing the influences of the food industry and politics in the making of public health policies about food.

2002   California jury awards $132 million to group of bakery workers from Hostess/Wonder Brands for racial discrimination in *Carroll, et al. v. Interstate Brands Corporation*.

2002   The initial filing of the first so-called obesity lawsuit, *Pelman, et al. v. McDonald's Corporation*, by several plaintiffs in District Court for the District of New York, alleging that McDonald's is responsible for plaintiffs' obesity.

2002   The decision by the U.S. Supreme Court in *United States v. Fior D'Italia, Inc.* that the Internal Revenue Service could place the burden on restaurants to correctly report the amount of tip income received by their employees.

2002   The Public Health Security and Bioterrorism Preparedness Response Act of 2002, also known as the Bioterrorism Act, is passed to empower the U.S. Department of Agriculture and the Department of Health and Human Services to regulate certain toxins that could affect the food and water supply of the United States.

2003   Announcement by the FDA that rules will be promulgated and will add trans fat content to the nutrition label required on all food products.

2003   An FDA statement makes it clear that food safety is an important national goal. It commissions the "Scientific Criteria to Ensure Safe Food," study released by the National Academy of Sciences.

2003   The FDA issues regulations banning use of downer cattle in the human food supply.

2003   The U.S. Court of Appeals, Second Circuit, strikes down as unconstitutional the kosher regulations of the State of New York in *Commack Self-Service Kosher Meats, Inc. v. Weiss* because they violate the separation between church and state.

2004   The Food Allergy Labeling and Consumer Protection Act requires special labeling of foods containing ingredients that come from high-allergy groups such as peanuts and wheat.

2005   In *Granholm v. Heald*, U.S. Supreme Court rules that laws in Michigan and New York banning the direct purchase of wine from out-of-state wineries and shipped to Michigan and New York interfere with interstate commerce.

2006   The City Council of Chicago passes an ordinance that bans the sale of foie gras in the city limits.

2006   Writer Michael Pollan's *The Omnivore's Dilemma: A Natural History of Four Meals* is published. It reflects the huge interest in healthy eating and the questioning of food produced by large corporations in the United States.

2007   The U.S. Department of Agriculture establishes rules for the use of the term "organic."

2007   New York's ban on trans fat in city's restaurants becomes effective.

2008   U.S. Department of Agriculture recalls downer beef from a slaughterhouse (Hallmark/Westland Meat Packing Company) in California that had been sent for use in the National School Lunch Program.

2008   California bans artificial trans fat in restaurants in food facilities.

2008   Marion Nestle writes *Pet Food Politics: The Chihuahua in the Coal Mine*, illustrating the interconnection between the human and pet food supplies.

2008   Farm Bill mandates that grocery stores and other retailers post or label country of origin of meat and produce.

2009   Sara Lee, maker of Ball Park Franks, sues Kraft Foods, maker of Oscar Mayer Franks, objecting to Kraft's claim that Oscar Mayer Franks are better than Ball Park Franks.

2009   President Barack Obama declares the U.S. food safety system a "hazard to public health" and promises to revamp it.

2010   California law banning artificial trans fat in restaurants takes effect.

A

ADDITIVES AND PRESERVATIVES

Food additives and preservatives are included in foods during the manufacturing process to help keep them fresh and inhibit growth of pathogens, as well as to enhance or maintain color. Additives can also improve flavor and texture. Food additives are listed on the label in the same way as other ingredients—in descending order by weight. Sometimes, the name of the additive is spelled out in full; however, when it is a standard additive that is used, the additive is represented by a number.

The U.S. **Food and Drug Administration** (FDA) is the agency appointed by Congress to monitor and approve food additives. According to the FDA there are three categories of additives. Indirect food additives are the package and the wrapping that touches the packaged food. These materials can include paper, glue, film, and plastic. Direct food additives are placed directly into the food. This type of additive can be preservatives, vitamins or other supplements, flavorings, and textures. Color additives are used to maintain or improve the color of food.

Almost all processed foods contain some sort of food additive. They are added to create additional value, to extend shelf-life, to keep the food safe for consumption, or to make the food more attractive. The FDA has identified more than 3,000 approved additives that appear on their lists and can be used without testing.

Preservatives are additives that preserve food and extend its shelf-life. There are three categories of preservatives. First are the ones that act to inhibit the growth of bacteria or the growth of fungi in food. An example of this inhibitor is the mold inhibitor, propionic acid, used in bread. A second type of preservative keeps food from oxidizing. Oxidation makes food darken and discolor, as well as become rancid. Nitrates and nitrites are used in meats to inhibit oxidation, which discolors meat, making it less attractive to the consumer and more prone to spoilage. The third type of preservative is used in fresh uncooked foods. This type of preservative can inhibit the ripening process. Benzoates inhibit bacterial growth.

Yet another category of additive is flavoring. Flavorings are either natural (made from natural ingredients) or chemical. They are used particularly in processed foods to enhance sweetness, add more of an inherent flavor (for example, fruitier), or introduce new flavors, such as butter flavor when no butter is used in the food.

In 1958 Congress passed the Food Additives Amendment to the Food, Drug, and Cosmetic Act. The amendment imposes the requirement that the FDA test and approve an additive before it can be used in food. When a manufacturer wishes to use an additive that is not pre-approved, the burden is on the manufacturer to prove that the additive is safe before the FDA can approve it for use in food. This means that an additive manufacturer is required to petition the FDA for approval before the manufacturer can market a new additive. No processer will use the new product without it being approved. The products that processors can use without further approval are found on the FDA's list. According to the FDA, manufacturers petition for about 100 new additives each year.

Most studies are done by dosing animals with the additive. These studies may cover extended periods of time to prove that the additive does what it is manufactured to do. It also must prove to be safe for humans when consumed at the normal and expected levels. The FDA will also accept human studies.

There is a set of criteria for examining additive petitions. The FDA reviews and examines the chemical composition of the additive. It determines the reasonable amount that will be consumed by humans in normal usage. It also examines the side effects and residual effects of consumption of the additive, and the intended use and the claims made for the substance are reviewed. There is no way to make a prediction of safety with absolute certainty, but the FDA can make a reasonable prediction based on the results of its testing. In making its determination, the FDA may take into consideration the record of the use of the additive in other countries, journals and scientific writings, and studies, trials, and opinions of food scientists and others.

When the FDA determines that an additive is safe enough to be included in the approved list, it determines the amount of additive and its ratio to other ingredients, the description that should be used on the label, and the use that can be made of the additive, including which foods may include the additive. Using the additives on the approved list makes it possible for a manufacturer to avoid waiting for approval of new additives.

The **U.S. Department of Agriculture** (USDA) has additional approval authority over additives used in meat and poultry. Even after approval, the agency continues to review and study the use of the additive and will reassess its approval criteria based on consumption studies and actual usage.

The Adverse Reaction Monitoring System (ARMS) of the FDA ensures that, as use of the additives changes or its interaction with other additives changes, the additive and its use remains safe. Complaints, made by individuals and physicians, that are related to additives of all types are investigated and a database is maintained. Use of the database helps determine whether reactions in different locations reveal a pattern of reactions or a pattern of lack of effectiveness. This ongoing safety check keeps the system under constant review.

Stephanie Jane Carter

The Assize of Bread

The Assize of Bread and Ale is credited with being the first consumer protection law related to food. Passed in the 13th century during the reign of Henry III of England, the law prohibited the use of adulterants in bread and ale. In addition, it regulated the weight of bread and the quality of beer. Bread and ale were generally not made at home. Ovens were expensive. Because the manufacture occurred outside of the view of the consumer, it was necessary to protect the consumer and set standards for the industry. Beans were used to increase the weight of the bread, because flour was expensive. The law prohibited this practice.

ADMINISTRATIVE PROCEDURES ACT

The Administrative Procedure Act (APA) creates a uniform system of rules and regulations needed to implement and enforce major legislative acts passed by Congress. These regulations are made by agencies that form part of the executive branch. The rules and regulations created by the executive branch are implementing in detail the more general action taken by the legislative branch.

The law is designed to provide a logical and consistent rubric that gives uniformity to the rule-making process of all federal executive departments and 55 independent federal administrative agencies such as the **Food and Drug Administration**, the **Environmental Protection Agency**, the **Interstate Commerce Commission**, and others.

The APA establishes a methodology for all types of hearings that may be necessary to ensure due process and public accessibility and transparency. These functions include those hearings necessary prior to rule making, as well as those that may be called for after rule making, challenging a rule. These are called adjudicative hearings. When there is a conflict between agencies, there is also a procedure for intra-agency review. Intra-agency review is important so that the public knows which rules are applicable. The public also needs a resolution of conflicts between and among rules. Finally it also establishes a procedure for judicial review, when agency review is insufficient to resolve issues. The APA also establishes rights, including rights of public access to administrative hearings, rights to counsel at hearings, and importantly the rights of an individual to privacy when information is collected by an agency. Not all information so gathered is public. It also ensures due process by providing a procedure in which federal courts can review decisions made by *agencies*. These agencies are making rules that have the force of law, so a transparent method that allows for input from the public is essential.

Congress passed the act in response to concerns about each agency's ability to safeguard individual rights and to shine a public light on the rule-making process. The APA has been referred to as a "bill of rights" for citizens whose lives are so impacted by federal regulation.

The APA is credited with bringing consistency, regularity, and principles of judicial review to what had previously been chaotic and unpredictable. For example, the APA established the requirement that proposed regulations need be promulgated in the *Federal Register* no less than 30 days prior to becoming effective. Also, all regulatory agencies must provide avenues for comment on proposed legislation, as well as objections and suggestions. These comments and objections become part of the public record of the rule making of the government. This public record can be referenced in case of judicial challenge of the rule making or interpretation.

The APA became law in 1946 following a decade of draft, revision, and debate and during a time of expanding federal government. Eighteen new regulatory agencies were created by the Roosevelt Administration as part of President Franklin D. Roosevelt's New Deal package to lift the country from the Great Depression. (Eleven new agencies were created between 1776 and the end of the Civil War in 1864; 6 were created between 1865 to 1900; 35 were created between 1900 to 1940.)

The APA passed after a contentious political battle. On the one hand, there were those who did not approve of what appeared to be an expansion in government. The advocates of the new law wanted to create a structure that made rule making open and less susceptible to control by political agenda. Once the act was passed on the federal level, most states followed suit and adopted similar legislation on the state level in the period from the late 1940s and early 1950s. Many other nations have passed administrative procedure acts as models for their own legislation.

The provisions of the APA require months and sometimes years of iteration and reiteration of proposed regulations, conciliation, and compromise to create landmark regulation such as that stemming from the Food, Drug, and Cosmetic Act, the **Clean Water Act**, and the Controlled Substances Act.

Individuals, businesses, and private and public organizations that violate federal regulations are subject to the same types of sanctions that may arise from the violation of legislation. These may include fines and cease-and-desist orders. Because the consequences of not following rules and regulations can be as serious as for violating legislation, it is now considered essential that the openness and specificity of regulation be promulgated to be enforceable.

See also: Appendix 1: *United States v. Fior D'Italia, Inc.*; Appendix 6: *United States v. Park*; Appendix 7: *In the Matter of McCormick & Company, Inc.*, Appendix 8: California Organic Products Act of 2003; Appendix 10: Senate Bill Introduced into the 111th Congress, Amending the Food, Drug, and Cosmetic Act; Appendix 13: Excerpts from the Code of Federal Regulations Regarding Cheese and Cheese Food.

William C. Smith and Elizabeth M. Williams

ADVERTISING OF ALCOHOL PRODUCTS

Alcohol consumption, such as of wine, spirits, and malt beverages, is promoted through a variety of media. Media outlets include, but are not limited to, television, print media, billboards, and the Internet. Along with tobacco advertising, alcohol advertising is one of the most highly regulated forms of marketing. The Alcohol and Tobacco Tax and Trade Bureau (TTB), the newest bureau under the Department of the Treasury, collects alcohol excise taxes; ensures that the products are labeled, advertised, and marketed in accordance to the law; and administers the laws and regulations to protect the consumer and revenue and encourage compliance. It promotes compliance with the Federal Alcohol Administration Act of 1935 and the Internal Revenue Code. The Federal Alcohol Administration Act was created in 1935 to regulate the alcohol industry after the repeal of Prohibition. Section 205 (f) pertains to advertising of alcohol.

Alcohol advertising, one of most regulated forms of marketing in the United States, is regulated along with tobacco. There are several reasons for this combination. First, there are age restrictions on purchasing both products. Under state and federal law, one must be at least 21 years old to purchase alcohol products. This restriction puts alcohol into a range of products that have been called "rite of passage products." These products are understood by consumers as a mark of adulthood, independence, and choice. There is also a risk of abusing both alcohol and tobacco. Although alcohol may be less addictive than tobacco, even short-term overuse of alcohol causes physical impairments. Long-term effects of over-use of alcohol are well-documented. Both tobacco and alcohol are highly taxed by the government.

As the regulatory agency that governs the marketing and sale of alcohol, the TTB enforces several restrictions on advertising these products. Like other advertised products, advertisements for alcohol must be truthful and their claims substantiated. The advertisements may not represent the use of alcohol as being therapeutic or curative. Words like "bracing" and "invigorating" must not be used. Advertisements may not suggest that their product will improve one's athletic ability. While sports imagery can be used in both advertisements and product labeling, the TTB investigates whether the messages created by the use of these images is misleading. If an athlete is used in the advertisement, the athlete cannot consume or appear to be preparing to consume an alcoholic beverage because that may imply that consuming alcoholic beverages improves athletic ability. Alcohol advertisements cannot be directed at underage consumers. Both the content and placement of the advertisements are regulated to prevent this.

In addition to federal regulations, some voluntary regulations are observed. Beginning in 1936, television networks have observed a voluntary ban of spirits advertising, although beer and wine are regularly advertised. Different television networks have different guidelines for beer advertisements. For example, NBC does not allow beer advertising to run during X games, otherwise known as "extreme games" like skateboarding, which are watched primarily by those under the legal drinking age. Now, many cable networks air spirits advertisements. Because there are so many networks, it may now be easier to isolate the acceptable demographic and aim the advertisements at adult consumers. Spirits companies have begun to produce products that fall under beer regulations for advertising. They are sweet, low-alcohol beverages such as Smirnoff Ice and Bacardi Breezer. This allows these companies to get their brand on most networks, even if it is not the product they are ultimately trying to sell. This enhances brand awareness while observing the letter of the current regulations. In the alcohol industry, these beverages are known as "flavored malt beverages."

These sweet, low-alcohol beverages are known to critics of alcohol advertising as "alcopops." Their sweet flavors are reminiscent of soda pop, with bright colors, and fun flavor names like "Razzberry," "Pomegranate Twist," and "Hard Lemonade." Moreover, since they are categorized as a malt beverage like beer, they avoid higher taxes. Still, they derive most of their alcohol content from added, distilled spirits. This keeps the price point lower, which makes the drinks even more appealing for youth. Since they are considered to be in the beer category rather than the spirits category, they are available wherever beer is available, making them easier to buy.

As they are so sweet, it is very difficult to taste any alcohol in them. They usually contain the same amount of, and sometimes more, alcohol as beer. Critics say that this makes these drinks a sort of gateway drink to alcohol consumption. In California, AB 346, a bill was recently passed that requires "alcopops" makers to put a warning label on containers stating "Attention: This drink contains alcohol."

Groups advocating against alcohol use by minors and younger adults have applauded the bill.

Critics also believe that some of the content in alcohol advertisements is particularly appealing to children. One of the most well-known characters was Budweiser's Spuds MacKenzie, a bullterrier introduced to sell Bud Light in the 1980s. Although critics said that Budweiser was using the loveable party dog to market its product to children, the **Federal Trade Commission** found that Budweiser was not violating any federal regulations. Still, the ad campaign was abandoned. A more recent ad campaign that was highly recognizable to children was the Budweiser campaign featuring the Budweiser frogs. Many alcohol advertisements appear in print magazines, such as *Spin* and *Rolling Stone*, that children read. On television, beer is most often advertised during sporting events, which are also popular with children. Critics believe that these campaigns get children to start drinking. Children are not the only groups that critics believe are wrongly targeted with alcohol advertisements. Some believe that inner-city residents, who demographically tend to be African American, are targeted. Critics believe that these individuals may not have access to health education that would prevent them from overconsumption of alcoholic beverages. Alcohol advertisers argue that they are not trying to get anyone to start drinking. Instead, they are trying to get legal drinkers to switch brands and to establish brand loyalty. Of course, alcohol is not the only factor that determines whether a person will drink. Banning, or further limiting, advertising limits communication aimed toward individuals who are old enough to drink and already do so. Moreover, the First Amendment is an issue here.

Another major issue in alcohol advertising is the types of imagery advertisers use. Advertisements portray alcohol as the magic potion that will make a person more attractive, more outgoing, more popular, and more fun. When athletic activities and sports imagery is used, the advertisements may deny the negative effects of alcohol consumption. After all, playing sports entails coordination and quick responses, the antithesis of what happens when one drinks alcohol. Advertising for alcohol is not limited to magazines and television. It includes naming rights of stadiums, logos on scoreboards, logos and names on racecars, and logos emblazoned on sports fields. Companies also advertise in more local ways. They sponsor local 5K and 10K races, as well as other sporting events. Beer advertising, in particular, has been heavily criticized for its propagation of hegemonic masculinity. Beer advertising has been criticized for how it represents, misrepresents, and influences the dominant male persona and women as the "other," which influences the construction of gender identities in a negative way. Miller Light was highly criticized for its "catfight commercials," which critics deemed sexist. The commercial featured two curvy women arguing over whether Miller Light is better because it tastes great or because it is less filling. They tear off each other's clothes and wrestle in wet cement. However, even when beer commercials forfeit the scantily clad women that have been a hallmark, the messages are still the same. Miller Light's next advertising campaign was "man laws." Man laws included "not fruiting the beer," an overt reference to homosexuality, and not clinking bottles with the tops of the bottles because it "could constitute kissing" another man, another reference to homosexuality. A man cannot leave his "fellow man" with "his" woman, unless his fellow man deems her attractive enough, which places male bonding above all else, portrays the woman as an object to be judged by her beauty, and portrays the woman as on object to be owned by a man. The woman as an object to be owned by a man was furthered with repeated references to another "man law," "You Poke it, You Own It." This one was used in reference to whether one man could stick a finger in the hole of another man's beer bottle when carrying a beer. It was also used in a "man law" commercial that argued when a man may date another man's ex-girlfriend. While the "man law" campaign was arguably wrapped around a core of hegemonic masculinity, it did call attention to one of the more pleasant aspects of drinking: figuring out the world over an alcoholic beverage. This image was commonly the beginning of most of the Platonic dialogues. Interestingly, the "man laws" campaign did not translate to higher sales for Miller Light. Judging from the parodies of the "Man Laws" on YouTube.com, blog entries, and FaceBook pages devoted to the "Man Laws," Miller Light did succeed in selling a particular brand of masculinity. That may be the real issue with sexist imagery in beer advertisements.

See also: Advertising of Food; Alcohol, In-State Distribution of; Children and Food; European Union Regulations.

Further Reading: Bosman, Julie. "Advertising; Beer Ads That Ditch Bikinis, But Add Threads of Thought." *New York Times,* May 1, 2006. http://query.nytimes.com/gst/fullpage.html?res=9A07E1DF113FF932A35756C0A9609C8B63&sec=&spon=&pagewanted=2; Sheehan, Kim. *Controversies in Contemporary Advertising.* Thousand Oaks, CA: Sage Publications, 2004; Wenner, Lawrence A., and Steven J. Jackson, eds. *Sport, Beer, and Gender.* New York: Peter Lang, 2009.

Stephanie Jane Carter

ADVERTISING OF FOOD

In the United States, advertising is regulated by the **Federal Trade Commission** (FTC). Under the Federal Trade Commission Act of 1946, advertisements must adhere to three general principles. Ads must be truthful, nondeceptive, and fair. Advertisers must have evidence to back up their claims. According the FTC's Deception Policy Statement, an advertisement is deceptive if it contains or omits information that is likely to mislead customers acting reasonably under the circumstances and if the information is relevant to a consumer's decision to buy or use the product. The Federal Trade Commission Act and the FTC's Unfairness Policy Statement define what makes an advertisement unfair. It is unfair if it causes or is likely to cause substantial consumer injury that could not be reasonably avoided. In addition, this injury cannot be outweighed by the benefit. According to the FTC, the advertisements that receive the closest scrutiny make claims about health or safety, such as, "This cereal reduces the risk of cancer." Advertisements that consumers would have trouble evaluating for themselves receive close scrutiny. An example is, "This food product is safe for the environment." According to the FTC, the advertisement claims that receive the least amount of scrutiny are subjective ones, such as, "This cola tastes great." Alcohol regulation is not determined by the FTC. The only power the FTC holds over alcohol advertising is the ability to take action if an advertisement is deceptive or unfair. Alcohol is regulated by the Federal Bureau of Alcohol, Tobacco, Firearms and Explosives and the Alcohol and Tobacco Tax Trade Bureau.

A major criticism of food advertising is that the amount spent on it is drastically more than the amount spent on nutrition education and related pursuits. According to a study published in 2003 on the Web site of the **U.S. Department of Agriculture** (USDA), food manufacturers spent $7 billion on advertising in the United States in 1997. The U.S. food marketing system is the second largest advertiser in the U.S. economy. The USDA spent a mere $333.3 million on nutrition education and related pursuits. The $333.3 million amounts to what the food industry spends on advertising for coffee, tea, and cocoa. Twenty-two percent of the amount the food manufacturers spend on advertising is used to promote processed, packaged foods. In 1999, McDonald's spent $627.2 million on advertising. Wrigley's Chewing Gum spent $117 million on advertising that same year. Critics of food advertising argue that it is impossible for nutrition education to compete with these numbers. Moreover, it is difficult to ask taxpayers for money to compete with these numbers.

Food advertising is important to the food manufacturers because people can only eat a limited amount of food. With so many foods marketed, manufacturers must compete for the customer. This fact also lends itself to an often-criticized attitude in the food industry, the "eat more" attitude. Food is a repeatedly purchased item, so every day is a new day and manufacturers have a new chance to compete for consumers' money. Of course, brand allegiance is one of the best ways to garner repeat buyers. Although Coke and Pepsi taste similar to many people, the companies have spent enormous amounts of time and money trying to get the customer to see them as different, to have loyalty to one brand. They have hosted taste tests and challenges to garner this sort of loyalty.

Both in and out of school, critics believe that the food advertising and alcohol advertising industries unfairly and unethically target children. Advertising industry publications emphasize that brand loyalty must begin at a young age, as early as age 2. In fact, research shows that children can recognize a brand logo before they recognize their own names. One of the most popular advertising campaigns with children was the Budweiser advertisements featuring the Budweiser frogs. Critics argue that "alcopops," (alcoholic beverages) are reminiscent of soda pop with bright colors and fun flavor names like "Razzberry," "Pomegranate Twist," and "Hard Lemonade." Critics say that this makes these drinks a gateway drink to drinking alcohol. California has passed AB 346, which mandates a warning label on "alcopops" stating "Attention: This Drink Contains Alcohol." Groups advocating against alcohol use by minors and younger adults have applauded this legislation. By creating a loyal consumer at an early age, companies create a loyal customer for life. This type of advertising is referred to as a "cradle-to-coffin" strategy. Another reason that children are attractive customers is what has been called their "pester power." Reportedly, children can control a family's purse strings by using one or more of the seven types of pestering to get their parents to buy something for them. Moreover, in cases such as fast food, if a child is getting a meal, chances are the companies have at least one more customer with them, such as a parent. McDonald's owns most of the playgrounds in the United States. They also give away toys. These elements help to establish a customer at an early age.

In 1978, the FTC unsuccessfully attempted to ban all television advertisements aimed at children. Currently, there are many people lobbying for a ban on advertising directed at children. However, as was apparent in the case of the Budweiser frogs, even advertisements that cannot legally be aimed at children are at times highly popular with them. The advertising industry has created a self-regulatory agency, the Children's Advertising Review Unit (CARU). The organization has written the *Self-Regulatory Guidelines for Children's Advertising*, which it uses to review advertising aimed at children. When it cannot resolve an issue, it refers the issue to the FTC. In school, children are the target of food advertising through agreements known as "pouring rights" contracts.

The foods most advertised are often the ones least recommended by the *Dietary Guidelines for Americans*. The advent of health claims in food advertising and on labels has made these heavily processed foods look healthier. The Nutrition Labeling and Education Act of 1990 forced the **Food and Drug Administration** (FDA) to start authorizing health claims for foods and supplements. Before this, health claims were forbidden. The claims had to be substantiated by significant scientific evidence. The **Food and Drug Administration Modernization Act of 1997** (FDAMA) required the FDA to permit nutrient-content and health claims for conventional foods when the claims are substantiated by published, authoritative statements by the federal public health agencies or the National Academy of Sciences. Although these rules apply to food labeling, they affect advertising as well. When a food is advertised as healthy, it has a tendency to sell. Consumers are overweight and they would like to change that without changing their diets. Health claims allow consumers to feel as if they are doing something good for their bodies, whether or not they are. A major breakthrough in food advertising is that the food could be marketed positively, instead of negatively. Instead of saying that a product is low-cholesterol, they could also say that a product promotes heart health. Critics argue that this form of advertising simply confuses an already confused public even more about healthy diets. Sugary breakfast cereals are even marketed with health claims. Others note that consumers should take responsibility for their own diets and actions. Over-regulation may stifle American freedom of choice. They note that it is the consumers' prerogative to choose a hamburger over a salad. Moreover, they point out that ultimately this is a game of supply and demand. If consumers did not demand these foods, companies would not supply them. Critics point out that irresponsible and unethical advertising creates the demand. In regulating the use of health claims in advertising, the FTC announced in 1994 that food advertising will be held to the same standards as food labeling set forth by the FDA. The goal of this policy is to make sure that food advertising messages are consistent with messages on food labels. The number of health claims makes it difficult to monitor all of them. Health claims in food advertising undeniably generate sales.

Self-Regulatory Guidelines for Children's Advertising

To avoid deceptive and/or inappropriate advertising to children involving product presentations and claims:

1. Copy, sound, and visual presentations should not mislead children about product or performance characteristics. Such characteristics may include, but are not limited to, speed, method of operation, color, sound, durability, nutritional benefits, and similar characteristics.

2. The presentation should not mislead children about benefits from use of the product. Such benefits may include, but are not limited to, the acquisition of strength, status, popularity, growth, proficiency, and intelligence.

3. Claims should not unduly exploit a child's imagination. Using techniques such as animation and computer-generated imagery, while creating fantasy, is appropriate for both younger and older children and should not create unattainable performance expectations nor exploit the younger child's difficulty in distinguishing between the real and the fanciful.

4. Advertisements should demonstrate the performance and use of a product in a way that can be duplicated by a child for whom the product is intended.

5. The advertisement should not mislead children about what is included in the initial purchase.

6. Advertising that compares the advertised product to another product should be based on real product attributes and be understandable to the child and the audience.

7. The amount of product featured should not be excessive or more than would be reasonable to acquire, use, or consume by a person in the situation depicted. For example, if an advertisement depicts food being consumed by a person in the advertisement, or suggests that the food will be consumed, the quantity of food shown should not exceed the labeled serving size on the Nutrition Facts panel; where no such serving size is applicable, the quantity of food shown should not exceed a single serving size that would be appropriate for consumption by a person of the age depicted.

8. Advertising of food products should encourage responsible use of the product with a view toward healthy development of the child. For example, advertising of food products should not discourage or disparage healthy lifestyle choices or the consumption of fruits or vegetables, or other foods recommended for increased consumption by current USDA *Dietary Guidelines for Americans* and *My Pyramid*, as applicable to children under 12.

9. Advertisements for food products should clearly depict or describe the appropriate role of the product within the framework of the eating occasion depicted.
   a. Advertisements representing a mealtime should depict the food product within the framework of a nutritionally balanced meal.
   b. Snack foods should be clearly depicted as such, and not as substitutes for meals.

Source: Children's Advertising Review Unit. The Children's Advertising Review Unit Self-Regulatory Program for Children's Advertising. http://www.caru.org/guidelines/index.aspx

Ultimately, food advertisements create confusion over diets. They often appeal to children, who do not have the ability to make the best choices for themselves or to know when to choose a salad over a hamburger. With so many health claims in advertisements, consumers have difficulty knowing what a healthy diet truly is. Education is important in combating the poor diets that advertisements intentionally or unintentionally create. Consumers must choose either to impose more regulation at the loss of some freedom, or to resist the urge to eat too much and to eat poorly.

See also: Children and Food; Diet Foods; Dietary Supplements; International Labeling; Kosher and Halal Labeling; Labeling Definitions; National Organics Standards Board; Portion Sizes; School Breakfast and Lunch Programs; Appendix 3A: *Pelman, et al. v. McDonald's Corporation*; Appendix 3B: *Pelman, et al. v. McDonald's Corporation*, Amended Complaint; Appendix 3C: *Pelman, et al. v. McDonald's Corporation.*

Further Reading: Gallo, Anthony E., John Connor, and William T. Boehm. "Mass Media Food Advertising," *National Food Review*, USDA Economic Research Service, NFR-9, Winter 1980; McNeal, James U. *Kids as Customers*. New York: Lexington Books, 1992; Nestle, Marion. *Food Politics: How the Food Industry Influences Nutrition and Health*. Berkeley: University of California Press, 2007; Schlosser, Eric. *Fast Food Nation: The Dark Side of the All-American Meal*. Boston: Houghton Mifflin, 2001; Sheehan, Kim. *Controversies in Contemporary Advertising*. Thousand Oaks, CA: Sage Publications, 2004; Wenner, Lawrence A., and Steven J. Jackson, eds. *Sport, Beer, and Gender*. New York: Peter Lang, 2009.

Stephanie Jane Carter

AGRICULTURAL DISASTER ASSISTANCE PROGRAMS

The United States government operates a variety of programs to assist producers and communities adversely affected by natural disasters, such as heavy storms, droughts, flooding, freezes, and infestations. The **U.S. Department of Agriculture** (USDA) conducts three major programs that assist agricultural producers—the Federal Crop Insurance Corporation (FCIC), the Noninsured Crop Disaster Assistance Program (NAP), and a program for emergency disaster loans. Since the late 1980s, the U.S. Congress has also regularly provided ad hoc agriculture disaster assistance following major natural disasters, often in the form of direct payments.

The **federal crop insurance** program began in the 1930s in response to the Great Depression and the Dust Bowl conditions in parts of rural America. The FCIC was created in 1938, and expanded and reformed by Congress in legislation in 1980, 1994, 1996, and 2000 to cover more crops in more regions and to require coverage to qualify for other disaster assistance. Since 1996, the FCIC has been housed within the USDA's Risk Management Agency (RMA), and since 2000 private-sector companies have expanded into the crop insurance business with support and regulation by the RMA. Federal funding for the crop insurance program provides premium subsidies to agricultural producers, covers program losses, and reimburses private insurance companies that offer crop insurance policies. Insurance is offered by crop type and by county and must cover a producer's entire crop within a county to prevent adverse selection of only the riskier areas by the insured.

The NAP provides assistance to producers of noninsurable crops when natural disasters cause lower yields or crop loss. Landowners, tenant farmers, and share-croppers are eligible as long as revenue is less than $2 million annually. A wide variety of food, feed, fiber, and seed crops are eligible, as are other crops including mushrooms, flowers, honey, and maple sap. The disaster must occur before or during harvest to qualify. The USDA requires annual acreage and crop reporting data to ensure that losses are actually incurred.

The USDA's Farm Service Agency (FSA) also provides emergency farm loans for 100 percent of the losses up to $500,000 to restore or replace property, pay production costs and living expenses, or refinance debt. To qualify, the president or secretary of agriculture must declare the local county a disaster area, and the producer must suffer a 30 percent or greater loss of crops, livestock, or other property. Again, USDA requires certain record keeping for a farm to qualify for loans and the local FSA office must also approve the farm plan. Furthermore, recipients of emergency farm loans are required to obtain crop insurance in the future.

Since at least 1990, the U.S. Congress has also often appropriated supplemental agricultural disaster assistance funding in response to certain significant disasters. This assistance comes in the form of direct disaster payments, livestock assistance, tree assistance, and conservation assistance. These payments usually apply within agricultural disaster areas and producers may qualify regardless of insurance. Livestock assistance usually provides help to livestock producers in purchasing feed, and the tree assistance program helps orchard, bush, and vine planters recover from disasters. The emergency conservation program provides funding to farmers and ranchers to rehabilitate farmland and conserve water during droughts.

To replace the ad hoc disaster payment program, the 2008 **Farm Bill** created the Supplemental Revenue Assistance Payments (SURE) Program to provide supplemental disaster assistance. To qualify, a farm must be located in a disaster county and see a production drop of 50 percent or more. There is an income limit of $2.5 million in annual income, which may be increased if farm income is over 75 percent of total income. In addition, producers must obtain crop insurance or NAP, with limited exceptions for forage crops. Socially disadvantaged or beginning farmers may waive this requirement. Although the SURE program aims to make agricultural disaster assistance more formal and predictable, Congress may continue to provide special ad hoc assistance as disasters occur. The 2011 Farm Bill will likely make additional changes to these programs.

Andrew G. Wallace

AGRICULTURAL PERSONAL PROPERTY, TAXATION, AND EXEMPTIONS

"Personal property" is the legal term used to describe property that is not real estate. Real estate is land and the things attached to the land like buildings or fences. Everything that is not real estate is personal property and includes tangible things like vehicles and intangible things like stock. Most states exact a tax on the personal property of businesses, collecting taxes on vehicles, equipment, and other personal property that is owned by the business and used to conduct business. However, to protect and encourage agriculture, many states make exceptions of some sort for agricultural personal property. These personal property exemptions usually do not extend to real estate or improvements to real estate.

Agricultural equipment and vehicles refer to equipment and vehicles that are used in planting or harvesting a crop. In addition it refers to those things directly used in raising or cultivating agricultural animals. The term also includes the collection of animals or farm products and their processing. The key to the definition and any application of exceptions has to do with direct use. Mowing equipment that harvests and collects grass for feeding animals is direct use. Mowing equipment that keeps the farm neat and may help keep the buildings looking attractive is not directly used in agriculture. In most states when the agricultural equipment and vehicles are purchased, the seller does not have to collect sales or use tax when the buyer fills out the appropriate form. The seller can then remit the form instead of the tax. The purchase of spare parts for the maintenance and repair of exempt equipment and vehicles is usually not exempt at the point of sale. The buyer must pay the tax and they can apply for a refund of the tax by the remission of the appropriate forms.

These exceptions also refer to commercial agriculture—crops must be cultivated, grown, and harvested or animals grown, and/or slaughtered for sale or processed into other products for sale. Thus, equipment that belongs to veterinary practices is not considered to be commercial agricultural equipment. Products stored off-site, whether in commercial silos or in other stockyards, are not applicable. Tree farms, nurseries, and traditional farms are engaged in commercial agriculture.

Sometimes qualified agricultural equipment is attached to or installed in buildings. Under normal definitions, once something is attached to or installed in a building in a permanent way, it loses its characteristic as personal property and becomes part of the real estate. However, some states make an exception to this rule when the equipment is being used in the direct conduct of commercial agriculture, even when it is attached to the real estate. The contractor who installs this equipment would usually collect sales tax from the property owner. However, under this exception, the contractor may accept the proper form in lieu of collecting sales tax. Examples of this equipment include tractors, combines, feeders, and crop dusters. The revenue departments will generally be expansive in determining what equipment qualifies for exemption.

In some states the animals are considered exempt from inventory even though they may be intended for resale. Some states require that the property be certified as agricultural land in order for certain exemptions to apply.

One type of exception has to do with sales and use tax. This is the tax that is imposed by state or local government on personal property when it is purchased. Sales tax is the tax paid by the buyer when a piece of personal property is purchased. This tax is collected by the seller at the point of purchase and is usually a percentage of the purchase price. Use tax is the tax paid on the transfer of property. Sales and use tax can also be collected on leased personal property. For example, if a vehicle is registered in one state and the owner wishes to transfer the registration to another state, the receiving state may impose a use tax on the registration. Some states exempt agricultural machinery and equipment for sales and use tax on sales and leasing. This encourages the purchase and leasing of agricultural equipment and vehicles and gives agricultural business a break. Nebraska is one of the states that has adopted this exception.

Personal property tax is the annual tax that is imposed by a state and/or local government on the depreciable personal property owned by a business. Depreciable personal property is property that can be used for more than one year and that is not consumed by use. This means that paper and fertilizer, consumed by use, are not subject to personal property tax. The Internal Revenue Service has tables that state the number of years certain types of equipment are considered useful, thus determining the rate of depreciation. Personal property tax, generally a percentage of the depreciated value of the item, is collected annually. Some states impose a personal property tax on agricultural vehicles and equipment but exempt the same property from sales and use tax.

Some states impose an inventory tax on those pieces of personal property that are stockpiled for resale or stockpiled for later use. The inventory of items for resale may not be applicable to agricultural business, such as a gift shop connected to a farm. Agricultural products such as jams and jellies made from harvested fruit could be considered agricultural inventory. Even without inventory, the stockpiling of consumables is something that a farm might do. Although inventory that is consumed is not subject to inventory tax, stockpiled goods may be.

Although there is a desire to encourage agriculture, states and local governments also want to received income from the businesses, even agricultural businesses, within their jurisdictions. Thus, different aspects of exemption will apply in those states where any exemption has been adopted. Inventory taxes, personal property taxes, sales and use taxes are within the areas of taxation traditionally imposed by state and local governments. Therefore, states that have expansive exemptions may find that large commercial agricultural operations become established there. The exemptions also provide some relief and encouragement to small farmers.

Elizabeth M. Williams

AGRICULTURAL REVENUE INSURANCE

Agricultural revenue insurance, or crop revenue insurance, refers to a type of federal crop insurance based on market prices and actual crop yield that protects revenue for farmers, as opposed to crop yields, by guaranteeing a certain amount of revenue and protecting the farmer from declines in crop prices during the growing season. While crops themselves fluctuate due to uncontrollable forces such as weather, revenue farmers can generate from even a healthy growing season can fluctuate wildly because of the volatility of the agricultural market. All agricultural revenue insurance is supported by the Federal Crop Insurance Corporation (FCIC), which is operated by the Risk Management Agency (RMA) of the **U.S. Department of Agriculture** (USDA). It is the USDA's decision whether insurance policies are available for specific crops and whether they are available in specific regions.

Agricultural revenue insurance is rooted in the Federal Crop Insurance Corporation (FCIC). The FCIC was created in 1938 in response to the negative economic effects on farmers resulting from the Great Depression and the decline in crop production due to the Dust Bowl. Originally, the insurance program was only applied to major crops and major producing regions. The program was expanded to include more crops and regions with the passage of the Federal Crop Insurance Act of 1980. The program has been expanded several times since then. In 1983, the Congressional Budget Office (CBO) explored agricultural revenue insurance as an option for farmers. The CBO stated that farmers were at more financial risk than they had been in the past. It noted that the global marketplace increased the volatility of the agricultural market and that farmers were increasingly dependent on that market. The Federal Crop Insurance Reform Act of 1994 mandated that the FCIC create a program that would offer revenue insurance to farmers. In 1997, agricultural revenue insurance began as a pilot program under the **federal crop insurance** program. The Agricultural Risk Protection Act of 2000 extended some agricultural insurance policies to include livestock. Agricultural revenue policies have become very popular since their inception in 1997, especially within certain industries. In 2006, the RMA reported that at least 75 percent of insured corn and soybean farms are covered by agricultural revenue insurance.

There are several types of crop revenue insurance, including crop revenue coverage, revenue assurance, income protection, and group risk income protection, and adjusted gross revenue. Agricultural revenue insurance accounts for about half of all crop insurance policies. Crop revenue coverage computes actual revenue by multiplying actual yield by an early season price or harvest market price. The guarantee is the higher of the two prices. An indemnity is provided when the actual revenue is lower than the guarantee. Revenue assurance is similar, but the harvest market price is based on a different period. For example, revenue assurance bases the average price of December corn futures on November rather than October, the month the crop revenue coverage uses. The coverage is based on a dollar amount of target revenue decided by the producer. It must be within a specified range of the expected revenue. Both crop revenue coverage and revenue assurance are based on a farmer's actual production. Both also use the Chicago Board of Trade futures prices as a basis for establishing guarantees. Unlike crop revenue coverage and revenue assurance, income protection's guarantee is not based on the harvest price. Income protection offers the producer protection of gross income when this income is lower due to a decline in crop price or yield during a growing season. Group risk income protection pays an indemnity when the revenue of an entire county is lower than the revenue the producer chose for a policy. Adjusted Gross Revenue does not insure individual crops, but insures the entire farm. The guarantee in this policy is for the average gross farm revenue. As of 2009, no revenue insurance policy can use a harvest market price that sets the guarantee higher than 100 percent above the base market price that is developed in February. The most popular types of revenue insurance are crop revenue insurance and revenue assurance.

According to some theorists, agricultural revenue insurance seems to be the solution to the issue of low participation levels in agricultural insurance programs often debated in the 1980s and early 1990s.

Stephanie Jane Carter

AGRICULTURE AND LIVESTOCK, URBAN

Urban agriculture refers to the practice of producing, processing, and marketing food and fuel in an urban or peri-urban setting. Animal husbandry or raising of urban livestock, horticulture, aquaculture, agriculture, apiculture, vermiculture, myoculture, and agro-forestry are all examples of types of agricultural practices that occur in urban and peri-urban environments. Urban farms represent a significant portion of new small farm registrations in the United States. In 1993, approximately 660,000 farms in the United States were located in urban areas. Many of the 15,700 small farms registered in the United States in 1998 were located in urban areas. The United Nations Development Program estimates that urban farms grow 15 percent of the food in the world. Urban agriculture can increase food security among insecure populations; conserve resources by decreasing the distance between food's origin and its destination in cities, where 80 percent of U.S. residents live; connect urban dwellers with food origins; provide access to fresh vegetables, meat, and eggs; produce income; and/or provide recreation, relaxation, and exercise. Additionally, urban agriculture can aid in waste management, land use, and broad health and economic issues. Urban agriculture crosses the income stratosphere, and the practice has become a popular proposal among city planners. Generally, there are three types of urban farmers: backyard gardeners, community gardeners, and commercial growers. These categories are not mutually exclusive. Even though urban agriculture continues to grow in its popularity, applications, and acceptance, government ordinances can be both supportive and hostile to the practice.

There are several main types of urban farming. Horticulture, the production of vegetables and fruit, is one of the most popular. The production of these crops can be done both with soil and without, with the popularity of hydroponics increasing. Aquaculture is the production of products that are raised in the water and includes fish, seafood, vegetables, and aquatic plants. Agro-forestry is most often seen in the developing world, where wood is used as fuel for cooking. Apiculture (bee-keeping), vermiculture (production of worms that can be used in composting and as fertilizer), and myoculture (production of mushrooms) are also types of agriculture seen in urban areas. Bee-keeping, for honey and wax, is praised for its applications in promoting biodiversity through pollination. Vermiculture creates products such as silk, compost worms, and fertilizer. Myoculture requires little land and water and can be carried out in both cellars and sheds. Snails are also raised in urban areas. Animal husbandry, or the keeping of urban livestock for food purposes, is a more contentious type of urban agriculture. In the United States, health codes were initially designed to reduce the public's contact with wildlife, thereby reducing the risk and spread of disease. Health codes and other city ordinances in many cities have not evolved to reflect the growing practice of urban agriculture, and urban animal husbandry is particularly affected by these legal restraints. However, many cities provide for the keeping of a specified number and type of animals in their city ordinances and zoning laws. Orleans Parish in Louisiana allows five domesticated animals per household. Neighborhoods also have their own codes. Animals that are raised in cities vary according to cultural food preferences and needs among different countries. Chickens, other poultry, sheep, pigs, goats, cattle, rabbits, and guinea pigs are all found living in cities. Common complaints about urban livestock include the smell, particularly from poultry, and the fear of disease. Proponents of urban livestock recommend rules to govern the practice, rather than forbidding the practice altogether. The number of chickens can be limited and they can be housed in cleaner sheds. Many diseases can be avoided with the proper disposal of animal waste, which can be used as fertilizer for other crops.

Even though urban farming has found new purpose in its conservation applications and its ability to satisfy the market for locally grown products, it is not a new concept. A 1649 map of Aachen, Germany, depicts farming both on the interior and exterior of the city walls. Salad was cultivated in the Marais district of Paris in the 1800s using horse manure from city horses. There is also evidence that urban gardening was popular in even earlier civilizations. Urban gardening has often been used in times of economic and social depression. In the late 1800s, Detroit, Michigan, asked the owners of vacant lots to let those out of work cultivate crops on the land in an effort to combat the negative effects of a Depression. In addition to providing subsistence and self-worth, the city did not have to contribute as much money toward unemployment. Similar measures were taken in Buffalo, Minneapolis, Chicago, and Denver. As populations increased and industrialization led to unhealthy and unsightly conditions in cities, some thinkers began to imagine greener, utopian cities. In 1902, Ebenezer Howard published *Garden Cities of Tomorrow*, a treatise on this type of city that was immensely popular in Britain. The concept also found followers in the United States with the City Beautiful Movement (1890 to 1910), though it was largely focused on ornamental urban gardens. Beautiful cities were thought to inspire civic virtue and morality. The National Mall in Washington, D.C., was born out of this movement. Though **rationing** among civilians was not imposed until World War II, World War I also created serious food shortages. In response to the shortages, the National War Garden Commission was formed. The purpose of the commission was to influence American citizens to increase food production through gardening on unused land. President Woodrow Wilson echoed this plea, saying that cultivation of a garden aided in the war effort. The urban gardens of World War I were called liberty gardens. Urban gardening gained followers again during the Great Depression, when they were known as relief gardens, welfare gardens, or subsistence gardens. They were to provide food and self-worth for those suffering the effects of the Great Depression. Federal, local, and nongovernmental organizations supported the effort. Between 1933 and 1935, the Federal Emergency Relief Administration gave funds in support of a work garden initiative, which actually paid gardeners. Urban gardening was again revived with World War II, when rationing was enacted. The War Food Administration created the National Victory Garden Program. These gardens had the same purpose and effect as the liberty gardens of World War I. Homemakers were able to help the war effort, have access to more food and a greater variety of food than the rationing program allowed, and use fewer resources. Additionally, the gardens offered homemakers greater flexibility in menu planning. All of these gardening efforts arose from great need, but the wartime gardens crossed class lines, although the Depression era gardens were typically reserved for the poor. Today, both developing and developed countries employ urban agriculture. In the United States, urban gardens became popular again during the economic crisis that began in 2008. Their popularity has also grown with the desire for local origin food and a movement away from processed foods.

Urban agriculture is used for various purposes and is done in various places. In September 1996, Chicago's Robert Taylor Housing Project, became the home of the first urban agriculture project in North America by Heifer International, an organization that develops projects to improve social and economic welfare. In one Heifer project, a youth group engaged in aquaculture and vermiculture in the basement of the housing complex, farming two barrels of fish, which they harvested every seven months for their families. They sold the worm products. By 1998, the Cabrini Greens (made up of residents of the remaining buildings of the Cabrini Green Housing Project) in Chicago farmed goats for milk and raw materials. California chef and restaurateur Alice Waters initiated the Edible Schoolyard project, which puts edible gardens on school campuses. Urban agriculture can be found in community gardens, some of which provide a shared product experience and others are divided into separate plots that are farmed and enjoyed by each gardener individually. Urban agriculture can also be found in community gardens, in compost facilities, in window boxes, on rooftops, at restaurants, and other locations.

In the United States, cities often made housing, agriculture, and industry distinct industries in an effort to minimize negative effects on human health. Cities have restricted urban agriculture because of competing uses of water and other resources, sources of nuisance complaints, and being detrimental to the city aesthetic. Some property owners have claimed that it decreases property values. Many policy changes have been made in recent years. On the federal level, there was no specific mention of urban agriculture in the 2008 **Farm Bill**. Section 4402 did provide monetary assistance for community food projects to establish "healthy urban food enterprise development centers" and for the Community Food Project. Urban agriculture proponents are hopeful about drafts of the 2012 Farm Bill, which may allow subsidies for more diverse crops. In recognition of urban farming, the **U.S. Department of Agriculture** (USDA) publishes the *Urban Soil Primer for Homeowners and Renters Planning Boards, Property Managers, Students, and Educators*. Many states are changing their policies toward urban agriculture. In March 2010, the Georgia State Legislature developed Bill 842, which deals with urban agriculture. In its original form, the bill would limit nuisance complaints against urban agriculture. However, many complained that the bill would allow no reprieve to neighbors who lived near loud roosters or other farming operations that can be offensive to urban residential living. While the bill will likely go through changes, it will establish the legality of urban agriculture. In 2010, Michigan interpreted the Right-to-Farm Act in relation to urban farming. The Right to Farm Act limits nuisance complaints against farming operations in existence prior to the residential housing. Michigan interpreted the act as not protecting farming operations from nuisance complaints when they move into a neighborhood that was previously residential. It further addressed urban farming by saying that all farms, including urban farms, should adhere to zoning and building regulations. If a city finds that the distance of a farming operation from other entities should be increased, the city has the power to increase the prescribed distances. Essentially, urban farming legislation takes place at the municipal level. Other forms of regulation occur through boards of health. Holyoke, Massachusetts, allows chicken farming with a permit from the board of health. In addition to support provided by some local and national authorities, urban agriculture finds support through international development agencies, research centers, nongovernmental organizations, and farmers groups. The USDA Small Farms/School Meals Program allows direct marketing for small farms. Community development corporations often are at the forefront of the development of many successful urban farms. The American Planning Association, a nonprofit organization, published a zoning publication in March 2010 to aid cities in changing zoning laws to allow urban agriculture.

Urban farming has many supporters and practical uses, but environmental, economic, organizational, social, and health issues are frequently cited. Some theorists cite environmental issues such as the lack of regulation regarding the use of pesticides and agrochemicals in urban areas. Other theorists point out that while regulation may reasonably be implemented, most urban farmers do so out of a preference for organic food, reducing the overall use of pesticides in urban areas to a nonserious level. Moreover, a lot of urban agriculture is performed on a small scale. City soil is typically contaminated with heavy metals such as lead-based paint, gasoline, cadmium, nickel, and mercury. Even though there is literature such as the USDA's guide, many critics worry that the importance of soil testing has not been communicated to urban farmers. Solutions to contaminated soil include raised beds filled with imported soil and compost, and phyto-remediation, which is the removal of heavy metals by plants. Also, compost keeps waste out of the city's system. Using it as fertilizer both decreases the extra resources that need to go into gardening and the waste that comes out of food consumption.

There are also land tenure issues because many urban farms are located on land, such as vacant lots, that does not belong to the farmers. Farmers can lose their investment when the owners take the land back. This problem can be circumvented with leases, land trusts that secure land for agricultural uses, conservation easements that reserve environmentally unstable land for agricultural uses, properties allocated to farming through city planning projects, and usufruct agreements that give farmers the right to use and profit from the public or private land so long as it is maintained.

Urban agriculture can be a source of income and nourishment for low-income families who participate, but food produced this way is not less expensive and it may not be accessible to everyone. The USDA **food stamp** program and the Women, Infants, and Children (WIC) Farmers Markets Nutrition Program have made farm products, urban and not, available to low-income consumers. Urban agriculture promotes activity through gardening and increases the consumption of fresh vegetables, aiding in the fight against poor nutrition, obesity, and obesity-related diseases. It has been noted that for urban agriculture to alleviate food insecurity, low-income people must have access to land and clean water. Additionally, there are some negative perceptions of urban agriculture. In many areas around the world, farming is considered a rural activity. The use of land for agriculture in the city can compete with more financially lucrative uses of the land. Others believe that urban agriculture is aesthetically undesirable. However, when urban agriculture occurs on blighted land or vacant properties, the activity can actually beautify cities. In 2010, Detroit businessman John Hantz argued for a Homestead Act approach for vacant land in Detroit, of which there is at least 50 miles. He wanted it to be easier to purchase the vacant land and use it for large, commercial, for-profit farms. The city was making changes to its master plan and zoning ordinances to support urban agriculture. Although some city residents were skeptical of large, commercial farms in the city, others argued that farming uses less government subsidies than other development projects, jobs and food could be provided for some of the 28.9 percent of unemployed individuals in Detroit, and the practice would eliminate some of the blight. Dickson Despommier, professor of public health at Columbia University, created the concept of a "vertical farm" with his medical ecology class in 1999. The class, which studies the intersection of human health and the environment, used the concept of hydroponic growing to propose farm towers and rooftop gardens. Sketches of the proposed buildings depict high-rise buildings covered in green plants.

Issues in developing countries include the perception that agriculture is not modern, is ill-suited for the city, and is a female activity. Urban farmers in developing countries have little access to post-production processes and may not benefit from the resources provided though official recognition. Many seeds and other aspects of farming are designed for rural use. Many experts note that urban agriculture increases food security among certain populations.

See also: Community-Supported Agriculture; Food Stamps; Soil, Organic; Appendix 9: Twenty-Eight Hour Law of 1873 as Amended in 1994.

Further Reading: Airriess, Christopher A., and David L. Clawson. "Vietnamese Market Gardens in New Orleans." *The Geographical Review* 84 (1994):16–31; Brown, Katherine H. *Urban Agriculture and Food Insecurity in the United States: Farming from the City Center to the Urban Fringe.* Urban Agriculture Committee of the Community Food Security Coalition, 2002; Howard, Ebenezer. *Garden Cities of To-Morrow.* London: Swan Sonnenschein and Company, 1902; Kaufman, Jerry, and Martin Bailkey. *Farming inside Cities: Entrepreneurial Urban Agriculture in the United States.* Lincoln Land Institute Working Paper. Cambridge, MA: Lincoln Land Institute, 2000.

Stephanie Jane Carter

ALCOHOL AND CAFFEINATED BEVERAGES

Cocktails combining both alcoholic spirits and caffeinated beverages such as tea or coffee have been prepared at home and at eating and drinking establishments for many years. Common cocktails of this type include rum and cola; Irish coffee, which combines coffee with Irish whiskey or Bailey's Irish Cream; and hot toddies, which combine an alcoholic spirit like whiskey or rum with tea. In addition, coffee-flavored liqueurs such as Godiva are also produced and contain caffeine as well as alcohol, and a variety of beers are brewed with coffee or chocolate additions. In recent years, beverage companies have increasingly sold pre-packaged beverage products combining alcohol and caffeine and have drawn legal and regulatory scrutiny.

In 2007, 29 state attorneys general urged the large brewing company, Anheuser-Busch, to warn buyers of alcoholic and caffeinated drinks about the danger of feeling less impaired and criticized the colorful marketing and similarity to popular caffeine-only energy drinks like Red Bull. In 2008, several state attorneys general entered into settlements with both Anheuser-Busch and MillerCoors to discontinue or remove caffeine from alcoholic beverages they were selling, such as Sparks, an orange-flavored malt liquor product that contained caffeine. Many other alcohol and caffeine drink combinations are also flavored malt liquor-based beverages.

In September 2009, 18 attorneys general further contacted the U.S. **Food and Drug Administration** (FDA) expressing concerns that caffeinated alcohol beverages were not legal for sale under FDA rules and could increase alcohol-related problems such as driving under the influence and violence. A number of studies have indicated that consuming caffeine along with alcohol may increase these problems, some of which were cited by the attorneys general. The FDA subsequently notified manufacturers of caffeinated alcoholic beverages in November 2009 that the FDA was reviewing the legality of such products and noted its concern with the drinks' popularity with college students.

Andrew G. Wallace

ALCOHOL CONTENT

The law of alcoholic beverages is one that is, in accordance with the Twenty-first Amendment to U.S. Constitution, which repealed **Prohibition** in 1933, a matter to be determined by each state. These states have set standards for the amount of alcohol that can be contained in various alcoholic beverages. Alcohol is measured by volume and stated as a percentage of that volume using the standard abbreviation ABV (alcohol by volume). Alcohol may also be expressed by use of the term "proof." Proof, as used in the United States, refers to two times the figure used in stating the alcohol content by ABV. Thus, beer that has an alcohol content of 6 percent ABV, is said to be 12 proof. But federal nutritional labeling standards could also be applicable to alcoholic beverages that would require more than "light beer" labeling. This would give caloric content and other nutrient information to consumers, treating alcoholic beverages as food. The Alcohol and Tobacco Tax and Trade Bureau (TTB) would issue labeling requirements—both nutritional and ingredient labeling.

Another method of measuring alcoholic content is to measure alcohol volume by weight (AVW). This method expresses total alcohol content as a percentage of mass. Some alcohol is labeled by AVW, especially in those states where this is the applicable measure and where the alcohol is sold within that state. This usually means beer. Low-point beer refers to the low percentage of alcohol percentage points. This beer is also called three-two beer or three point two beer, because it contains 3.2 percent alcohol AVW—equal to 4 percent ABV. Several states, notably Kansas, Oklahoma, Colorado, and Utah, allow low-point beer to be sold in groceries, but beer of a higher alcohol content can only be purchased through **alcohol beverage control** (ABC) **stores**.

Alcohol content has a number of repercussions and implications. One of these is the taxation of alcohol content by volume in some states. Another implication, as discussed, is the defining of the type of alcohol that must be sold at an ABC store or state-licensed store. New Hampshire and North Carolina, for example, actually place a limit on the alcohol level by ABV of beer that can be sold in their respective states. Ohio sets a maximum alcoholic beverage level on beer and on wine sold in the state.

Ohio provides a limited number of licenses to certain stores to sell spirits of over a stated alcohol level of over 21 percent ABV. There is an easier way to obtain a license for those who sell spirits at a level of 21 percent or less. This level is obtained by dilution with water. Vermont also has a special license for higher-volume alcohol content. In Oklahoma, beer with a higher than low-point level of alcohol cannot be sold cold. It must be sold at room temperature. West Virginia prohibits the sale of pure grain alcohol, generally 95 percent ABV.

But alcohol content of beer, wine, and spirits does not tell the entire story. The federal definition of an alcoholic beverage is any beverage of .5 percent ABV. Some states are dealing with a controversy over so-called "alcopops." These are beverages with an alcohol content of low-point beer that are often sold in groceries where the law bases the sale of alcoholic beverages in ABC stores or groceries based on the alcohol content. "Alcopops" are made of near-beer, a malt beverage with a miniscule percentage of alcohol and then flavored with alcohol-based flavorings to bring them up to the 3.2 ABW level. Because they are often sweet, they are treated as sodas by the drinkers and tend to attract underage drinkers. Many alcoholic beverage commissioners wish to keep these drinks out of groceries, even though their alcoholic content is equivalent to low-point beer.

Certain flavorings, such as vanilla extract, have a high alcohol content, yet are not always covered by the general state alcoholic beverage laws. The **Food and Drug Administration** (FDA) controls the alcohol content of vanilla extract. It requires that the extract contain 35 percent ABV and 13.35 ounces of vanilla bean per gallon. This solution can be labeled "pure" vanilla. This is a labeling law and not a law that controls where and whether the substance can be sold within a state. Certain over-the-counter pharmaceutical products, such a Nyquil, also have a high alcohol content (25 percent ABV). Similarly some mouthwash contains a high alcohol content. There is no consistency about whether these products can be sold in pharmacies or whether they fall within the general alcoholic beverage laws of a given state. Most states, however, make an exception for extracts that are commonly used for cooking and not intended for sale as a beverage.

Some states also regulate the sale of bakery products and candies that contain alcohol. Those states that regulate these products generally do so when the amount of alcohol contained in the products exceeds a certain minimum threshold. In some of these states a special license must be contained by the retail outlet where the product is sold, such as a bakery or confectionary shop or grocery. Some states require the purchaser to be 21 years old to purchase these products. In other states, there is no minimum age for purchase of confectionary products that have alcohol as an ingredient. In other states, confectionary products that contain alcohol are prohibited. Interestingly "simple extracts" are exempted, making it possible to use vanilla extract or other similar flavorings. There is no prohibition against the use of liquor-flavored extracts, however, just the use of the liquor itself. Thus, rum flavoring can be used in a cake, for example, but not in rum. Minnesota has a specific exception for liqueur-filled candies. They are specifically not alcoholic beverages.

Labeling of alcohol products and products containing alcohol is controlled by the various states. While most consistently require labeling for alcohol content of alcoholic beverages, the labeling required on confectionary products varies from no labeling or warning required to a specific prohibition of sale to minors under the age of 21.

See also: Labeling, Nutrition; Lite Labeling.

Elizabeth M. Williams

ALCOHOL, IN-STATE DISTRIBUTION OF

Since the repeal of Prohibition in 1933, most states have had what is known as a three-tiered system of distribution for alcoholic beverages. The three tiers are the producer, the distributor, and the retailer. In some states the retailer is tightly controlled by state-run **alcoholic beverage control** (ABC) stores. Most ABC stores sell only alcohol. In other states a retailer can be licensed to sell package liquor. In these states alcohol can be purchased in any licensed retail store.

The reason for this three tiered system is to control the producers, give the government a way to collect taxes, and to limit the abusive marketing and investment by producers that existed before prohibition. The middle tier, the distributor, is a buffer between the retailer and the producer.

In some states the producers of wine are an exception to the three-tiered system. Wineries may sell their own wines to consumers in on-premise retail stores. In California, for example, visitors can drive from winery to winery tasting and buying wine. Some states require wineries to sell only through distributors and others also allow wineries to ship directly to consumers.

A similar exception has been made for brew pubs in some states. These are restaurants or breweries that sell beer directly to customers to be drunk immediately on the premises. In some states brew pubs may also bottle their product. In other states a brew pub can only sell directly to customers in open containers and bottling is not allowed.

Most producers enter into distribution agreements that are exclusive for defined geographic areas. Since the 1950s there has been a great reduction in the number of distributors. Some estimates made the reduction from 6,000 to 600

Prohibition

From 1920 to 1933, the Noble Experiment occurred in the United States. The Eighteenth Amendment to the U.S. Constitution barred the manufacture, sale, and transportation of alcoholic beverages in the United States. Alcohol was still made for certain industrial purposes. This amendment kicked off the experiment, which became increasingly unpopular, especially doing the Great Depression. Speakeasies, places where alcohol was served illegally, flourished. In 1933 the Twenty-first Amendment ended the Noble Experiment to the joy of many. The failure of the Experiment is an excellent example of how important the support of the citizenry is in civil obedience.

distributors nationwide. The three-tiered system, which was originally designed as a reaction to conditions that existed before Prohibition, has changed into a system which gives distributors an enormous amount of power in the control of alcohol sales. The distributors benefit from the tight regulation of sales and delivery of alcoholic beverages.

With a shrinking number of distributors there is greater control over pricing and thus less competition. Profit is taken by the producer, the distributor, and the retailer. The need to have a distributor makes it very difficult for small producers to enter the market, because distributors find it unprofitable to represent small producers. This further limits competition.

The three-tiered system has been under attack in the courts by consumer groups who claim that the conditions that created the need for the multi-tiered system no longer exist. Some argue that the power that was additionally held by producers is currently shifting to the distributors. Although these are state laws, the federal courts have been the forum of choice, because consumers are arguing that the current system violates the commerce clause and restricts competition.

Some states also have laws that allow each county to determine whether it should be dry. This choice could be made by a countywide referendum or by a county governing body. Those counties that elect to be dry do not allow the sale of alcoholic beverages within their geographic limits.

See also: Alcohol, National Distribution of; Alcoholic Beverage Control Stores; State Legal Systems.

Elizabeth M. Williams

ALCOHOL, NATIONAL DISTRIBUTION OF

Interstate distribution of alcohol is a complex system based on the crazy quilt of state laws. The basic distribution system is a three-tiered system made up of producers, distributors, and retailers. Each state has its own rules as to who may sell directly to consumers. In addition to licensed retailers, the distributor must be licensed in a given state. Not all distributors are licensed in each state, so some producers are represented by different distributors depending on the geographic area that the distributor may cover. Sometimes the distributors have cooperative agreements that relay the distribution from one distributor to another to cross state lines.

This three tiered system was instituted after the end of Prohibition in 1933. Prior to prohibition producers had a great deal of power in their relationship with retailers. They had tying agreements that forced retailers, bars, and restaurants, to buy only from them. They not only threatened to withhold the alcoholic beverages if the retailers used another producer, but in many cases they also had invested in the business and could call loans and shut down the retailer for violating the tying agreement.

Distribution and Antitrust Laws

Antitrust laws are applicable only in situations where interference by government is necessary to curtail noncompetitive business practices that are so unreasonable as to be illegal and without justification. The Ninth Circuit Court of Appeals **in California** in *Costco v Hoen* (2008) supported the distribution system in the case in which box-store Costco challenged the three-tiered distribution system as being a violation of federal antitrust law finding that the distribution system was justifiable.

After the repeal of Prohibition states instituted a system that included a distributor to create a buffer between the producer and the retailer. In addition, the additional regulation allows for more control in the collecting of taxes. In some states the retail sales of package liquor is only allowed in state-owned or **alcoholic beverage control** stores (ABC stores). Since Prohibition this tiered system has remained the same, while the conditions that created it have changed.

Some states allow in-state wineries to sell directly to consumers. These states have had protective laws that have prohibited out-of-state wineries from selling directly to consumers in that state. The U.S. Supreme Court ruled in 2005 that Michigan and New York could not prohibit out-of-state wineries from selling directly to consumers, since those states allowed in-state wineries to do so. The high court held that the disparity in treatment between in-state and out-of-state vintners was a prohibited violation of the Commerce Clause of the U.S. Constitution.

Wineries and consumers of wine have been very active in challenging the requirement of using a distributor to purchase wine. As barriers to direct sales have been eroded, wineries have created sales on the Internet and through wine clubs, which has extended the reach of the wineries without the need of a middle party. But where wine sales in-state still require a distributor, the Twenty-first Amendment (the constitutional amendment that repealed Prohibition) allows for state regulation.

Although states can set their own policies with regard to sale of alcohol, the federal government has adopted legislation that authorizes the withholding of state highway funds from those states that allow the sale of alcoholic beverages to persons under the age of 21. Federal pressure influences policy set by the states. The federal government levies taxes on the sale of alcoholic beverages. And where there is federal jurisdiction in a geographic area, such as a military installation, the federal government can make policies that regulate the sale of alcoholic beverages.

See also: Internet Sales.

Elizabeth M. Williams

ALCOHOLIC BEVERAGE CONTROL STORES

Alcoholic beverage control stores (ABC stores) are stores in certain states where package alcoholic beverages may be sold. The stores are either run by the state or specially licensed by the state. They are not general retail stores and other stores in those states cannot sell package alcoholic beverages. In recent times, some states allow wineries to sell directly to consumers or brew pubs to sell beer made on premises even when there are ABC stores in the state.

Privatization of Alcoholic Beverage Control

Bob McDonnell, a 2009 gubernatorial candidate in Virginia, put forth in July 2009 a proposal to privatize alcoholic beverage control (ABC) stores:

As Governor, Bob McDonnell will evaluate other government assets that can be leveraged for additional revenue for the Commonwealth's transportation needs. Privatizing the commercial operations of the Virginia Department of Alcohol Beverage Control is one such asset that can be used to help fund transportation infrastructure. Virginia ABC operates over 300 retail liquor stores throughout the Commonwealth, and is one of only 18 states that does not permit the private retail sale of alcoholic beverages within its borders. Beer and wine are already sold by private entities and the sale of other alcoholic beverages is also best handled by the free enterprise system.

Governor Mark Warner's Commission on Efficiency and Effectiveness, chaired by former Governor L. Douglas Wilder, recommended to "acquire sound business assessments of the real value of a privatized ABC retail operation and develop an RFP [request for proposal] process to realize this value and authorize legislation." The report went on to say that "privatization should be structured so as to provide at least as equal a revenue stream to the localities and to the state activities that are presently supported by ABC earned income."

Source: Excerpt from "End Gridlock, Create Jobs: Get Virginia Moving Again." http://www.bobmcdonnell .com/images/site_images/PDF_Forms/End_Gridlock _Create_Jobs_Get_Virginia_Moving_Again_FINAL_3 .pdf.

The ABC stores are a way of controlling the sale and consumption of alcohol. (The role of ABC stores in some states has been broadened to also control the sale of tobacco products.) The ABC stores in a given state all charge the same amount for the same beverages. This eliminates competition. The lowered price that competition might create and the additional alcohol that might be purchased at the lower price cannot happen under the ABC store system. The ABC store revenue is a source of revenue for those states that operate their own stores. It allows the state to make money on vice and keeps the citizens out of the vice business, as when a state operates a lottery.

In addition to controlling sales through uniform pricing, ABC stores control access to alcohol by controlling the hours and days when alcohol is sold. Some states have ABC stores that are not open on Sundays or only operating limited hours on Sunday. The ABC stores are also thought to be the only reliable way to ensure that package alcohol is not sold to minors.

In those states in which the ABC agency licenses or contracts with individuals or corporations to sell package liquor for consumption off premises, those stores are known as package agencies. The prices are regulated by the state and the package agency is not operating an independent business. Money is still being earned by the state. Often these stores are located in communities that the ABC agency considers too small for a regular ABC store to be operated by the state. Keeping in mind that these stores are operated in part to provide revenue for the state, some package agencies are located in resorts or hotels where money can be earned from out-of-state visitors.

In some states ABC stores and the agencies that control them have the responsibility for licensing distribution, licensing those who sell liquor for on-site consumption, as well as consumer and youth education about alcohol consumption. The agency may also have enforcement powers.

The ABC stores were originally a reliable method for states to begin to regulate the sale of alcohol in post-Prohibition times. The Twenty-first Amendment to the Constitution not only repealed Prohibition, but it also empowered the states to control the production, sale, and distribution of alcohol within the state. States wanted to ensure that consumers received a safe and unadulterated product. And in addition the states wanted the control over sales that allowed them to collect taxes and to regulate the amount of alcohol to which consumers had access.

Not all states use ABC stores for the sale of alcoholic beverages. Some states simply issue package sales licenses to individual retailers. In those states, there is no regulation of prices or limitation of types of liquor sold.

See also: Advertising of Alcohol Products; Alcohol, In-State Distribution of; State Legal Systems.

Elizabeth M. Williams

ALLERGENS

The legal issues surrounding food allergens are related to a number of laws and practices—food labeling and advertising, for example—economics, law suits, and public health. As the society learns more about allergy and allergens, there are more ways to respond to them. The way an allergen should be handled by the food industry (for example, restaurants and manufacturers) depends on the number of people who suffer from the allergy and the severity of the reaction caused by the allergen.

Peanuts, for example, can cause a severe reaction, even death, even in minute quantities. Thus, it is reasonable that products containing peanuts or peanut products, such as peanut oil, or that may have been manufactured in a facility that uses peanut products, should be so labeled. It may be prudent in some instances to refrain from serving peanut products in confined places. Restaurants that serve dishes that may contain peanuts should clearly note such a fact either on the menu or in the restaurant.

On the other hand, other types of allergens, such as strawberries or mustard or cilantro, may not be as damaging or as pervasive. The balance of responsibility of the person with the allergy and the obligations of care that are owed by the manufacturer or by the preparer of food will be determined by a court when a person has been harmed by the ingestion of or the exposure to a food allergen.

A person who is allergic to monosodium glutamate (MSG) is wise to ask whether food in an Asian restaurant contains MSG. A prudent restaurant will also likely note on its menu or in the restaurant that is uses MSG. It is presumed that the restaurant will tell the truth about serving an allergic person MSG-free food. But the responsibility of the allergic patron to ask about the use of MSG is lessened, because there is less reasonable expectation that the patron would know that the restaurant uses MSG.

Another issue of liability, especially in restaurants, is related to the practices of the kitchen. The information is a relay from the patron to the wait staff to the kitchen. If the allergen is egg, which might be found in mayonnaise, or mustard, the wait staff must relay this information to the kitchen. The kitchen, omitting the mayonnaise or mustard from the sandwich, has to do more than just hold the mayo. Using the same knife that had been previously used to spread mustard on a sandwich, even if it has been wiped on a napkin, may be sufficient to spread mustard on a sandwich of a patron who simply does not want mustard. If the patron is allergic to mustard, that small amount of mustard that is left on the knife may be enough to trigger the allergy. The kitchen staff must be trained, must know that it is an allergy and not simply a person who doesn't like the allergen, and the wait staff must relay the proper information to the kitchen. When the allergic patron informs the restaurant of the allergy, but is nevertheless served the allergen, it is the fault of the restaurant.

See also: Food Allergen Labeling and Consumer Protection Act of 2004.

Elizabeth M. Williams

AMERICANS WITH DISABILITIES ACT AND RESTAURANTS

The Americans with Disabilities Act (ADA) is a federal law that protects the rights of people who have disabilities. In essence it is a civil rights law recognizing that some people might be discriminated against in employment because of a disability. In addition, the law requires certain accommodations to the physical space to make spaces accessible to those with disabilities. The anti-discrimination aspect of the law is administered by the **Equal Employment Opportunity Commission** (EEOC), the same agency that administers other civil rights laws. Although the ADA applies to restaurants and others in the food service industry, restaurants and the industry also have the strictest health and sanitary requirements to uphold. This can make for a difficult balance.

Any business that employs 15 or more employees, whether full- or part-time, is subject to the provisions of the ADA. From the perspective of the employee, the ADA protects the potential employee or applicant who has a disability and who is qualified to perform the job. There is no list of covered disabilities; however, there is a three-part test for disability. The person must have an impairment, that is, a medical condition or disorder; the person must be "substantially limited" by this impairment; and the limitations must be to "major life activities." There are examples of disabilities that are recognized, such as limited hearing or vision, limited use of limbs, or loss of a limb. The types of daily tasks that are considered major life activities include walking, lifting, sitting, and even thinking.

The ADA does not give an advantage to the person with the disability, as, for example, extra points on a civil service test may be given to veterans of the armed services. The business may hire the most qualified person, even if that means that the person with the disability does not receive the job. To be considered qualified, the person with the disability must meet or exceed the job requisites, such as educational, experience, and skill levels. And the person has to be able to perform the "reasonable functions" of the job without or with reasonable accommodations. Employers are allowed to consider the cost of making an accommodation, in determining whether the accommodation is reasonable. Cost and other efforts to provide accommodations are measured by whether making the necessary accommodation would be an undue hardship on the employer.

Factors to be considered in determining whether an accommodation imposes an undue hardship include the disruption of the running of the business or incurring great difficulty or great expense; and actually requiring the business to be changed to make the accommodation. These factors are decided on the degree of difficulty that they impose. For example, determining whether making an accommodation would create a financial difficulty to an employer would be a judgment call related to the financial size of the employer.

The ADA also applies to current employees who may become disabled after employment. An employer may terminate an employee who becomes a direct threat. This means that within the workplace a person's disability may cause the person to harm himself or others.

One question that has been settled is that even in businesses such as the restaurant business, where wait staff and front-of-house personnel must interact with the public, a disability such as a disfiguring scar that might make customers uncomfortable will not be considered one that disqualifies the applicant or employee.

The Food Code, published and updated by the **Food and Drug Administration**, contains a list of pathogens that are food-borne as well as the symptoms of someone suffering from them. The **Centers for Disease Control and Prevention** publish a list of diseases that are food borne. The ADA does not allow a person to be asked about these diseases until after it is determined whether the person is qualified. If it is determined that a person is qualified and is conditionally offered the job, then asking about symptoms and the use of Food Code Model Form 1-A can determine whether the person may take the job. An employer may require a physical exam, but all similar job candidates must be treated in the same manner. If applicants are not qualified, probing into their health is not appropriate under the law.

Once it is determined that an applicant is ill and that the illness causes the disability, the ADA applies. Then whether the job is a food-handling job that disqualifies the person must be determined, including whether a reasonable accommodation can be made to allow the person to still perform the job. If the person is not disabled, then the ADA is not applicable.

The ADA does not prohibit the restaurant or food service establishment from requiring current employees to fill out Model Form 1-A. The law requires the disclosure of certain symptoms, disclosure of past diagnosis of certain high-risk conditions, as well as the disclosure of a current diagnosis. A person can be required to be screened medically before returning to a food handling position. The law requires that person who has symptoms of food-borne illness must be excluded from food handling. The public health requirement overcomes any other considerations. If the employee is not disabled by the covered pathogens, the ADA does not apply. However, when the business is covered by the Family and Medical Leave Act, there may be a requirement to allow the employee to use leave under this act until the employee has recovered and can legally return to a food handling position.

The ADA also has accessibility requirements. These requirements apply to patrons of the facility and do not pose the special and particular problems in the restaurant industry that food handling by employees may pose. The discrimination that is prohibited by the ADA includes public accommodations and commercial facilities. This means that these facilities must be made accessible by people with disabilities, so that the lack of accommodation does not prohibit the disabled person from using the facility. The U.S. Architectural and Transportation Barriers Compliance Board has issued ADA Accessibility Guidelines for Buildings and Facilities (ADAAG). The law outlines the applicability of the guidelines to new construction, as well as existing structures, historic structures, and other special cases. Restaurants, bars, and other food service facilities open to the public are considered public accommodations under the law.

Accommodations depend on what amenities exist and do not require duplicative amenities. For example, if there is a water fountain in a lobby of a restaurant, a wheel-chair accessible accommodation may be as simple as the adding of a cup dispenser to allow the wheel chair user to fill a cup with water to get a drink. Today, most building codes have adopted the ADAAG requirements, so complying with local building codes, especially in new construction, will result in ADA compliance.

Elizabeth M. Williams

ANTITRUST LAW AND FOOD MANUFACTURING CONSOLIDATION

Antitrust law is designed, in the simplest of terms, to prevent monopolies from forming and to preserve competition. The body of laws that collectively form the antitrust laws support competition and prohibit anti-competitive behavior, such as price-fixing and the forming of illegal cartels to allocate markets. This is based on the presumption that if many businesses, rather than a single business, act in concert to control a market, they are more likely to succeed. The Sherman Act makes it illegal to form a monopoly through prohibited means. After some litigation resolved by the U.S. Supreme Court, Congress passed the Clayton Antitrust Act in 1914. The **Federal Trade Commission** (FTC) and the Justice Department are given authority to enforce Clayton. The Federal Trade Commission Act of 1975 provided the authority to the FTC to enforce the antitrust laws and safeguard competition.

Antitrust laws are a balance between behavior, which through competition forms a monopoly and thus destroys competition and working together to stop competition. The law recognizes the need to protect competition for the benefit of consumers and also recognizes that competition itself can produce a winner who should not be penalized.

When companies in the same industry begin to merge or be purchased, the government has an interest in approving or prohibiting mergers or sales that would result in a market share so large that it would restrict or eliminate competition, leaving consumers with little or no choice. The Hart-Scott-Rodino Antitrust Improvements Act of 1976 requires that certain mergers must file a notice with the FTC and the Justice Department. Filing is required when companies with a net revenue, sales, or assets of over a certain threshold amount and when the other party has assets, sales, or net revenues of over threshold amount and where the sale price or the value of the acquired company is more than a certain threshold amount wish to merge or purchase or be purchased. Thresholds are set each year under the act by the FTC. The thresholds were reduced in 2010, so now smaller transactions fall into the net of the notice requirements. The law also establishes a waiting period, giving the government time for review of the proposed action. Although it is not prohibited, it is unlikely that the government will file an action to challenge a merger or acquisition, if it has not objected during the waiting period. This gives business a sense of security in its actions. When the government objects to the merger, it is referred to as not cleared. The two snack companies, Snyder's of Hanover and Utz Quality Foods, called off a planned merger in 2009 reportedly as a result of the objection of the FTC during the waiting period and the filings. Parties complained that having to respond to a "second filing" and answering all of the questions and providing the requested information could be cost prohibitive.

To further the seamlessness of the transaction, the National Association of Attorneys General has provided a Voluntary Pre-Merger Disclosure Compact that allows the merging parties to not only provide information to the FTC, but also share that information with the states that are parties to the compact. Because the states may also object to a merger under state law, this compact can facilitate a smooth transition to merger when there is no objection.

For example, the Justice Department brought an action in 2010 to force Dean Foods to dispose of the part of the company it obtained when it purchased Foremost Foods. The acquisition took place in April 2009. The Justice Department asserts that there is no competition in the sale of milk to grocery stores and to schools in multiple states. Because competition was destroyed in this particular area, prices are not competitive and there is no choice. The action also prays for a notice to the Justice Department before other mergers by Dean in milk production and sales. Dean has argued that because of the merger dairy farmers have a better business environment, making sales of their milk to the processor more profitable and secure. As Dean grows, it will need more milk from the dairy farmers. In addition, the economies of scale created by the merger should reduce costs and thereby reduce prices for consumers.

In 2009 the chocolate industry faced antitrust threats from the government. Mars, Hershey, Cadbury, and Nestle were accused of fixing the price of chocolate. These four companies control up to three-quarters of the chocolate candy market in the United States. A comparison of their prices makes it appear that the companies raised their prices in concert, to destroy competition, giving consumers no alternative price choices. Consumers had to settle for the higher prices. This group of candy companies faced many separate antitrust actions that were consolidated. They were accused of price-fixing on three separate occasions. Contributing factors could be market saturation and a flat demand, causing the parties to collude to raise prices. The chocolate manufacturers claim that they did not collude, but simply paralleled each other.

The European Commission of the European Union also has an antitrust provision in its laws. Many foreign countries have antitrust laws as well. Canada and Germany have brought antitrust actions against the chocolate industry. In Canada there is a class action lawsuit that alleges 10 years' worth of price-fixing in the industry, causing the citizens of Canada to have paid too much for chocolate candy because of lack of competition. Also alleged are secret meetings to plan the price-fixing. The parties are said to have punished those retailers who wished to discount the product. Cadbury agreed to pay money to be dismissed from the suit and agreed to cooperate with the plaintiffs. In Germany, meeting to fix prices in the chocolate market has been admitted by some parties.

See also: Appendix 7: *In the Matter of McCormick & Company, Inc.*

Further Reading Clayton Antitrust Act in 1914, 15 United States Code section 12 and following. The Federal Trade Commission Act of 1914, 15 United States Code section 45 and following; Hart-Scott-Rodino Antitrust Improvements Act of 1976, 15 United States Code section 18; Sherman Antitrust Act of 1890, 15 United States Code section 1 and following.

Elizabeth M. Williams

ANTITRUST LAW AND GROCERY STORE CONSOLIDATION

Antitrust law has the purpose of preventing monopolies and preserving and protecting competition. Protecting competition includes the prohibition of combining to fix prices and to enter into other agreements that would restrict competition. Just as in the food manufacturing business, the grocery business has been guilty of practices that tend toward creating a monopoly or to limiting or restricting competition.

In 1941 six groceries that belonged to the Connecticut Grocery Council, the Council, and a number of individuals were brought to trial under the Sherman Antitrust Act for combining to fix prices. The parties were fined and ordered not to combine. The Great Atlantic and Pacific Tea Company (A & P), a large grocery chain in the mid-20th century, was considered a threat to competition because of its buying power and practices. It was considered such a threat that the U.S. Attorney General was approached by an organization of independent grocers in 1949 with the proposal to bring an antitrust action against the A & P as a monopoly.

Grocery stores that become very large through merger or acquisition of other stores reduce competition by reducing consumer choice. In addition, because of economies of scale of large purchases and buying power that can result in lower costs to the grocer, it can become hard for independent stores and other smaller chains to offer competitive pricing. It may be easy to cry monopoly to try to regain the advantage, as did the grocers in 1949. But today the power of the large store is even greater than in the past.

The case that best represents this power is Wal-Mart. Wal-Mart has grown so large and powerful that it can demand concessions from suppliers, it puts local retailers out of business just by virtue of its size, and its sales are greater than the combined earnings of the next six businesses. Although Wal-Mart has plans to grow, the failure of these large, powerful companies can also have a serious effect on the economy, as there are no businesses left to absorb the employees who may be let go. It has been argued that Wal-Mart does not operate within the market with market rules. Wal-Mart controls and manages the market. That a large concern has this power and can control the market does not mean that it is doing anything illegal. The Cato Institute, for example, considers Wal-Mart a lower price alternative that gives consumers what they want at the price they want. The balance between intentional price fixing and anti-competitive behavior and having anti-competitive results of legal behavior is the balancing act that courts must engage in when trying to resolve complaints against a monolithic power. The power of a company in this position is called monopsony.

Wal-Mart has been sued in several states, notably Arkansas, Wisconsin, and Oklahoma, either by the state attorney general or private concerns, alleging various types of antitrust complaints such as lowering prices to eliminate competition and selling below cost to eliminate competition and thus obtain monopoly status. The Supreme Court of Arkansas ruled in favor of Wal-Mart, which is headquartered in Arkansas. In other states, cases have been settled rather than being finally determined by a court. Wal-Mart was accused of monopolistic pricing in both Germany and in Mexico. Wal-Mart successfully defended itself in both venues.

In 2007 the Federal Trade Commission (FTC) challenged a proposed merger between Whole Foods Company and Wild Oats. The FTC and Whole Foods reached a settlement in 2009 in which Whole Foods agreed that it would divest itself of a number of Wild Oats properties as well as one Whole Foods store. Whole Foods would also not maintain the Wild Oats brand, although the settlement allows Whole Foods to sell the brand. The FTC abandoned its pursuit of dissolution of the merger, which had been in the courts for several years. The FTC had taken the position that the merger would reduce competition in the natural and health foods marketplace.

The FTC asserted that natural, health, and organic foods were not the same market as regular groceries, and since Whole Foods and Wild Oats were the only two national chains competing in this special market, their merger could not be allowed. If this merger were to be analyzed in the larger grocery market, Kroger, Winn Dixie, Wal-Mart, and many other grocery chains would dwarf even the combined Whole Foods and Wild Oats, making the merger insignificant in the grocery store world. Many of the larger chains are now carrying organic products and it seems that that trend is increasing, thus the merger between Whole Foods and Wild Oats has even less impact on the overall market. This is curious, because the FTC usually relies on price data to make an objective case when describing market share and carving out what it calls a "distinct" market. It did not do so in the case of Whole Foods.

The FTC's failure to approve a merger or lawsuits by states to address charges of anti-competitive activities places a heavy burden on the businesses in question. They have the burden, whether the actual legal burden or the de facto burden, of showing that their actions or intentions are not anti-competitive. This can be very expensive and time-consuming for the business. Settlements in these matters commonly are entered into to avoid continued litigation and to allow businesses to move on. The stalling of activities because of litigation or threat of disapproval by the government can be very expensive also. The time value of money, increased interest payments, and loss of financing all greatly affect the ability of a business to continue to defend its position.

See also: Antitrust Law and Food Manufacturing Consolidation; Laws, Enforcement of; Appendix 7: *In the Matter of McCormick & Company, Inc.*

Further Reading: Bradley, Robert L. "On the Origins of the Sherman Anti-Trust Act." *Journal of Legal Studies* (January 1985): 14; *Wal-Mart Stores, Inc. v. American Drugs, Inc.* 319 Ark. 214, 891S.W.2d 30 (1995).

Elizabeth M. Williams

APPELLATION D'ORIGINE CONTRÔLÉE

Appellation d'origine contrôlée (AOC) is a French term that means "controlled name of origin." The French apply this term to a legal certification system that grants the use of a particular name based on geographic indicators. Thus certain wines, cheeses, and other food products may be named with the name of their region. This certification system reflects a belief that the soil, culture, and environmental conditions affect the flavor of a product. Similar products produced by a similar method but in a different location will not have the same flavor. Examples of AOCs are Champagne, as opposed to sparkling wine, and Roquefort, as opposed to blue cheese.

The French Department of Agriculture not only polices the use of the AOC in France to see that other products do not use the protected names, but also monitors the standards that are required of those producers within the designated geographic regions. Italy and Spain have similar laws. Their controls, *denominazione di origine controllata* and *denominación de origen*, respectively, apply to wines, cheeses, and other products. Other countries that have foods protected by certification systems are South Africa, Portugal, Germany, and Austria.

These fierce protections have greatly influenced the position of the European Union (EU) on this point. The EU regulations refer to the Protected Designation Point of Origin (PDO), also the Protected Geographical Indication (PGI), and the designation Traditional Specialty Guaranteed (TSG). The law that is currently enforced within the EU is being extended outside of the EU as a part of the EU's protection of its member states. The law is being extended through treaties and other agreements that are being negotiated between the EU and other nations.

This law has several purposes. The first is to protect the reputation of the products that have been traditionally produced in these areas from inferior imitators who might try to use the name. These are products known by the name of the place where they are produced, for example, Parma ham. Also the products are usually produced according to certain standards, and the law helps to maintain those standards from deteriorating by removing the privilege of using the designation from those who do not maintain the standards. And finally, the law is a form of consumer protection so that those people who want to buy the special products are assured that others cannot use the name.

The rules in the EU rely, to a great extent, on the specialized laws already adopted in the various member nations that have these traditional products to protect. However, the EU also has created an overarching regime to manage these laws. That regime is called the general regime. Within the general regime are separate rules regarding different types of foods, such as spirits and wine.

The designation PDO means that a food stuff comes entirely, that is processed and totally produced, in the region named. The designation PGI refers to traditional products produced within a given geographic area. For example a special traditional cake made from local ingredients may include flour that is not actually from the area, because flour may not be grown in the area and has traditionally been brought in for the product. The designation TSG refers to the traditional method of making a product. It is not a geographic designation.

The United States does not really have an analogous system, but has relied on the trademark system to protect products and to protect consumers. This has caused some conflict with the EU and certain member countries who object, for example, to the sale of products labeled "champagne" produced in the United States. Without a deep tradition in the United States to protect traditionally produced products, but rather to rely on trademark and the free market to protect products, there has often been conflict with more traditional nations.

The question of whether Parmesan cheese can actually be produced in Wisconsin or whether it is only a Parmesan-style cheese is one with which the United States is grappling. However, the list of

Genuine Roquefort

On August 31, 1666, the Parliament in Toulouse, France, declared that "the only genuine Roquefort comes from the cellars in the town bearing its name." This is considered the first assertion of *Appellation d'origine contrôlée*.

Counterfeit Wine?

In *Koch v. Christie's*, 10-cv-2804, U.S. District Court, Southern District of New York (Manhattan), fine wine collector William Koch sued Christie's auction house in 2010 for allegedly selling wines that because of its experience it knew or should have known were counterfeit. In 2005, Koch purchased wines at Christie's that were purported to have belonged to Thomas Jefferson, dated 1784 and 1787. Koch claims that the auction house knowingly inaccurately attributed the wine to Thomas Jefferson.

products that have trademarked the name of their product, which includes the name of a product protected by an AOC or other controlled name, is long. The trademark laws and many other U.S. laws would have to be changed to stop this practice. Currently, the EU can stop the importation into the EU of these products with offending names; however, sometimes this merely means a relabeling for the EU market. As the EU expands its influence, especially with other European nations that wish to join it, those nations may also begin to control the importation of offending products.

See also: European Union Regulations; Trademarks; Appendix 16: World Trade Organization Ministerial Conference Decision.

Elizabeth M. Williams

B

BABY FOOD

Baby formula is regulated by the Center for Food Safety and Applied Nutrition (CFSAN) of the **Food and Drug Administration** (FDA). The CFSAN oversees nutritional requirements, labeling, and packaging. The regulations that oversee infant formula are found at 21 Code of Federal Regulations sections 106 and following. Manufacturers of baby formula must register their formula with the FDA and produce formula that conforms to the stated FDA nutritional requirements. As a part of its regulatory function, the agency annually inspects facilities that manufacture infant formula. The agency takes samples and analyzes them to ensure that the formulas meet the nutritional requirements and contain no harmful contaminants. New facilities are inspected. Any necessary recalls are handled by the agency.

There are three types of infant formula: powdered formula that is intended to be mixed with water, a concentrated liquid that is intended to be diluted with an equal amount of water, and a ready-to-drink formula that can be fed directly to infants.

Because formulas must be prepared for infants for feeding and may require the addition of water, the FDA has an interest in the instructions that are given to the preparer. These instructions are considered safety instructions and inform the preparer how to prepare the water and mix the formula. In addition, since the product will be administered with a bottle and nipple, instructions for preparing the nipple and bottle are given. Warnings about using the correct amount of water, the temperature of the formula when serving, and the correct storage of prepared formula are required and regulated.

Federal regulations compel a "use by" date be placed on infant formula and other foods intended for consumption by infants. Infant formula may retain its nutrient value if used beyond the use-by date; however, liquid formula may separate and powdered formula may clump and not dissolve. In either case, old formula may not pass through the hole in a nipple, clogging it, thus, the use-by date not only refers to nutrient retention, but also ability to be properly used, that is, pass through the hole in the nipple. For other infant foods, the use-by date refers to retention of nutrient levels as stated on the label and maintenance of texture and color of the food.

In late 2008 there was a controversy when the FDA found contaminants in baby formula manufactured in the United States but did not immediately inform the public or propose a plan for removing the contaminants. The contaminants were melamine and cyanuric acid, which is used in the sanitizing of the equipment used to make infant formula. Melamine was found previously in infant formula manufactured in China. Melamine is used to elevate the level of protein in diluted formula to make it appear to comply with nutritional requirements. Several children in China died as a result of drinking this formula and thousands were hospitalized. After the FDA found contaminated formula manufactured in the United States, the agency called the manufacturers and notified them of the agency's findings. The agency did not say when it would inform the public.

The FDA did not believe that the U.S. melamine contamination was intentional, but it was a part of the manufacturing process. When discussing the melamine contamination in the Chinese formula, the FDA scientists did not consider any level of melamine safe. Several days later the FDA issued minimum levels of melamine considered safe. The controversy raised by the way the FDA handled the finding of melamine in U.S. manufactured formula has made the FDA more sensitive regarding infant formula.

Recently the FDA has warned baby food manufacturers that they could not make unverifiable health claims. Health claims on labels and in advertising are based on dietary guidelines established by the government and promulgated through the administrative process. There are currently no such guidelines for infants under two years of age. Other objections to labels have also been challenged as being misleading. The manufacturers have 15 days to either challenge the FDA's claims or to give the FDA a response as to how they will comply and change their labeling. The agency has notified manufacturers of its intention to propose new guidelines for labeling and nutritional content.

The administration of the organic label being applied to baby food is controlled by the **U.S. Department of Agriculture** (USDA) as are other organic labeling matters. There has been some controversy regarding what additives are actually organic. There are two synthetic fatty acids that are at the heart of the controversy: DHA and ARA. Some studies have shown that these acids may encourage neural development. In 2006 the staff of the USDA stated that because the fatty acids are synthetic, baby formula that contains these substances cannot be labeled organic. They were not on the list of approved substances. There was general belief that if an application was made through the usual procedure, they would be denied inclusion on the list. The fatty acids are produced in a procedure that some consider potentially dangerous, utilizing hexane. A USDA administrator has overruled the staff's position of these additives.

An attorney for the formula makers had argued that leaving the two substances off of the approved list was actually an oversight. The USDA administrator agreed. The reasoning was that vitamins and minerals were on the approved list. Fatty acids are not considered vitamins and minerals. Fatty acids are accessory nutrients. That category was not included on the approved list. Hexane is the substance that is banned from being used in processing organic food. The USDA official has stated that it isn't specifically banned in processing synthetic additives.

Several consumer groups have challenged the USDA's position, saying that the additives are synthetic, and thus they should not be approved in organic baby food. They also argue that by approving these additives by finding an "oversight," the administrator is making rules unilaterally and thus illegally in absolute violation of the rule-making procedure established in the **Administrative Procedures Act**.

See also: Administrative Procedures Act, Food and Drug Administration, U.S. Department of Agriculture.

Elizabeth M. Williams

BANKRUPTCY

Bankruptcy is the remedy for indebtedness that allows the bankrupt party to seek relief and protection from creditors. A recognition of bankruptcy as a federal protection stems from Article 1, Section 8 of the U.S. Constitution. The law is federal, although there are some state-based protections. The most recent revisions of the Bankruptcy Code are found in the Bankruptcy Abuse Prevention and Consumer Protection Act of 2005. (Cases filed after October 17, 2005, are handled under the new law. Those that continue their proceedings, but were filed before that date, continue under the provisions of the previous law.) The law reflects the principle that a person or business can be in debt from which it is impossible to recover. The bankruptcy law allows the debtor to recover, either by legally discharging debts—allowing the creditor to take the debt as a loss for tax purposes—or by allowing the debtor to reorganize the debts to allow him or her to be better able to repay them.

Bankruptcy can apply to individuals, such as farmers, those involved in the food industry as either employees or owners, or businesses. Downturns in the economy, oversaturation of markets and changes in the real estate market are among the types of factors that affect the economic health of the restaurant industry, for example, and thus affect the number of restaurant bankruptcies. Benningan's and Black Angus are two restaurant chains that filed for bankruptcy protection in 2008 and 2009, respectively.

The different types of bankruptcy are traditionally known by the chapter numbers in the Bankruptcy Code. Chapter 7 is also known as liquidation. This refers to the takeover of the debtor's estate by a bankruptcy trustee, under the aegis of the bankruptcy court, which liquidates the debtor's assets and applies them to the debts. The remaining debts are discharged on completion of the liquidation. If the debtor is an individual, the law requires that a means test be applied to determine whether the debtor is eligible for liquidation. Not all debts are dischargeable in bankruptcies. Student loans and back taxes, for example, may not qualify for discharge.

Chapter 13 is also known as debt adjustment. This provision is applicable to those debtors who have a regular source of income, but who have amassed debt that cannot be paid in accordance with the agreed-on schedule. For example, an escalating mortgage amount might make it impossible to keep making mortgage payments on time. A debtor who files for bankruptcy under this chapter submits a plan for repayment. Under an approved plan the debtor remains in control of his estate and may keep those assets, such as a house, while making payments under the approved plan. Those whose income does not pass the means test to qualify for Chapter 7 may also file under Chapter 13.

Chapter 11 is known as Reorganization. This chapter is used by businesses that are unable to pay their debts on schedule but desire to continue to operate and do business to earn money to pay their debts. The business continues to operate under a court-approved plan to repay debts. The creditors can have input in the reorganization plan. This is the chapter usually selected by companies that are having trouble paying debt without the protection of the court from seizure and suit. It provides a great deal of latitude in the court to affect leases and debt payment and other business contracts.

Chapter 12 is a form of reorganization for family farms and fishermen. If the farm or fisherman has regular income, the provisions are very much like the ones applicable in Chapter 13. Similarly Chapter 12 provides for a trustee who approves a plan, while the farmer or fishermen continue to operate the business. Both Chapter 12 and Chapter 13 bankruptcies may last up to five years, so a discharge may be delayed until the completion of the plan.

There are also other special provisions for members of the armed forces whose finances are adversely affected by their service, as well as other provisions for special circumstances.

A discharge in bankruptcy is a specific type of elimination of the debtor's legal liability for certain debt. As stated, not all debts are eligible for discharge in bankruptcy. But when the discharge is granted, creditors may not proceed against the debtor for the collection of the debt. The creditor may not take legal collections action and is also prohibited from telephoning or writing letters or in any other way attempting to collect the debt. The discharge is a permanent injunction against the collection of the debt. When a lien has not been avoided by the court, however, a creditor may enforce the lien on the termination of the bankruptcy. This means, for example, a mortgage that remains on the property after the bankruptcy will allow a mortgagee to recover the property from the debtor but not collect on the debt.

Discharge occurs as soon as is practicable depending on the provision under which the bankruptcy was filed. This could be after the time for filing an objection to the discharge in a Chapter 7 filing or as long as five years after filing in a Chapter 13 or 12. In filing a petition for bankruptcy, the debtor must list all debts, all assets, and all income. A failure to comply with this requirement could result in a refusal by the trustee to discharge the debt. Besides most tax debt, other types of debt generally not dischargeable include court-mandated spousal and child support, fines and penalties that are due to a branch of government, debts caused by a deliberate and intentional act causing injury to a person or property by the debtor, debts that resulted from a personal injury caused by the debtor while intoxicated, debts owed to co-ops or condominium associations for regular fees, and overpayments made by the government to the debtor that the debt has not yet refunded. Other types of debt that involve fraud or alleged fraud may not be discharged by bankruptcy; however, this is dependent on objection by the creditors. Creditors may make other objections to discharge. There are some types of debts that are allowed to be discharged in a Chapter 13 filing, but not a Chapter 7 filing.

Once a discharge has been made in a Chapter 7 bankruptcy, a debtor may not receive another discharge if a new case filed is less than eight years from the previous discharge. There are additional limitations on second filings and the timing of second filings depending on the type of bankruptcy.

Bankruptcy Damage Control

Press Release Issued by New World Pasta Company in 2004 upon Filing for Bankruptcy Protection and Made a Part of the Securities and Exchange Commission Record:

New World Pasta Company obtains commitment for $45 million in financing
Company files for voluntary Chapter 11 Reorganization
Company is conducting business as usual and looks forward to the future

HARRISBURG, PA—May 10, 2004—New World Pasta Company announced today that the Company (and its U.S.-based subsidiaries) has filed a voluntary petition seeking reorganization under Chapter 11 of the U.S. Bankruptcy Code. The filing in the U.S. Bankruptcy Court for the Middle District of Pennsylvania will enable the Company to operate under the protection of the Court while it reorganizes and reduces its debt, strengthens its financial position and restructures its balance sheet. In connection with the filing, the Company also announced that it has obtained a commitment for a $45 million debtor-in-possession financing facility from a financing group led by one of its current banks. New World Pasta Company is conducting business as usual in the United States, and throughout the world. New World Pasta Company's subsidiaries in Canada and Italy are not part of the Chapter 11 filing.

Upon Court approval, which is expected within the next few days, up to $20 million of the financing facility will be available immediately on an interim basis. The Company believes that the $45 million financing facility, together with internally generated cash from operations, will be sufficient to operate its business, including the payment of all post-filing obligations to suppliers and vendors.

Wynn Willard, the Company's Chief Executive Officer, commented,

This action by our Company to file for reorganization under Chapter 11 was taken only after much review by the Company's Board of Directors and our senior executive team, and after consultation with advisors expert on these matters. We concluded that it was the right step to improve our business for the future.

Now, we have the opportunity to reduce our debt burden and to strengthen our financial and marketplace position. We expect our core business activities to continue unimpeded. We will manufacture and ship our products in the normal course, and our consumers will continue to enjoy our great products on a daily basis.

"This filing will help our efforts to emerge as a stronger, more financially stable competitor," added Ed Lyons, the Company's Senior Vice President and Chief Financial Officer. "We will continue to work on strengthening our business, reducing costs, and becoming more efficient. We at the Company will be talking to our stakeholders, and we look forward to working productively with them through the reorganization process."

"This reorganization will allow us to better position our Company and, importantly, our trusted brands for future growth," said Doug Ehrenkranz, the Company's Senior Vice President of Sales and Marketing. "We expect there to be no business interruption during this process. Our reorganization process should be invisible to our customers and consumers."

Employees are being paid in the usual manner and employee benefits will continue, subject to Court approval, which the Company believes it will receive within the next few days.

New World Pasta Company is a leading marketer and supplier of dry pasta in the United States and Canada, with well-known brands such as Ronzoni, Creamette, San Giorgio, American Beauty, Skinner and Prince. Headquartered in Harrisburg, Pennsylvania, New World Pasta Company has over 1,100 employees in the United States, Canada, and Italy.

Forward-Looking Statements

This Press Release Includes Forward-Looking Statements within the Meaning of Section 27a of the Securities Act of 1933 and Section 21e of the Securities Exchange Act of 1934, As Amended, Which Represents the Company's Expectations and Beliefs Concerning Future Events That Involve Risks and Uncertainties Which Could Cause Actual Results to Differ Materially from Those Currently Anticipated. All Statements Other Than Statements of Historical Facts Included in This Release Are Forward-Looking Statements. Forward-Looking Statements Include But Are Not Limited to the Intent, Belief, or Current Expectations of the Company and Members of Its Senior Management Team with Respect to the Timing of, Completion of, and Scope of the Company's Reorganization Plan, Strategic Business Plan, Financing Arrangements, Debt Market Conditions, and the Company's Future Liquidity, as Well as Assumptions upon Which Such Statements Are Based. Factors That Could Cause Actual Results to Differ Materially from Those Expressed or Implied in Such Forward-Looking Statements Include but Are Not Limited To Approval of Plans and Activities by the Bankruptcy Court, Risks Associated with Operating a Business under Chapter 11 Protection, Obtaining and Complying with Terms of Debtor-In-Possession Financing, Future Adverse Developments with Respect to the Company's Liquidity Position or Operations of the Company's Various Businesses, Adverse Developments in the Company's Efforts to Renegotiate Its Funding, and Adverse Developments in the Financing Markets for Debt, Adverse Developments in the Timing or Results of the Company's Business Plan, Including the Timeline to Emerge from Chapter 11, the Completion of the Company's Financial Statements, Which Could Uncover Adjustments in Presently Unknown Areas, the Preparation of Restated Historical Financial Statements, If Necessary, as Well as Those Factors Set Forth in Our Periodic Reports Filed with the SEC. Consequently, All of the Forward-Looking Statements Made in This Press Release Are Qualified by These and Other Factors, Risks, and Uncertainties.

A debtor who has been discharged from a debt may pay the debt, although the creditor cannot legally collect the debt. There are many reasons why a person or company may wish to do this, for example, to protect a reputation or to repay a family member.

The law is very clear about discrimination against debtors. This is particularly important in a transient industry, like the restaurant industry, where people come and go. Discrimination based on filing bankruptcy or for not paying a discharged debt is prohibited.

See also: Bankruptcy, Business Liquidation; Bankruptcy, Business Reorganization.

Elizabeth M. Williams

BANKRUPTCY, BUSINESS LIQUIDATION

Bankruptcy is a process by which debts can be discharged and a business reorganized. When a business has suffered losses that make it impossible to continue to reorganize, a liquidation is the course of action that allows the business to resolve its debts and close. In such a bankruptcy, which is also known as a Chapter 7 filing, because it is defined in Chapter 7 of the Bankruptcy Code (Title 11, United States Code), the business is actually liquidated under the control of the trustee. The trustee assesses the debt, liquidates the assets, and uses the funds created through the liquidation to pay the debts in the statutorily defined order of priority.

For example, Tom's Foods, Inc., defaulted on approximately $60 million owed to creditors, and it filed for bankruptcy protection. Although it originally attempted to reorganize, this effort was not successful. The bankruptcy court approved the liquidation of the company through purchase of the assets by Lance, Inc. The debts of Tom's were discharged by the court, so Lance received the assets of the company without its debts.

Although a debtor may be forced to file a petition for bankruptcy relief, there are times when creditors can put the debtor into bankruptcy. This is known as involuntary bankruptcy. In either case the business must cease operations until the business is taken over by the bankruptcy trustee. A trustee is appointed as soon as feasible after filing so that the business does not further deteriorate and so that assets can be safeguarded. The trustee assesses the assets of the business and determines the best method of liquidation to obtain the most money for the payment of creditors. The best method may be by selling assets to another similar business in one parcel or the trustee might determine that selling the assets piecemeal will yield more lucrative results.

Selling the business to another similar business or selling a division of the debtor business as a unit may result in the employees retaining their jobs. This may be something that the trustee takes into consideration when deciding how to proceed.

Once the business is liquidated, the trustee pays the creditors in the order of priority enacted into the Bankruptcy Code. All of the claims in one class of priority are paid before the next lower class is satisfied. The first priority is to pay the administrative expenses of the bankruptcy. This ensures that the trustee can be paid and expenses of the trustee are reimbursed. Other priority claims to be paid are to employee benefit plans. There are limits to what is due to employees as wages. The funds must be for income earned in the 180 days prior to filing the bankruptcy and with a limit to the dollar amount that can be paid per employee. On a limited basis, claims based on sales of grain to producers of grain and sales of fish owed to U.S. fishermen form the next class of priority. Priority creditors without a security interest in the assets of the debtor are known as unsecured priority creditors. The other unsecured creditors are known as general unsecured creditors. Priority unsecured creditors are paid until the funds are depleted.

Only after the priority creditors are paid will the general unsecured creditors be paid. When the liquidation of the assets results in insufficient funds to pay the general unsecured creditors, they may not receive anything in a bankruptcy. Alternatively they may receive only a proportion of the funds owed to them. All general unsecured creditors would receive an amount proportional to the debt owed.

Secured creditors may receive all or part of the secured property from the trustee in a bankruptcy. The determining factor will usually be the value of the security interest in proportion to the value of the asset. For example, when there is a recent mortgage on a building, the building may not sell for more than the amount owed. The trustee may allow the secured creditor to foreclose on the property. However, if the amount still owed on a mortgage is substantially less than the value of the building, the creditor may have to pay the excess to the bankrupt estate to obtain the asset. Alternatively, the trustee may sell the asset and pay the debt to the secured creditor and use the difference to pay other creditors. On the other hand, where the secured amount is more than the value of the asset, the debt can be divided into the amount that is secured and the excess that is general unsecured debt. From the standpoint of the creditor, the amount owed is referred to as the claim.

Creditors may file for involuntary bankruptcy, forcing the debtor into bankruptcy, when the creditors think that the debtor is not administering the payment of its debts to their advantage or the priorities of payment would favor the creditors in bankruptcy, but not out of bankruptcy. For example, if a restaurant is paying its employees and its suppliers, but not its landlord, its bank debt secured on fixtures, or its payments on sales tax, the creditors might decide that as the city might file a lien for back sales tax, thus creating a priority, creditors might fall into a higher priority in the bankruptcy than outside the bankruptcy. Forcing the debtor into involuntary bankruptcy would protect the creditor.

To protect employees and retirees from loss when a company files for bankruptcy, bills were introduced into Congress in 2010 by Assistant Senate Majority Leader Dick Durbin and House Judiciary Committee Chairman John Conyers. Their proposed law, titled Protecting Employees and Retirees in Business Bankruptcies Act, would apply to Chapter 11 bankruptcies. The proposed law would increase the amount that an employee can receive as an unsecured priority creditor. It also would allow a second amount for the same employees for contributions to employee benefit plans. It provides for employees or retirees to claim a loss in value to the retirement plan due to fraud or by the company's breach of fiduciary duty.

See also: Bankruptcy, Business Reorganization.

Elizabeth M. Williams

BANKRUPTCY, BUSINESS REORGANIZATION

Bankruptcy is a process by which debts can be discharged or a business reorganized. A small business that is a sole proprietorship cannot file bankruptcy separately from its owner, so discussing a business bankruptcy applies to a business that is a corporation, a formal partnership, or a limited liability company (LLC).

For a business that is not able to pay its debts, but that is making money, reorganization of the business under the protection of the bankruptcy court could be an option that can allow the business to pay its debts in a different fashion. Bankruptcy may also be a business strategy for businesses where creditors are unable to renegotiate debt.

When there are changes in the economic climate, a high interest rate, which may have been reasonable at the time entering into the loan, may make payment of a debt a struggle for a business even when the business is still making money. Invoking the protection of the bankruptcy court could provide additional cash for operations, allowing the company to perhaps reduce the interest rate it was paying on its debt. The filing will invoke the automatic stay that will stop any creditors from going to collections or being brought to judgment. The filing could allow the business to be freed from onerous contracts.

A bankruptcy could allow the business the ability to prune the business and create more advantageous loans. Paying the debts under the approved reorganization plan and coming out of bankruptcy could create a new and viable company that can either continue to operate and make money for its owners or could present an attractive company that can be sold by its owners. It is not an immediate solution, but a company that owners desire to sell might need the transformation of bankruptcy to become attractive enough to sell in a relatively short time.

A reorganization usually allows the business to remain under the control and operation of the management. This situation is known as a debtor-in-possession. The bankruptcy court can appoint a trustee to operate the business, when it considers this is in the best interest of the creditors, as when there is gross mismanagement of the business. Even when the court allows the owners or managers to continue to operate, they do so under the power of the court. However, the reorganization also requires the business to work with creditors to negotiate the plan, to comply with the reporting requirements of the bankruptcy law, and to cooperate with lawyers who represent the business. Bankruptcy filings are a public document, so that becomes an issue to be considered by the business. The business is required to disclose to the court and thus to creditors the actual financial position of the business. It is often a revelation to the creditors to see the position of the business. Sometimes this causes the creditor to be willing to change the terms of a debt to ensure that it is repaid. Sometimes the creditor is not able to renegotiate a debt itself, even if it would like to, and filing bankruptcy is the only way to change the terms of a debt under orders from the bankruptcy court. The business is the fiduciary of the creditors, operating the business on their behalf, during the bankruptcy. Success in coming out of bankruptcy is dependent on following a realistic plan.

The creditors in a reorganization have to vote to approve the plan. A committee of creditors is appointed. The creditors committee can accept the plan or negotiate with the debtor until it can approve the plan. If the plan cannot be accepted by the creditors, the court can convert the reorganization to a liquidation. The threat of this conversion of the bankruptcy is a powerful pressure on the debtor company to negotiate with the creditors. When the creditors do not accept the plan, it is still up to the court to decide whether to accept the plan after hearing the input of the creditors and the debtor. The court must believe that the debtor can realistically achieve the plan and pay back creditors.

In a Chapter 11, the short-term plan is proposed by the debtor. After 120 days the creditors can also propose a plan. The term for approval of the reorganization plan is to say that the plan is confirmed by the court. It the plan is not approved, the bankruptcy can be converted to a liquidation or the bankruptcy can be dismissed. When the bankruptcy is dismissed, the automatic stay is lifted. After dismissal the creditors may pursue their remedies for collection of any remaining debt in methods available to them in ordinary out-of-bankruptcy proceedings.

Bankruptcy provides for relief from executory contracts. Executory contracts are those in which the parties have not yet taken substantial action in fulfilling the obligations to each other or where there are continuing obligations between or among the parties. The contracts can be terminated when doing so would be in the best interest of the company and the creditors. Examples of the types of contracts that can be terminated are leases and supply contracts. When these are terminated, no additional payments are due. Monies that are past due from a period before the contract is terminated are general unsecured debts.

When a publicly traded company files a bankruptcy, those traded on the New York and the American Stock Exchanges and the NASDAQ will be delisted. Delisted stock can still be traded as over-the-counter stocks. For many businesses, the stock is left without value by the termination triggered by confirmation of the reorganization plan.

Issues covered by the reorganization plan include the best way to prune or dispose of assets, whether to recapitalize, whether to merge with another business, and whether imprudent contracts should be terminated. Assuming new debts during the bankruptcy—as in recapitalizing—is problematic in a plan, because debts acquired after filing for bankruptcy are usually not able to be discharged. If the debtor does not make a full disclosure of debts or income, it may not be fully discharged or even find the bankruptcy dismissed. Creditors, too, can be dismissed if they do anything fraudulent or conceal certain information from the court.

See also: Bankruptcy, Business Liquidation.

Elizabeth M. Williams

BEEF, ORGANIC

The **U.S. Department of Agriculture** (USDA) adopted organic standards for beef under the authority of the Organic Foods Production Act (OFPA), which was part of the 1990 Farm Bill. The bill authorized the National Organic Program (NOP) under the USDA to promulgate regulations defining what is organic in all areas including the production of beef. To be labeled organic under federal regulations, the food, including beef, must be produced in accordance with the OFPA.

Organic standards for beef include raising cattle without the use of growth hormone, antibiotics, or steroids. Feed given to the cattle, including any grains, must be organic. There is an exception in the organic feed requirement in that the organic feed must be available. This means that, if it is not available, the beef can be labeled organic even if the animal was fed nonorganic feed. And the soil on the pasture land used by the cattle must be certified as organic. The processing plants where the cattle are butchered must also be organic. There can be no irradiation.

There is still some dissatisfaction regarding the adequacy of enforcement of the federal regulations. And state standards for organic beef are often more stringent than federal standards. In some cases other associations and organizations have been formed to certify standards across state lines that are higher than those of the NOP.

In addition the question of the practice of feeding cattle with grain as opposed to grass-fed cattle is one that is often of interest to those consumers who want to eat organic beef, but that is a separate issue from that of organics. Some consumers prefer to eat grass-fed beef, because they believe that grass-fed cattle are healthier and that these cattle are allowed to roam freely to graze. Grass-fed beef are also not "finished" in feed lots where they are fed grain. There are currently no federal standards for use of the term "grass-fed," so even a small amount of grass feed may give rise to the label grass-fed. Other consumers prefer grain fed beef, because the beef produced is thought to be healthier and raised under more humane conditions.

Another term that is used in connection to beef is "natural." This generally means that the beef does not contain hormones, additives, or preservatives. This term is not regulated by the USDA. There is no standard or consistency about what natural means.

Another issue that is not covered by the organic standards is whether animal products are fed to cattle.

Grading of beef by the USDA is also separate from organic standards. Such terms as "Prime" and "Choice" are regulated by the USDA and have to do with the level of marbling of the beef. Other organizations that have added phrases to the production of beef include the Animal Welfare Institute with its phrase "animal welfare approved."

See also: Growth Hormones; Humane Slaughtering Practices; "Natural" Labeling; Appendix 8: California Organic Products Act of 2003.

Elizabeth M. Williams

BERMAN, RICHARD (1943–)

Richard (Rick) Berman, a high-power lobbyist who has worked on behalf of corporate food giants, was born in 1943 in New York City. He grew up working during the summers in his father's gas stations and car washes before attending the William and Mary School of Law in Williamsburg, Virginia. He graduated in 1967 and soon after began his career in law at the Dana Corporation in Ohio. He then moved to Washington, D.C., in 1972, to work as the labor law director of the U.S. Chamber of Commerce until 1974. He then moved to the private sector of food and beverage companies as an employee of the Steak & Ale restaurant chain. For the next decade he continued to work for large food and beverage corporations, including serving as vice president of Pillsbury Restaurant group before he started his own company, Berman and Company, in 1986.

Berman is now the president of Berman and Company, a lobbying firm based in Washington, D.C. This company manages several nonprofit, educational companies that advocate for personal freedom and less government control over aspects of daily life. Berman and his company use these entities, with names like the Center for Consumer Freedom and the Center for Union Facts, to fundraise and run media campaigns that discredit popular regulatory campaigns from organizations such as Mothers Against Drunk Driving (MADD) and the **Centers for Disease Control and Prevention**. Most of the campaigns undertaken by Berman champion personal choice and seek to prevent a "nanny state." Berman is usually in the forefront of campaigns against regulation in food and beverage as well as personal freedom debates.

Although his clients prefer to remain anonymous, many big names in the corporate food and beverage world have reportedly employed Berman, including the Coca-Cola Company, Tyson's Chicken, and Wendy's. Tobacco company Phillip Morris funded the organization of a campaign against nonsmoking sections in restaurants. By employing Berman's companies, the larger corporations can avoid having their names directly linked to publicity counterattacks while benefiting from the messages Berman releases. He uses television, the Internet, and physical advertisements to drive his points home, which range from discrediting the concerns of mercury levels in tuna to arguing that no policy can or should be made to take away a person's choice or to regulate those choices, even in an attempt to address the high levels of obesity in the United States.

His counterattacks and controversial advertising have made it harder for people to sue organizations for personal issues. The aggressive campaigning undertaken by the Center for Consumer Freedom and its partners helped Congress to consider the American Personal Responsibility in Food Consumption Act, otherwise known as the "cheeseburger bill," in 2004 that would have prevented Americans from forming class-action lawsuits against fast-food companies. The House of Representatives passed the bill, but the Senate did not, and thus the bill did not become law. The bill stated that food suppliers and manufacturers that were legally selling food should not be held responsible for a consumer's obesity or health-related issues. This was a great victory for the corporate food industry, many of who may have employed Berman to advocate for their position.

Berman also participated in challenging the positions of MADD on several issues from lowering the legal blood alcohol content in most states to raising taxes on alcoholic beverages. His companies created campaigns pointing out the flaws in the studies MADD used to justify their claims, leading in part to a Congressional panel's decision that raising taxes on alcoholic beverages would not reduce underage consumption. Berman also attacked the organization's high bureaucratic costs and its contradictory positions on proposed laws such as California's proposition that drunk-driving accident victims could sue the drunk driver's insurance company for compensation. Berman has also made it part of his cause to discredit MADD's push for what he calls the "nanny state."

Other significant campaigns led by Berman and his companies include fighting what he sees as fear-mongering by organizations discussing the risks of eating fish with high mercury content or beef that could be tainted with Mad Cow disease. These counter-campaigns may have not directly influenced policy changes, but they present another argument for consumers to consider, and they seem to have done their part in what they see as keeping the public hysteria under control.

Berman consistently uses the same scare-tactics and makes what some see as outrageous claims of the kind that he accuses his opponents of making, but his response to criticism is that it is only fair to respond in kind. He sees himself as fighting the "nanny state" of government that would limit the freedom of choice that Americans now enjoy. He wants people to think twice about the claims of all organizations, and his campaigns have demonstrated the ability to do so in some cases in the halls of Congress.

See also: Appendix 3A: Pelman, et al. v. McDonald's Corporation; Appendix 3B: Pelman, et al. v. McDonald's Corporation, Amended Complaint; Appendix 3C: Pelman, et al. v. McDonald's Corporation.

Further Reading Berman, Richard. "BBB's New Rating System Draws Fire." January 10, 2009 http://www.consumeraffairs.com/news04/2009/01/bbb.html; Graham, Nicholas. "Rachel Maddow Confronts Notorious Corporate Lobbyist Rick Berman." *Huffingtonpost.com.* October 7, 2009, http://www.huffingtonpost.com/2009/10/07/rachel-maddow-confronts-n _n_312334.html; Zernike, Kate. "The Nation: Food Fight; Is Obesity the Responsibility of the Body Politic?" *New York Times,* November 9, 2003, http://www.nytimes.com/2003/ 11/09/weekinreview/the-nation-food-fight-is-obesity-the-responsibility-of-the-body-politic .html?sec=health.

Kelsey Parris

BEVERAGE CLOSURES AND CONTAINERS, ALTERNATIVE

Cork is the outer bark of the oak cork, *Quercus suber*. Traditionally grown in Portugal, Spain, France, and Italy in Europe and in Morocco, Tunisia, and Algeria in Africa, the bark is harvested about every nine years without killing the tree. The trees live for almost 300 years. Corks have been used for hundreds of years to stopper wine.

In an era of sustainability awareness, cork forests make up millions of acres of forests and support many species of animals, including endangered species. The forests can be managed by their owners, who benefit by maintaining the forests, thus benefitting the forests. In addition, cork recycling programs are being promoted to produce flooring, footwear, aggregate stoppers, and other products from former wine stoppers. The cork forests are argued to be important in maintaining the health of the environment.

The use of cork has been threatened recently with the use of plastic synthetic corks, which stopper a wine bottle in a fashion that mimics a natural cork. The synthetic cork can be removed from a wine bottle with a corkscrew. Many wine enthusiasts consider the ritual of opening the bottle of wine, uncorking it, a part of the pleasure of drinking wine. Such people prefer the use of synthetic corks, as a substitute for natural cork, over the use of aluminum screw caps.

Aluminum screw caps were once considered a sign of a cheap wine, eschewing tradition, and eliminating the ritual of uncorking. However, today, wineries are adopting the screw caps, and the use of screw caps is not an automatic signal of cheap wine. Studies have shown that, although not perfect, screw caps fail less frequently than synthetic corks and natural corks, making the loss of wine through cork taint less frequent. Cork taint is caused by 2,4,6 trichloroanisole in the cork, making the wine smell like wet paper and reducing the natural aroma of the wine. For those wines that are particularly affected by cork taint, such as from Switzerland, alternate closures have been adopted more readily. Besides the aesthetic objection, traditionalists argue that aluminum screw caps are not recyclable. Both screw caps and synthetic corks take more energy to manufacture than natural cork stoppers, making the natural cork stopper the more ecological choice.

Cork forests are abundant and the development of alternatives to natural cork was not due to a shortage of cork, but to address the issues of cork taint and ease of removal of the cork, as the plastic cork does not crumble or break in the bottle. It is argued that a plastic cork is better used with a wine that will be drunk quickly, as the plastic cork does not breathe. That means that there is no air exchange with a plastic cork, as there is with a natural cork stopper. The air exchange helps develop the aging of wine. But many traditionalists and environmentalists simply fear that the adoption of synthetic corks and aluminum screw caps will lead to the reduction of the cork forests unless other uses for cork are quickly developed. Screw caps do not allow for the air exchange either. But cork taint is said to affect as much as 5 percent of bottled wine, which is a significant impact on product. This affects manufacturers as well as sellers of the product.

Another type of closure is the vino-seal, which is a glass stopper that has an o-ring made of an inert material. Some European wineries have adopted this type of stopper.

In 2006 in Spain, where many cork forests are found, the government adopted laws in their *Denominación de Origen* (DO) regulations that do not allow the use of alternate closures, making the tradition of manufacture and bottling a part of the overall process. The laws do not ban the use of alternative closures. It denies DO status to those wines that use alternative closure methods but that would otherwise qualify for DO status. There are movements in other countries in Europe, notably Italy, to adopt similar rules. Portugal has been slow to consider any closure method other than cork as about half of world cork production is from there. The cork industry has been gathering evidence to pressure the European Union to adopt regulations that would limit or prohibit the use of noncork stoppers in wines that receive an **Appelation d'origine contrôlée** as a way to protect cork forests and ensure their continued economic viability.

Cork is an organic product that has historical bases for use, but it does have drawbacks because of its nature, primarily cork taint. Alternate wine closure of all types, whether synthetic cork, aluminum screw caps with plastic inserts, or glass stoppers with an o-ring, must all comply with the food safety requirements of materials suitable for use with food. They must also not deteriorate when in contact with alcohol. Some wine experts claim that the plastic cap imparts a slightly chemical taste to wine.

The exploration of alternative closures and their widespread adoption by all levels of the world wine industry has caused the cork industry to explore improvements and work toward the elimination of cork taint.

As alternatives to cork as a closure for wine bottles develops, there is additional exploration of other alternatives, including alternatives to glass bottles. Legally there is no requirement that wine be packaged in glass, merely in an appropriate container that will stand up to the alcohol. A box containing a collapsible bladder that allows wines to be resealed without exposure to air—a problem with bottles—is an example. Other examples are the Tetra-Pak, which is akin to a children's drink box, and aluminum cans. Individual cans and drink packs can be served in places like stadiums and at concerts where glass containers are not allowed because of safety regulations. These containers are opaque, which also provides an additional protection to the wines, by keeping light away from the wine. In single-serving containers, the wines do not require a glass and can be opened without special equipment, like a corkscrew.

See also: Appelation d'origine contrôlée, Corks.

Elizabeth M. Williams

Zork Patent Abstract from the patent application

Inventors: John Brooks
Agents: AKERMAN SENTERFITT
Assignees: Zork Pty Ltd.
Origin: WEST PALM BEACH, FL US
IPC8 Class: AB65D4132FI
USPC Class: 215256
Patent application number: 20100012615

Abstract:
The present invention describes a bottle closure for bottles containing liquids at high pressure, such as bottles of sparkling wine, the closure having a first part and a second part, the first part having a portion adapted to receive a portion of an upper section of a neck of the bottle, and a second part that fits substantially over the first part, which is relatively movable with respect to the first part and has at least two positions, a first of which is in a free position and a second of which is in an interlocking position whereby a portion of the second part urges against a portion of the first part receiving the upper section of the neck of the bottle so as to be engaging against an outer side of the said first part to hold it thereby to resist release from its interlocking position with respect to the said neck of an industry standard bottle.

BIOLOGICAL WARFARE AND FOOD

Biological warfare uses biological agents such as bacteria, viruses, or other pathogens to produce casualties in humans, animals, plants, or supplies, or the defense against the use of such pathogens. The biological weapons may be either infectious diseases such as small pox, or biologically produced chemical compounds such as *botulinum* toxin produced by the bacteria *Clostridium botulinum*. They may be delivered by a variety of mechanisms such as specialized military munitions or infected items, animals, or persons dispersed in the enemy population, or by directly dispersing the biological weapon through means ranging from a small aerosol spray to a crop dusting aircraft.

Practitioners of biological warfare have used poisoned water and food supplies as a way to inflict disease on large numbers of enemy soldiers or civilian populations. Biological warfare attacks have been recorded since ancient times, and, therefore, may have also been practiced in prehistoric times as well. Both the Assyrians and the Greeks used well poisoning dating back to the 6th century BCE and used rye grain poisoned with the ergot fungus and the poisonous plant known as black hellebore, respectively, in separate recorded incidents.

Poisoning water wells or other water sources with dead bodies of humans or animals or fecal matter was a common historical military tactic that would cause disease among enemy soldiers and populations. These tactics were repeatedly used during Greek, Roman, and medieval times, although there was some varying degree of stigma attached to the practice. In more modern times, in World War I, German undercover agents infected Allied livestock with the bacteria *Burkholderia mallei,* which causes glanders, a disease that can also affect humans. To this day, biological attacks on food, agriculture, or water supplies remain a potential threat, given the ability to destabilize a society or government, particularly one dependent on agriculture or specific commodities.

In 1925, the Geneva Protocol banned the use of bacteriological methods of warfare as well as chemical poison gases as a form of attack for its signatories. The Protocol did not ban the production or stockpiling of such weapons, however, and the United States did not fully join the Geneva Protocol until 1975. During the international Disarmament Conference in the 1930s, there were several efforts to reach an additional agreement to ban such weapons, but they were unsuccessful. In World War II, neither the Axis powers of Germany and Japan nor the Allied powers of the United States and Great Britain chose to use biological weapons of any kind on a large scale against each other. In 1942, President Franklin D. Roosevelt warned Japan against the use of such weapons and committed the United States not to use them unless in retaliation. Japan used biological weapons against China during World War II, and there were reports of infected water supply wells and ponds.

In 1969, President Richard M. Nixon announced U.S. policy to unconditionally renounce all methods of biological warfare. In 1972, many nations including the United States signed the Convention on the Prohibition of the Development, Production, and Stockpiling of Bacteriological (Biological) and Toxin Weapons and on Their Destruction, often known as the Biological Weapons Convention, and the U.S. Senate ratified the treaty in 1974. The convention went into force in 1975 and fully prohibits the development, production, or stockpiling of biological weapons, other than in small quantities for purely defensive research programs.

Article I of the Convention specifically prohibits potential biological weapons in quantities that have no peaceful purpose or the means of delivery of such biological agents for hostile purposes. The language of the treaty is broad enough to prohibit the production or stockpiling of biological agents regardless of the focus of the attack—the human population directly or the agricultural base on which a population depends. The particular targeting of agriculture with biological weapons is not specifically addressed in the text of the Convention. The 1925 Geneva

Protocol prohibits the use of bacteriological methods of warfare, which again is broad enough to include all types of attacks, both human and agricultural, although it was drafted prior to the full knowledge of viruses and certainly before the development of genetically modified plants and animals, neither of which are related to bacteria.

Although the Protocol and Convention prohibits biological attacks by nation states, individual national laws also criminalize biological attacks by individuals or groups within nations. There is some concern that economically interested individuals, speculators, or corporations could use an attack on agriculture to generate a windfall profit. In the United States, 18 U.S.C. § 175 prohibits the use of biological weapons within the United States and carries a penalty of up to life in prison. In addition, § 175a permits the attorney general to request the secretary of defense to provide military assistance within the United States to enforce the domestic prohibition in an emergency situation, an exception from the Posse Comitatus Act (1878), which generally prohibits U.S. military action on domestic soil.

Despite the international bans, both the United States and the United Nations consider biological attacks on agriculture and food supplies a significant threat. The U.S. Department of Homeland Security operates the National Biosurveillance Integration Center to compile the data from the biomonitoring efforts of numerous other government agencies to detect and provide early warning of a biological attack on human, animal, plant, or environmental health, in addition to pandemics. The Department of Homeland Security also coordinates Food, Agriculture, and Veterinary Defense for all disasters related to food and agriculture, including potential biological or hostile contamination attacks.

The **U.S. Department of Agriculture** (USDA) is also heavily involved in the protection of food and agriculture from biological and other attacks. In 2006, USDA published the Pre-Harvest Security Guidelines and Checklist for farms, covering areas such as awareness, planning, barriers, inventory control, law enforcement, locks, and visitor control. The security checklists are detailed for specific operations including dairy, crop, cattle, and poultry. For example, the guidelines urge that aerial applicators, or crop dusters, be kept locked with anti-theft devices. The USDA's Food Safety Inspection Service (FSIS) further monitors the food supply to detect acts of intentional contamination, assesses the food industry's vulnerability, and offers food defense guidance.

The FSIS specifically conducts vulnerability assessments of meat, poultry, and egg producers and develops countermeasures to protect the food supply from intentional attack. Along with the USDA's Food Nutrition Service and other federal agencies, FSIS also provides food defense awareness training for other regulators, law enforcement, and food program administrators. The FSIS also provides guides for facility operators to develop Food Defense Plans at slaughterhouses, processing plants, warehouses, and distribution centers, including for small and very small operations. The USDA requires suppliers for its feeding programs, such as federal school meals and disaster relief programs, to have food defense plans.

The **Food and Drug Administration** (FDA) in the **Department of Health and Human Services** is responsible for food security outside the farm, meat, or poultry operation. Those areas are under the jurisdiction of the **Department of Agriculture**. As a result, the FDA regulates 80 percent of all food in the United States. Food processors and transporters are encouraged to provide food defense training, control visitors, inspect incoming and outgoing vehicles, and limit access to food handling and storage areas. The guidelines also recommend background checks, perimeter security, and segregation of imported and domestic products.

The 2009 U.S. National Infrastructure Protection Plan (NIPP) includes a chapter on agriculture and food. Both the USDA and FDA submitted their plans for their areas of jurisdiction and state departments of agriculture also participated in its development. Under the NIPP framework, both agencies set goals for the agricultural and food production sectors, identify key assets and functions, assess risks, prioritize infrastructure, develop protective programs, and conduct research and development. The Department of Homeland Security, USDA, and FDA jointly lead a Government Coordinating Council for the food and agriculture sector to manage food defense activities on a day-to-day basis. The food and agriculture private sector participates in a self-governing body, the Sector Coordinating Council, which is divided into sector-specific subcouncils.

See also: Embargoes; Food and Drug Administration; Importation of Food; U.S. Department of Agriculture; World Trade Organization.

Andrew G. Wallace

BIOTERRORISM ACT OF 2002

The Public Health Security and Bioterrorism Preparedness and Response Act, often referred to as the Bioterrorism Act of 2002, was passed in reaction to acts of terrorism against the United States. In anticipation of future acts, the law attempts to protect against what is generically called bioterrorism. This refers to terrorism that attacks and threatens the food and water supplies, as well as other systems.

The Act was created in the aftermath of September 11, 2001, during the administration of President George W. Bush. The Act requires the development of local plans for security and the identification of vulnerabilities. The Bioterrorism Act has five major parts that cover the safety of various biosystems. They are Title I—National Preparedness for Bioterrorism and Other Public Health Emergencies; Title II—Enhancing Controls on Dangerous Biological Agents and Toxins; Title III—Protecting Safety and Security of Food and Drug Supply; Title IV—Drinking Water Security and Safety; and Title V—Additional Provisions.

Protection of the Food Supply

The Bioterrorism Act of 2002 forms the basis of the authority of the U.S. **Department of Health and Human Services** (HHS) in matters that protect against bioterrorist activity. This means that the safety of the food supply and the regulations that ensure this are in the control of HHS. The **Food and Drug Administration** (FDA), essentially the food subdivision of the HHS, carries out this obligation and mission by creating a four-part process. To monitor the food processors in the country, the FDA requires that all companies, whether foreign or domestic, that are part of the chain of food making and production, register with the FDA. This includes food made for human and animal consumption. There was a "registration by" date of December 12, 2003, for existing facilities. New facilities must register before beginning to operate. Before a shipment of food can come into the United States, the FDA must have received notification.

The FDA is required by the act to establish regulations that would require that records be kept by the companies and individuals in the chain of the food system, which would be available for review by the FDA. This allows the FDA to know where the food came from, who processed it, and where it went after a particular facility has finished its contribution. If the FDA needs this information to trace a problem, in particular, the problem of intentional contamination, the records will facilitate getting to the source of the problem.

The Administrative Detention provisions of the act give the FDA the power to seize and sequester food when there is a belief, based on serious information, that there is a problem with food in some part of the food chain that represents a danger to the food supply of food for either animal or human consumption.

Protection of Drinking Water
The act also concerns the safety of the drinking water supplies throughout the United States. The provisions of the act are applicable to areas that serve and provide drinking water with populations of 3,300 people or more. Each community must provide the FDA with a self-assessment of the safety of the drinking water and identify areas that are weak links in the system subject to intentional sabotage or attack, whether violent or covert.

The Bioterrorism Act requires that the **Environmental Protection Agency (EPA)** coordinate with those companies that provide drinking water, process it, or otherwise form a part of the drinking water supply so that each has a response plan that is approved by the EPA that can be put into action in case of a terrorist attack. These include a determination of the weak points of the safety system; certification of the report of the self-evaluation to the EPA; creation of a plan that addresses all of the problems that were spotlighted by the self-evaluation, which can include corrective action or a plan of action that is implemented on attack; and certification to the administrator that this plan is created and ready to be put into action when needed.

Further Reading FDA Bioterrorism Act, http://www.fda.gov/oc/bioterrorism/bioact.html; Homeland Security, USDA http://www.usda.gov/wps/portal/!ut/p/_s.7_0_A/7_0_CJ?navid= HOMELANDSECU&navtype=CO.

William C. Smith and Elizabeth M. Williams

BOYCOTTS
A boycott is an action by consumers who refrain from buying a product, usually so as to induce a change in the product, to protest the product itself, or to induce

change in the way the product is produced. The activism may be motivated by health concerns as well as other political concerns. A boycott has been enacted on numerous occasions in the food industry. It is contrasted with a strike, which is an employee action. It is often argued that a boycott is a peaceful form of consumer coercion; however, especially when combined with strikes and market interference, the boycott can trigger violence. A famous boycott was the Boston Tea Party, in which prerevolutionary citizens of Boston dumped a shipment of tea in Boston Harbor in protest of what they considered unfair taxes being levied by the British crown on the colonies. This boycott not only called on consumers to not drink the tea, but actually destroyed the product to prevent its consumption. This boycott is often cited as the first action of the American Revolution.

The United Farm Workers, in an effort led by Cesar Chavez in the mid-1960s, encouraged consumers to boycott grapes and lettuce in solidarity with migrant farm workers to protest their conditions of employment. Because the farm workers had little political power, the appeal to consumers to pressure farmers to improve conditions was seen as a more effective method of making the farmers conform to the desired improvements. Eventually the grape workers obtained a union contract with the grape growers of California. These boycotts were supported and widely publicized by singer Joan Baez. These boycotts were criticized because often consumers did not know which lettuce growers or grape growers were involved in the practices that were being protested by the boycott, so sympathetic consumers boycotted all grapes and lettuce, causing harm to all growers. Some groceries, in response to this concern, began to label the produce with the name of the farm or grower.

In the 1970s the Swiss food company, Nestlé, was the subject of a boycott. The company marketed powdered baby formula to countries in Africa, encouraging mothers to abandon breast feeding in favor of using formula. The women did not have access to clean water and sometimes mixed the formula with unclean water, causing the infants to become ill, and in some cases to die. Often the mothers could not resume breast feeding if they stopped producing milk and thus were forced to continue using the powdered formula. In response to the practice of encouraging the use of powdered formula, especially in places that lacked access to clean water, where cleaning bottles and boiling water were impractical, and where there was no refrigeration, many people in developed nations worldwide began to boycott Nestlé products in protest. Some groups continue to boycott Nestlé products.

In the 1980s, Operation PUSH, a civil rights organization led by Jesse Jackson, held several boycotts of the products of Coca-Cola, Kentucky Fried Chicken, and Anheuser-Busch. These boycotts encouraged African Americans and others who supported their cause not to consume the products of these major companies until the companies made strides in employment of African Americans, especially in positions of leadership. It is not clear whether the economic effect of the boycotts or the negative publicity that was received when spotlighting the business statistics of these companies actually caused the companies to meet with Operation PUSH. However, these companies entered into agreements to change their business practices in response to the boycotts, thus ending them.

Because the right to engage freely in business and commerce is protected, the corresponding right not to do business with certain businesses or to refrain from purchasing certain products is also protected. Individually deciding what products to purchase and what stores to patronize makes a boycott an individual action. There may be an illegal action when a labor union engages in what is called a secondary boycott, the encouraging of its members to boycott companies that supply a boycotted company. However, individuals may make their own decisions.

The Export Administration Regulations (EAR) prohibit citizens of the United States from participating in the organized boycotts sponsored by foreign governments. The purpose of this law is to keep American citizens from being used by foreign governments. The provisions of the EAR cover import and export activities, financing, and forwarding of import and export freight. The provisions only apply to boycotts that are initiated by foreign governments, not those boycotts that are initiated in the United States or by the United States government.

As companies expand around the world, the complexities of world politics affect boycotts in different companies. For example, when the United States attacked Iraq in 2003, India called for a boycott of American companies such as Coca-Cola and McDonald's. In another instance, Burger King, in response to a boycott in Arab countries, withdrew a restaurant from a West Bank settlement in Israel. In response to this action, pro-Israel forces in the United States began a boycott of Burger King. Although not directly involved, McDonald's offered to make a donation of hospitals serving Palestinian children for every hamburger sold.

In April, 2010, the Coalition of Immokalee Workers rallied to bring attention to their boycott of Publix, a large supermarket chain, for poor labor practices in the tomato industry of Florida, where Publix obtains its tomatoes for sale.

In late 2009, students at Medford (Massachusetts) High School, as reported in the *Boston Globe*, pledged on Facebook to boycott the lunch at the school cafeteria for being unhealthy. The school claimed that it was in compliance with the federal school lunch program guidelines and did not serve fried foods or other unhealthy foods. In addition, it always offered a salad and vegetable.

See also: Farm Labor Laws and Regulations; Appendix 15: Uruguay Round Agreement on Agriculture; Appendix 16: World Trade Organization Ministerial Conference Decision; Appendix 17: World Medical Assembly Declaration on Hunger Strikers.

Further Reading Glickman, Lawrence B. *Buying Power: A History of Consumer Activism in America.* Chicago: University of Chicago Press, 2009.

Elizabeth M. Williams

BUSINESS MEALS TAX DEDUCTIONS

Under the U.S. Internal Revenue Code (IRC) § 162, businesses and self-employed individuals can deduct costs incurred in the course of running a business or a trade to make a profit. Businesses deduct these eligible costs, under certain conditions, from the amount of federal income tax that a business or sole proprietor owes in a given tax year, thus reducing their overall tax burden and increasing net income. To deduct these costs, business income tax filers report the expenses on their returns and keep records to justify the deductions.

The IRS Publication 463 explains that federal income tax deductible expenses can include business-related entertainment such as providing meals and recreational activities to employees, clients, or customers of a business. Meal expenses include food, beverages, taxes, and tips. Lavish or extravagant entertainment and meal expenses are not deductible. The IRS does not use a fixed dollar limit or prohibit deduction of expenses incurred at luxury hotels, restaurants, or other entertainment establishments, or for alcohol, on a per se basis, but instead applies a reasonableness standard to judge allowable expenses. An income tax filer may divide a specific expense at a restaurant into a reasonable expense that may be deducted and a lavish expense that may not.

Business meal and entertainment tax deductions are generally justified for their encouragement of business activity and recognition of the essential role that meals play in the conduct of many business activities, such as the "power lunch" or a dinner as part of the closing of a business deal. Congress also provides the deduction to encourage the patronage of food service businesses, many of which are small businesses that collectively employ well over 10 million people.

To qualify, meals must fall into one of two categories, either meals provided as part of business activity, or necessary meals as part of travelling away from home on business. The deduction may be made either by the employees or by the employer. These deductions differ depending on whether the business reimburses their employees and whether such reimbursements are subtracted from an employee's pay.

To be deductible as business activity expense, entertainment expenses such as meals must be ordinary and necessary, and the expense must also be either directly related to business or meet a lesser standard—associated with business. Ordinary expenses are those that are common and accepted in a given line of business. Necessary costs are those that are helpful and appropriate for business, but they do not need to be required or mandatory expenses. Meals are often ordinary and necessary business expenses if they occurred in a clear business setting, such as a board meeting lunch on company property.

An expense is directly related to business if the following criteria are met: business activities are the main purpose behind an event that also includes entertainment, actual business is conducted during the entertainment, and there was a clear expectation of income or other business goal in the future. Examples include meals to develop and solicit clients or sales, determine contracts and other business agreements, or other conducted substantial, bona fide, business work. An entertainment or meals expense is associated with business activity if it has a clear business purpose or is conducted directly before or after the tax filer actively engaged in a substantial business discussion or meeting. A business trade show or convention is considered a substantial business meeting if the schedule includes a program of business activities that is the main activity of the convention.

Reimbursed employer expenses and unreimbursed employee expenses for meals when on business travel outside the tax home area are also deductible. To qualify as a deductible business travel meal, the employee must travel outside the city or general area where the business is located substantially longer than an ordinary day's work and there is a need to sleep or rest significantly as a part of the work trip. These expenses do not need to meet the separate business entertainment related criteria to be deducted.

As a general rule, IRC § 274(n) sets a 50 percent limit for deducting qualifying business-related meal and entertainment expenses or business travel-related meals. Therefore, if a company reimburses its employees for $2,000 worth of meals provided to clients of the business as part of business lunch meetings, only $1,000 would qualify as a deductible expense from income on federal income tax filing. Similarly, if employees are only reimbursed for part of their eligible expenses when buying client meals, they may deduct 50 percent of the remainder from their personal income reported to the IRS.

The 50 percent rule deduction limit does have several exceptions, however, which permit full 100 percent deduction of meal expenses. In the transportation industry, meal reimbursements may be deducted at an 80 percent level for fully accounted for and reimbursed meal expenses in the airline, barge, bus, ship, train, or trucking industries. To qualify, the expenses must be incurred by employees while away from their tax home and subject to the Department of Transportation Hours of Service rules, which limit the amount an employee may work to prevent fatigue and improve safety, but may delay a return to their tax home.

If an employer reimburses its employee for business expenses but does not account for actual expenses with receipts, then these reimbursements are considered employee wages, and the business may fully deduct them. If an employee is reimbursed for an expense, and the reimbursements are not reported as wages, then they may not be deducted at all. Reimbursements provided to nonemployees that are also reported on the recipients' 1099-MISC as miscellaneous income are fully deductible. Self-employed individuals may also fully deduct meal expenses when three criteria are met: the individual is an independent contractor; the customer or client reimburses or provides an allowance for the expense; and the individual provides adequate records of the expenses.

Outside of the reimbursement context, meals in certain business contexts are also exempt from the 50 percent limit. Meals that are provided for sale to customers are fully reimbursable as clearly essential business costs for the restaurant and food service industry. In addition, meals provided to employees as a minimal fringe benefit, such as the costs of meals for staff at a restaurant, are also fully reimbursable up to 100 percent. Free food given away to the general public as part of an advertising or promotional event is also reimbursable and not subject to the 50 percent limit. Free food provided for the recreational benefit of employees, such as the employee picnic or office holiday party, is also fully reimbursable.

The general 50 percent business meal deduction level was reduced from 80 percent by the Omnibus Budget Reconciliation Act of 1993, and legislation has been introduced in the U.S. Congress in 2010 to raise the deduction level back to

80 percent. Legislative proponents such as the National Restaurant Association argue that such legislation would increase employment and overall economic activity.

See also: Appendix 1: *United States v. Fior D'Italia, Inc.*

Andrew G. Wallace

CARSON, RACHEL (1907–1964)

Biologist and writer Rachel Carson is best known for writing *Silent Spring*, a 1962 book that exposed the harmful effects of pesticides and other chemicals on the earth. Her books have often been cited as influential in the push for more environmentally friendly policies. In recent years, though, there have been questions regarding the soundness of Carson's conclusions and the effects her books might have had as well.

Rachel Louise Carson was born in Springdale, Pennsylvania, on May 27, 1907, to Robert Warden Carson and his wife, Maria McLean. Carson spent much of her childhood in the outdoors, exploring the shorelines of the Allegheny River and the acres of farmland that her family had. It appears that she was a naturally talented writer; she was first published at the age of 11 in the *St. Nicholas Magazine* with her story, "A Battle in the Clouds."

Carson continued to pursue a writing career as she entered the Pennsylvania College for Women, majoring in English and writing for the school's newspaper, *The Arrow,* as well as their literary magazine, *The Englicode*. However, on reaching her junior year, she discovered a new passion: biology. She graduated magna cum laude in 1929 with a degree in science, and received a scholarship to study zoology at Johns Hopkins University. She spent time there and at Woods Hole Marine Biological Laboratory in Massachusetts before graduating from Johns Hopkins with her master's degree in zoology in 1932. Unable to continue her education due to family obligations, Carson moved quickly into part-time teaching jobs, one at University of Maryland and the other at Johns Hopkins.

In 1935, Carson accepted a position with the U.S. Bureau of Fisheries, writing radio scripts for a scientific program entitled *Romance under the Waters* that sought to interest the public in the agency's work. This job led to promotions within the Bureau until she became the chief editor of publications in 1949. Carson continued to write articles for the science section of the *Baltimore Sun* throughout this time to supplement her income. Carson's first book, *Under the Sea Wind,* came out in 1941, but she was not a nationally recognized writer until her second book, *The Sea around Us*, was finally published in 1951. Both books focused on oceanography, marine biology, and the delicate ecosystems built throughout the world and its waters. The success of the books allowed her to retire from the U.S. Bureau of Fisheries, and she was free to pursue topics of her own interest. After finishing a third book about the sea, *The Edge of the Sea*, in 1955, she began to work on what would be her most controversial and influential piece of writing.

The increased use of synthetic pesticides and chemicals to control pests on farmland and in communities following World War II caught Carson's attention at that point. She found other scientists and authors who were interested in documenting and alerting the public of the effects of the insecticides. They followed the outcomes of campaigns of the pesticide DDT against mosquitoes, gypsy moths, and red ants, noting the aftermath of widespread spraying on the local ecosystems. Further research continued through the Library of Medicine, the National Institutes of Health, and the work of Wilhelm Hueper, who believed that pesticides could prove to be carcinogenic. After four and a half years of research, Carson was finally ready to publish her book documenting the many reasons to be wary of many of the most popular pesticides. She wrote that the widespread use of these chemicals was upsetting the balance of nature, poisoning not only the pests they targeted, but everything else, including wildlife, water, soil, food, and eventually people.

Carson called her book *Silent Spring*, a metaphor for the possible extinction of life and the natural world if the use of chemicals continued. With the publishing of the book in 1962, Carson made many enemies in the corporate world of pesticide production. She claimed that the chemical industries were deliberately spreading misinformation and not paying heed to the problems of their products, while the government enacted policies that enabled the continuation of the corporations. Spokespeople for the companies decried her research and her writing, claiming that she was a crazy environmentalist, with unsound research and faulty conclusions.

However, the public was intrigued and worried by the book and its message. President John F. Kennedy was convinced by the public's concerns to form a committee to investigate the allegations, and in 1963 they reported that pesticides should be used in moderation, and that more research had to be conducted to examine the potential harmful effects. The Chemical Pesticides Coordination Act was put into motion by Congress to regulate the sale and use of pesticides, and the **Environmental Protection Agency** (EPA) was formed to represent a separate commission that could make decisions to protect the environment without political or industrial pressure. Although Carson died before any serious regulation was put into effect, DDT and similar chemical insecticides and pesticides have subsequently been banned for most uses by the EPA since 1972.

One of the more controversial issues surrounding the banning of DDT is the control of malarial mosquitoes in the malaria-prone areas of the world. DDT was proven to be one of the more effective chemicals in killing these mosquitoes, and the difficulty of obtaining DDT can be detrimental for countries struggling to control the malaria outbreaks. The chemical is still being observed for long-term effects to people, food sources, animals, and the environment at large. Carson was one of the first people to draw attention to the potential threat posed by widespread pest elimination, and it was her work in the sciences that helped to lead to the creation of the EPA and new, environmentally conscious policies.

Further Reading Carson, Rachel. *Silent Spring*. New York: Mariner Books, 2002 (Reprint); Darby, William J. "Silence, Miss Carson." *Chemical & Engineering News* 1 Oct. 1962: 60–63; McDonnell, Lawrence and Sarah F. Bates. *Natural Resources Policy and Law: Trends and Directions*. Washington, D.C.: Island, 1993.

Kelsey Parris

CATERERS, REGULATION OF

Catering is an area of the retail food service business that provides for food to be stored and prepared in one location and transported and served in another. Personal chefs who prepare and deliver food to those who order it and cooks who are hired to prepare meals in the home of the employer can be considered caterers for purposes of regulation. In addition, those who have trucks from which they sell food that has been prepared elsewhere, although partially assembled in the truck, can be considered caterers.

Catering is regulated by the same laws that cover food handling operations in restaurants and other food service facilities. Food must be prepared in licensed kitchens and transported according to state and local government rules and regulations. Food that must be kept cold, must still be kept cold, although caterers may keep things cold in ice chests and portable coolers and not in a refrigerator. The temperature at which the food must be held does not change because the food is being transported. The **Hazard Analysis Critical Control Point** and other Food Code rules apply.

Because caterers are harder to identify, however, they often operate without being licensed or inspected. Thus, there is no way to ensure that they always comply with appropriate regulations. In 2005, the Mississippi Hospitality and Restaurant Association complained that although Mississippi did have appropriate laws and inspection procedures in place, the state chose to allow unlicensed and thus uninspected catering businesses to operate in the state. The Mississippi Code gives the power to the Mississippi Department of Health to create regulations and set standards, license, inspect, and otherwise regulate food service, including caterers in the state. But although the Department of Health in the state had the authority to require a license, it had no enforcement authority. Thus, it could not issue a citation or issue a cease-and-desist order. Its only authority was to go to court and request that the court issue the order to close the unlicensed business.

A person or business that hires an unlicensed and uninsured caterer is likely to be unable to collect damages for the liability of the unlicensed caterer should the failure to follow the food service food handling standards cause illness. However, simply informing consumers that they should only use licensed caterers shifts the burden of enforcement from the state or local government to consumers. Other caterers who are licensed argue that allowing unlicensed caterers to operate creates unfair competition, because unlicensed caterers do not pay sales tax, may not pay income taxes, and may not be properly paying their employees.

Generally, chefs who cook in people's homes do not need special licenses if they are employees of the homeowners. However, those who operate as independent contractors may need a general business or occupational license from the state or local government. Locales differ in their regulation depending on the number of personal chefs operating in the area with more regulation in places where many personal chefs operate. Generally, where food is prepared at the home and food is stored at the home, there is little regulation beyond business licensing of the chef.

See also: Hazard Analysis Critical Control Point, State Legal Systems.

Elizabeth M. Williams

CENTER FOR CONSUMER FREEDOM

The Center for Consumer Freedom (CCF) is a nonprofit organization associated with Berman and Company, a lobbying firm based in Washington, D.C., operated by **Richard Berman**. This company was founded in 1996 and a part of its mission is to promote consumer freedom of choice, advocating personal responsibility and nonregulation by governmental entities. The group raises funds and runs media campaigns that discredit popular media campaigns from organizations such as Mothers Against Drunk Driving (MADD) and the U.S. **Centers for Disease Control and Prevention.** Most of the campaigns undertaken by CCF and Berman champion personal choice and seek to prevent a "nanny state" of government. Many of the issues that the CCF monitors are related to the regulation of food by government. In particular the group has monitored obesity lawsuits and attempts to control what people might be allowed to eat.

The CCF is supported by a range of multinational companies, although many choose to remain anonymous. Phillip Morris and other restaurant and tobacco companies reportedly funded the Guest Choice Network in 1995, which was the original organized attempt to prevent the laws creating nonsmoking sections in restaurants. Philip Morris was a major contributor, giving the start-up $600,000, and they have continued to fund the Network, along with the restaurant groups Host Marriott Corp. and Brinker International, Inc. In 2001 the Guest Choice Network became the Center for Consumer Freedom, as Berman and his clients decided to change the focus of the organization to more general food and beverage policies. The company is now concerned with broad food issues that are often debated in the United States, such as obesity prevention, alcohol control, and genetically modified products.

Large food manufacturers concerned with the effects of legislation on their food and beverage products often employ the CCF or one of its smaller related organizations to create advertising campaigns to counter the published studies on everything from deaths caused by obesity to the levels of mercury in fish. Sometimes the studies can be discredited by pointing out flaws with the study. At other times, studies may be refuted as misguided or not having a sound scientific basis. Using the CCF allows the large, well-known corporations to avoid a direct connection with the advertisements, while at the same time having their positions broadcast. Known sponsors have included the Coca-Cola Company, Wendy's, and Tyson Foods, each of which has had an interest in preventing certain regulatory proposals of either local, state, or federal government.

The CFF uses television, the Internet, and physical advertisements to drive their points home. Past advertisements have used popular figures such as the *Seinfeld* character the "Soup Nazi" to shout ridiculous judgments at people (for example, "Nothing for you! Come back when you're thinner") as well as an advertisement posing the choice, "Big Apple or Big Brother," with regard to certain food regulations proposed in New York City in 2009 and 2010.

The counterattacks and controversial advertising have made it harder for people to sue organizations for personal issues. The aggressive campaigning undertaken by the CCF and its partners helped Congress to consider the American Personal

Responsibility in Food Consumption Act, otherwise known as the "cheeseburger bill," in 2004, that would have prevented Americans from forming class-action lawsuits against fast-food companies. The House of Representatives passed the bill, but the Senate did not, and the bill did not become law. Under the bill, food suppliers and manufacturers that were legally selling food could not be held responsible for a consumer's obesity or health-related issues. This was a great victory for the fast-food industry and for the issue of personal responsibility. While this was a great success of CCF, it is difficult to know which companies have employed Berman to advocate for their side. Besides personal responsibility, and the "nanny state" arguments, there was concern that no single nexus could be established between the foods and health issues and that fast-food companies were being singled out for their deep pockets.

The CCF has also participated in challenging the positions of MADD on everything from lowering the legal blood alcohol content in most states to raising taxes on alcohol. Advertisements and campaigns pointed out the flaws in the studies MADD used to justify their claims, leading in part to a Congressional panel's decision that raising taxes on alcoholic beverages would not reduce underage consumption. The techniques of the organization include two tracks seeking to find internal contradictions and inconsistencies in the positions of the organizations they are disputing, appeal to legislators to continue the arguments to the logical end, and to appeal to principles of freedom of the marketplace. The second track is the more public and raucous media fight that continues to emphasize the dangers of the "nanny state."

The CFF claims to be primarily concerned with making sure that every American can "choose how they live their lives, what they eat and drink, how they manage their finances, and how they enjoy themselves," without having to deal with "food police" and excessive taxes on food and drinks. The company is criticized by many advocates of governmental regulation like the Center for Science in the Public Interest. However, the CFF Web site also seems to support the freedom of people to choose to be vegetarians and make other personal choices, while it seems to oppose the imposition of conduct or limitations on conduct by governmental entities.

See also: Center for Science in the Public Interest; Obesity Lawsuits; Appendix 3A: *Pelman, et al. v. McDonald's Corporation*; Appendix 3B: *Pelman, et al. v. McDonald's Corporation*, Amended Complaint; Appendix 3C: *Pelman, et al. v. McDonald's Corporation*.

Further Reading Center for Consumer Freedom. http://www.consumeraffairs.com/news04/2009/01/bbb.html; Source Watch. http://www.sourcewatch.org/index.php?title=Center_for_Consumer_Freedom

Kelsey Parris

CENTER FOR SCIENCE IN THE PUBLIC INTEREST

The Center for Science in the Public Interest (CSPI) is a controversial nonprofit consumer-advocacy group headquartered in Washington, D.C. It was co-founded in 1971 by the group's still-current executive director, **Michael Jacobson**, an

MIT-trained microbiologist. The group's tagline claims it is "[t]ransforming the American diet." Its mission statement describes the group as dedicated to "research and advocacy programs in health and nutrition, and to provide consumers with current, useful information about their health and well-being." The CSPI's $17-million annual budget is funded by members and, to a lesser extent, by foundation and grant money.

While CSPI strives to appear as a benevolent watchdog focused squarely on influencing nutrition through the court of public opinion, much of CSPI's divisive work over its nearly four decades of existence has centered instead on efforts to use the courts to shape public and private behavior. The CSPI has sued to ban or limit calories, fat, salt, food coloring, and even some vegetarian foods. The group advocates in favor of stricter government oversight of food and food safety, increased labeling standards for packaged foods and restaurant foods, anti-obesity measures, and mandatory reductions in or warnings regarding the contents of various foods and beverages. Two of the biggest CSPI targets are the restaurant- and packaged-foods industries. The CSPI's loudest support comes from those in the neo-public health field. This recent school of public-health advocates looks beyond traditional notions of public health, those grounded in preventing the transmission of communicable diseases, and instead looks to manage human decisions—such as the choice to eat or not eat certain foods—that have nothing to do with pathogens. In addition to drawing support from some in the public health community, CSPI backers also include members of the modern alcohol-temperance movement, activist vegetarians and vegans, and anti-corporate and anti-caffeine advocates. Opponents of CSPI often accuse the group of favoring "nanny state" legislation and of employing questionable science as part of an effort to limit consumer choice. The Center for Consumer Freedom is the primary group working to oppose CSPI.

The CSPI publishes reports on a variety of food-related topics. Previous CSPI reports have targeted Chinese food, soda, salt, and restaurant cleanliness. Others have also advocated in favor of menu labeling, stricter oversight of food additives, and limits on food marketing to children, and alcohol marketing to college-age students.

The CSPI also publishes the monthly *Nutrition Action Healthletter*. Issues in the newsletter typically contain an editorial by Jacobson; a cover story highlighting a food-health issue; an additional feature story; brief summaries of recent nutritional studies; a series of product comparisons; a list of CSPI-endorsed recipes; and a back-cover story promoting one food ("right stuff") and attacking another ("food porn"). It also includes the well-known list of the 10 "best" and "worst" foods. The newsletter now boasts 900,000 subscribers, comprised of CSPI members whose annual membership fees makes up the bulk of CSPI's funding.

Although a good deal of the newsletter's content is uncontroversial, it helps CSPI raise funds to carry out a litigious agenda that may not be readily apparent to any casual reader. Throughout its history CSPI has targeted government and corporate parties in a variety of legal actions. The group's varied legal actions have come in the form of petitioning government agencies, supporting existing lawsuits as an amicus party, filing lawsuits against government and corporate parties, joining existing suits against government and corporate parties, providing legal counsel to plaintiffs suing corporate parties, seeking plaintiffs willing to work with CSPI to sue government or corporate parties, and threatening to sue corporations with which CSPI subsequently settled out of court. In the 1970s, CSPI's legal action consisted largely of petitioning government. In the 1980s, CSPI shifted its approach and sued the federal government. In the 1990s, though CSPI continued such suits, it mostly joined others' suits by filing amicus briefs.

In the mid-2000s CSPI launched a "Litigation Project," a project for managing its many legal actions. This legal arm is headed by former Texas state consumer protection official Stephen Gardner. With its Litigation Project in place, CSPI now routinely sues or threatens to sue some of the country's largest food chains in an effort to force these restaurants and food makers to change their products, packaging, and marketing practices more to CSPI's liking. The Litigation Project has launched several controversial lawsuits since its inception. In 2005 CSPI sued the maker of Quorn for deceptive labelling, a nutritive meat substitute, and Whole Foods Market, which sells Quorn. The suit came three years after CSPI's newsletter had given Quorn a "Best Bites" award. Probably the best-known controversy to plague CSPI was its advocacy in favor of foods cooked with **trans fats** as a safer alternative to those cooked in animal fat. After food makers bowed to pressure from CSPI, the group later became a staunch opponent of trans fats—going so far as to sue Burger King and KFC for cooking with the same trans fats CSPI had urged food companies to adopt in their cooking. In addition to the Quorn, Whole Foods, Burger King, and KFC suits, CSPI has recently sued or joined suits against Denny's, MillerCoors, Airborne, Aurora Dairy, and Coca-Cola. The group recently threatened to sue numerous parties, including Quaker Oats, Sara Lee, Starbucks, and Anheuser-Busch.

In spite of its many legal actions, few if any of CSPI's suits have resulted in courtroom victories for the group. But these losses have not dampened its support. The media, food writers like Michael Pollan, and nutritionists like Marion Nestle often cheer the group's efforts.

See also: Litigation; Obesity Lawsuits; Appendix 3A: *Pelman, et al. v. McDonald's Corporation*; Appendix 3B: *Pelman, et al. v. McDonald's Corporation*, Amended Complaint; Appendix 3C: *Pelman, et al. v. McDonald's Corporation.*

Further Reading Center for Science in the Public Interest. "Wok Carefully: CSPI Takes a (Second) Look at Chinese Restaurant Food," http://www.cspinet.org/new/200703211. html; *Nutrition Action Healthletter.* http://www.cspinet.org/nah/index.htm.

Baylen J. Linnekin

CENTERS FOR DISEASE CONTROL AND PREVENTION

The Centers for Disease Control and Prevention (CDC) is an organization that coordinates information about disease and prevention, disseminates information to local and state departments of health as well as CDC regional offices, investigates causes of new diseases and epidemics, and remains ready to act in case of epidemics and pandemics and other threats to public health. Areas of concern include food borne illnesses, food pathogens, and toxic substances.

The agency was formed in 1946 as the Communicable Disease Center. Its original purpose was to fight malaria, and much of its early efforts centered around that struggle. To fight the mosquito that caused malaria, the CDC sprayed DDT, the powerful pesticide that was later exposed in the work of **Rachel Carson**. Most of the early staff members were entomologists, and only a few staffers were medical officers. The CDC is an agency of the Department of Health and Human Services. Its headquarters are located in Atlanta, Georgia. The agency was located in the southern United States because the belt of malaria was located in the South. The CDC has regional offices in 10 other cities in the United States and Puerto Rico.

In the global community of health organizations the CDC is distinguished by the fact that its mission is not only to conduct research, but to apply the results of its research to improve the public health and the health of individuals. It also responds to health disasters and participates in the forming of a public plan for containment and cure.

In the early part of the 20th century, there were advances in public health. Although many food-borne pathogens had not been eradicated, food handlers both in slaughterhouses and on farms began to use more sanitary practices. The work of **Upton Sinclair** exposed many unsanitary and alarming practices. With the establishment of the CDC, such practices were encouraged and coordinated with state offices of public health. The **Food and Drug Administration** as well as state health offices kept records of food-related illness, a practice that is continued by the CDC to this day.

Bacterial pathogens and pesticides contained in foods were also areas of public health and safety that have been monitored by the CDC. The CDC was involved in the process that resulted in actions by the **Environmental Protection Agency** to ban the use of the pesticide DDT.

In 1998, epidemiological studies conducted by the CDC made it possible to trace a particular strain of *Listeria* by use of DNA markers. The CDC was thus able to associate seemingly unrelated cases. There were 22 deaths and more than 100 cases of *Listeria* infection. The source of the infection was a manufacturing plant that produced delicatessen meats and hot dogs. In another case in the same year the CDC was able to identify that imported parsley was the source of shigellosis infection in several states.

As more raw agricultural products were being imported into the United States to supply the demand for fresh vegetables and fruits during times when they were not available from U.S. growers, the CDC was identifying the need for regulation and control over those foods that might harbor food-borne pathogens, because of the agricultural practices in those supplying nations. The CDC also saw new pathogens being brought in through imports. This is of particular importance when the food is eaten raw, as is much fruit and salad, or where the food is not easy to wash well, such as curly parsley.

The CDC has been central in the prevention of chronic disease. The Framingham Heart Study is an example of the CDC studying eating habits, as well as other cultural habits, to determine the influence of these factors on heart health. The Study began in 1948 and is an on-going project of the National Heart, Blood and Lung Institute and the University of Boston. The National Cancer Institute, a part of the CDC, has been active in disseminating information, especially dietary information, about how to reduce the incidence of cancer.

Currently the CDC has concentrated some effort on the study of obesity in the United States. The CDC has studied obesity by race, by social class, and by geographic region, yielding interesting trends and information that is still being interpreted. It has issued statistics that indicate the level of obesity in the country and its impact of longevity and morbidity, and more. These studies have been widely quoted and were influential in the awareness of this condition. However, these studies are not without controversy. The CDC has been criticized for overstating numbers for effect and with not applying good scientific method to its review of studies. This is important when the statistics published by the CDC are used as facts in support of lawsuits brought by people who seek to obtain damage awards for their obesity, the so-called **obesity lawsuits**. The CDC claims that obesity costs over $100 billion each year. Recently the CDC studies have shown a slowing or even an end of the growth of obesity.

The CDC also provides information for travelers on food and water safety in other countries. It provides suggested medications to ask for based on certain symptoms that might arise during travel and suggestions to avoid certain problems. In addition to food-related issues, the CDC studies sexually transmitted diseases, cancer, and most recently has been active in various influenzas that are expected to infect many Americans.

See also: Department of Health and Human Services.

Elizabeth M. Williams

CHICKEN, ORGANIC

Federal laws regarding organics are developing, but the most stringent laws are primarily found in state laws. In general, to qualify as organic, the chicken must be raised on soil that has been certified as organic. The life of the chicken must be reviewed, considering its food, its housing, its exercise, and its medical treatment.

Federal organic rules are found in the Organic Foods Production Act (OFPA), which was part of the 1990 **Farm Bill**. The bill authorized the National Organic Program (NOP) under the **U.S. Department of Agriculture** (USDA) to promulgate regulations defining what is organic in all areas including the production of chicken. To be organic under federal regulations, the food, including chicken, must be produced in accordance with the OFPA.

The various issues that must be certified include the chicken's feed. The feed must be organic and any additional scraps that it is fed must the organic. There have been some exceptions made in the requirement of all organic feed, in that organic feed should be readily available and of a cost not considered too expensive under a stated formula. An organic chicken cannot have been dosed with antibiotics routinely. (In some states sick chickens can be treated with antibiotics.) It must be free-range, thus not confined to close quarters. In addition, no hormones can be administered to the chickens.

These high standards are controversial. The definition of "free-range," for example, is not necessarily as free and open as the term implies. In some states, it means that the chicken has access to a yard or a larger cage than standard mass-produced chicken producers use. It is easier to make this requirement more quantitative by limiting the number of chickens that can be raised in a specific measured area. Stating that a chicken is hormone-free or antibiotic-free is an easier standard to measure than the use of the term free-range.

The USDA has been taken to task because the NOC, which requires that organic chickens have access to a yard, have approved regulations that consider the addition of a "porch" on a chicken house sufficient to allow the chickens adequate fresh air and access to the outdoors for exercise and sunlight. The USDA was further criticized because consumers assume that organic chickens have access to an actual yard and not only a small "porch."

Organic standards also extend to eggs produced by the chickens. In addition, many issues of humane treatment of the animals can be listed on the label. These terms are defined by the USDA and include the terms "cage-free" and "free-range." The term "pasture-raised," which is found on some egg cartons, is not regulated.

The Animal Welfare Institute (AWI) also certifies certain treatment of chickens raised for eggs. The AWI uses the phrase "animal welfare approved" and requires that hens are raised outdoors and not have their beaks trimmed. Humane Farm Animal Care and the American Humane Association are both organizations that certify certain standards and give approval for the use of certain phrases on labels.

See also: Appendix 8: California Organic Products Act of 2003; Appendix 11: Bill AB 1437 Introduced into the California Legislature Dealing with Shelled Eggs.

Elizabeth M. Williams

CHILDREN AND FOOD

Health professionals believe that the human body is more adept at gaining weight and storing fat than shedding it because of humanity's historic struggle to provide itself with enough food. Although lack of nutrients in food is still an issue for many individuals, a more common issue is the health problems caused by the luxury and burden of too much high-calorie food. This change in diet is relatively new and is a particularly important issue with children.

The **National School Lunch Program** has shifted its focus from its original focus, providing children with enough calories, to preventing children from consuming too much food and too many of the wrong types of food. Obesity in children can be a precursor to serious health issues such as Type 2 diabetes. The potential diseases include high blood pressure, asthma, and other respiratory problems, metabolic syndrome, sleep disorders, early puberty or menarche, eating disorders, liver disease, and skin infections. Since children spend so much of their time in school, teaching healthy food choices is, arguably, very important. However, budget considerations have influenced some schools to allow **vending machines**, "pouring rights" contracts with soft drink companies, less nutritious foods that compete with the lunch program, and the **advertising of food** in schools.

Moreover, both in and out of school, critics believe that the food advertising and alcohol advertising industries unfairly and unethically target children. Advertising industry publications emphasize that brand loyalty must begin at a young age, as early as age 2 years. In fact, research shows that children can recognize a brand logo before they recognize their own names. One of the most popular advertising campaigns with children was the Budweiser advertisements featuring the Budweiser frogs. By creating a loyal consumer at an early age, companies create a loyal customer for decades after that. This type of advertising is referred to as a "cradle-to-grave" strategy. Another reason that children are attractive customers is what has been called their "pester power." Children can control a family's purse strings by using one or more of the seven types of pestering to get their parents to buy something for them. Moreover, in cases such as fast food, if a child is getting a meal, chances are the companies have at least one more customer with them, such as a parent.

In 1978, the **Federal Trade Commission** (FTC) unsuccessfully tried to stop advertising on television that was aimed at children, including breakfast cereal and candy. Currently, there are many people lobbying for a ban on advertising geared at children. However, as is apparent in the case of the Budweiser frogs, even advertisements that cannot legally be aimed at children are at times highly popular with them. The advertising industry has instituted an agency to monitor and regulate itself, the Children's Advertising Review Unit (CARU). The organization has written the *Self-Regulatory Guidelines for Children's Advertising*, which it uses to review advertising aimed at children. When it cannot resolve an issue, it refers the issue to the FTC.

See also: Advertising of Alcohol; Advertising of Food; Allergens; Diet Foods; School Breakfast and Lunch Programs; Trans Fats.

Further Reading McNeal, James U. *Kids as Customers.* New York: Lexington Books, 1992; Schlosser, Eric. *Fast Food Nation. The Dark Side of the All-American Meal.* Boston: Houghton Mifflin, 2001; Sheehan, Kim. *Controversies in Contemporary Advertising.* Thousand Oaks, CA: Sage Publications, 2003.

Stephanie Jane Carter

CLEAN WATER ACT

The Federal Water Pollution Control Act, more commonly referred to as the Clean Water Act (CWA), enacted in 1972 and overseen by the **Environmental Protection Agency** (EPA), essentially ensures water quality in the United States by governing water pollution. The CWA has several objectives. Its mission is to rehabilitate the nation's waterways by preventing pollution from various sources. Point source pollutants come from a single, identifiable source. They are easier to regulate. More difficult to regulate are non-point source pollutants, such as polluted runoff from storm drains and snowmelt. The CWA also helps public treatment works improve the treatment of wastewater and helps to maintain wetlands.

Originally, the goal of the act was to eliminate the discharge of pollutants into waters and to have the waters fit for swimming or fishing by 1985.

Agricultural nonpoint source pollution is a major contaminant of U.S. waters. Causes include poor management of animal feeding operations; overgrazing; over-plowing; and too much, improper, or poorly timed application of pesticides, irrigation, and fertilizer. Sediment is a major pollutant resulting from farming and ranching. Soil washes off fields and into nearby lakes and streams. This clouds the water, inhibiting the ability of sunlight to reach aquatic plants. It can also harm fish. The soil often contains other pollutants such as fertilizers, pesticides, and heavy metals. Other pollutants from the runoff are nutrients such as phosphorus, nitrogen, and potassium. These pollute when they are overapplied or applied just before it rains. According to the EPA, the contamination of drinking water is one of the harmful effects of these pollutants. High concentrations of nitrates can cause methemoglobinemia, also known as blue baby syndrome. Other pollutants from agricultural runoff are pathogens from animal waste, which puts bacteria and viruses in the water. Agricultural runoff can cause a number of food-borne illnesses, such as intestinal cryptosporidium. Pesticides from runoff and toxins in the atmosphere can poison fish and wildlife and contaminate food sources. In May 2002, President George W. Bush signed the Farm Bill, which increased the amount of funding for conservation programs to prevent polluted runoff by 80 percent.

Critics of the CWA claim that the EPA rarely enforces it, that the EPA is too often swayed by lobbying groups, and that the regulations are too weak to make much of a difference. Many critics believe that large, corporate farms are treated with too much leniency. Another issue related to the CWA is the popular use of bottled water. Critics of bottled water claim that it makes the enforcement of unpolluted water less mandatory since people get their water out of bottles, rather than taps. If enforcement of water supplies were lacking, those who had to drink tap water and who would most likely be economically disadvantaged, might lose access to clean drinking water. Opponents of bottled water claim that drinking the water that CWA is charged with protecting offers more reasons to enforce these regulations. Other opponents of bottled water consider the packaging to be environmentally wasteful. The restaurant industry has been criticized for pushing bottled water and charging high prices for it, when clean tap water is inexpensive and readily available.

See also: Runoff, Agricultural.

Stephanie Jane Carter

CLONING

Cloning refers to a scientific process by which a genetic twin is created using cells or embryos from the desired organism. Essentially, cloning creates an identical twin with a different birth date. In discussions about the food system, cloning specifically refers to the cloning of mammals.

The three methods by which an animal can be cloned are embryo splitting, blastomere nuclear transfer, and somatic cell nuclear transfer. When an early stage embryo is divided, cells are made available that can be developed into

embryos and implanted into surrogates. This process is known as embryo splitting. In the blastomere nuclear transfer method, blastomeres, which are multiple
cells produced by later-stage embryos, are produced from a fertilized egg and
implanted into eggs, which are scientifically made devoid of a nuclei. These are
then implanted into a surrogate. Somatic cell nuclear transfer is the most popular
type of cloning for animals. This method allows the scientists to take cells from
adult animals. The cells taken from the adult are grown and preserved in a culture until the nuclei can be inserted into eggs devoid of a nucleus. These eggs are
tricked into producing embryos by electric spark or a chemical and then are
implanted into a surrogate. Since the cells are taken from adult animals, this
method is more useful when trying to identify and replicate the most desirable
animals. The United States currently allows certain cloned animal products in the
food supply, but the policy is controversial.

The first time scientists successfully used somatic cell nuclear transfer to clone
a mammal was on July 5, 1996, with the birth of a sheep named Dolly. The success was announced to the public in 1997, sparking the controversy regarding
whether products from these animals should be allowed in the food supply. The
Food and Drug Administration (FDA) tentatively said that the products were safe
for human consumption in 2003. The FDA drafted a 678-page risk assessment
repeating that conclusion in December 2006. The report was widely perceived as
a victory for biotechnology. However, the 2007 **Farm Bill** delayed a formal approval by the FDA by including in it the Mikulski-Specter Amendment, which
required that effects of cloned animals on human health and the economy be
reviewed before those products were released into the food supply. By 2008, the
FDA formally declared with a risk assessment, risk management plan, and written
guidance for the industry, that cloned animals and their offspring were safe for
human consumption. The declaration only applied to cows, pigs, and goats. As
the FDA decided that cloned animal products were essentially the same as their
conventional counterparts, no special labeling requirements were imposed for the
cloned animal products.

The approval sparked controversy within the U.S. government and internationally. The **U.S. Department of Agriculture** (USDA) responded to the FDA approval with a requested moratorium on the sale of clones into the food supply.
The Center for Food Safety condemned the FDA determination, saying that the
research came from cloning companies, a biased source. They also criticized the
ruling for not requiring tracking systems. The same year, the European Group on
Ethics in Science and New Technologies concluded that cloning caused suffering
to animals sufficient to keep those products off the European Market. Specifically,
the group noted that the surrogates could suffer and that clones had higher than
normal rates of health problems. Also in 2008, the European Food Safety Authority in Parma, Italy, concluded that products from cloned animals appeared to not
pose a threat for humans consuming them. California, in particular, is a state that
has proposed bills to require labeling on cloned animal food products. The bill
was known as SB 1121.

Some theorists point out that there is no difference in the offspring of a cloned
animal and the offspring of a conventionally bred animal, eliminating the need

for labeling or restrictions on the food products derived from these animals. In fact, artificial insemination is another reproductive technique that was originally viewed with skepticism. Now it is commonly used to impregnate animals. Theorists who support cloned animal products in the food supply also point out that this technique improves the quality and consistency of meat and dairy products, actually speeding up the reproduction of the most desirable animals. However, other theorists note that this is a threat to diversity that could make entire herds disappear from one disease. Moreover, it remains questionable whether scientists truly understand what the desirable traits are. While quality is important to consumers, many argue that the drive toward consistency destroyed the flavor in many vegetables commonly found on grocery store shelves, as seen in the market for heirloom varieties. Cloning may accelerate and intensify monoculture in animal agriculture. Proponents of cloning point out that the process could also create lines of animals that are resistant to certain diseases. Of course, diseases constantly evolve and diversity has proven to be a way to circumvent some of the harm caused by disease in a group of animals. When a disease is no longer successful in replicating, it attempts to evolve into one that will succeed. If an entire herd is too similar, none may survive the mutated disease. Proponents of cloning, not specific to the food system, point out that the process can also save animals from extinction when applied to endangered species. Cloning has faced opposition from specific industries, such as the organic food industry. Although food derived from cloned animals may not have to be labeled "cloned," it should not be labeled "organic" according to the Organic Trade Association, because only natural breeding and raising of animals is accepted in their definition of the organic system. Another criticism of cloning is that the cloned animals often suffer higher than normal rates of health issues than conventionally bred animals, making it questionable whether these animals or their products should enter the food supply. Proponents argue that the health issues are not passed on to the offspring of the cloned animals and that they are the same as conventionally bred animals and that it is those animals that enter the food supply. The birth defects are mostly due to the genes being turned off and on at the wrong times.

Consumers too have been reported to be hesitant about cloned animals, especially in the food supply. A December 2006 report by the Pew Initiative on Food and Biotechnology found that 64 percent of Americans were uncomfortable with cloning while only 22 percent were comfortable with it. In addition to the arguments that theorists make, many consumers are opposed to cloning for ethical, religious, or emotional reasons. Theorists like Paul Thompson, W.K. Kellogg Chair in Agriculture, Food, and Community Ethics at Michigan State University in 2007 in an interview with the American Veterinary Association, thought that the opposition to animal cloning stems from the more intense opposition to human cloning and that people view cloning animals as treating the animals as things rather than creatures. A Consumers Union study in 2008 found that 89 percent of Americans want cloned food labeled. However, if cloned animal products were labeled, consumers may be more likely to choose the noncloned food, essentially killing an industry that some believe is an advancement for the food industry. The fact that the FDA is perceived to have disregarded the wishes of the public has sparked a criticism not only of cloning, but also of the mission of the FDA. In fact, the FDA's own Center for Veterinary Medicine, in a study titled "Focus Groups on Public's Perception on the Health Risk Associated with Products from Animal Clones," found that people do not want to eat cloned animals or have their children eat such meat or drink milk from cloned animals.

It is currently unlikely that an actual clone would enter the food supply since a cloned animal is very expensive. Instead, cloned animals are usually reserved for breeding purposes. What enters the food supply would be the progeny of the cloned animals and products from them.

See also: European Union Regulations.

Further Reading The Stakeholder Forum on Biotechnology, Pew Charitable Trusts (2003) http://www.pewtrusts.org/uploadedFiles/wwwpewtrustsorg/Reports/Food_and_Biotechnology/ PIFB_StakeholderForum_Process.pdf; Fact Sheet: State Legislative Activity Related to Agricultural Biotechnology in 2005–2006, Pew Initiative on Food and Biotechnology http:// www.pewtrusts.org/uploadedFiles/wwwpewtrustsorg/Reports/Food_and_Biotechnology/ PIFB_State_Legislature_2005-2006Session.pdf; Consumers Union Cloning Poll (2008) http://www.consumersunion.org/campaigns//notinmyfood/005685indiv.html

Stephanie Jane Carter

CODE OF FEDERAL REGULATIONS

The Code of Federal Regulations (CFR) is a codified version of the final versions of rules and regulations that have been promulgated in the *Federal Register*, which is the daily publication of the **executive branch** and contains final and proposed regulations. These provisions are the rules and regulations of the agencies of the executive branch of the federal government. These rules are promulgated based on the procedures outlined in the **Administrative Procedures Act** and are in furtherance of enabling **legislation** passed by Congress. The CFR contains 50 divisions, called Titles, which are the various subjects that the regulations cover. Organics standards, for example, are part of the CFR, as are social security regulations and the rules and regulations of the **Food and Drug Administration**.

The CFR is available online and in print. The CFR is updated annually and one-quarter of the entire code is updated each quarter of the year. Thus, the Code is constantly in revision.

Titles are divided into Chapters. The Chapters are named for the agency. Sometimes a subject is affected by more than one agency, so there may be several Chapters per Title. Chapters are divided into parts and then, when there is much material, into subparts.

The CFR is the source of the detailed rules and regulations affecting the environments, organics, food production and safety and a myriad of other subjects related to food. This Code is as important as any other source of law in that it contains the specific requirements of law, not the more general principles that may be found in the enabling legislation. As the CFR is revised, it is released to the Government Printing Office Access (the online version) at the same time as the paper copy is released. The out-of-date versions are kept as part of the historical record of the law and the agency. Often previous volumes must be referenced because if a question occurs about applicable regulations from a previous time, research in the current CFR would not be useful.

To determine whether there have been changes in the CFR since the most recent publication, researchers can access the List of Sections Affected. This list will refer to CFR sections that have been amended since the last publication. It is vital to check this list to find the most current rules.

For reference to the CFR in effect prior to 1996, it is necessary to refer to the paper version, as the online version begins in 1996. Federal Depository Libraries maintain older versions of the CFR for research and historical purposes. Before reaching the CFR, but being published for comment, the information about public comment can be accessed through the Regulations.gov Web site. For those regulations that are needed regularly, single or multiple volumes of the CFR can be purchased from the Government Printing Office.

See also: Appendix 6: *United States v. Park*; Appendix 10: Senate Bill Introduced into the 111th Congress, Amending the Food, Drug, and Cosmetic Act; Appendix 12: Excerpts from 21 United States Code Sections 341 and Others; Appendix 13: Excerpts from the Code of Federal Regulations Regarding Cheese and Cheese Food.

Elizabeth M. Williams

CODEX ALIMENTARIUS

The **Food and Agriculture Organization** (FAO) **of the United Nations** and the World Health Organization (WHO) have a number of food programs that they operate together. Together they have created the Codex Alimentarius Commission, which has promulgated rules, standards, and procedures that are applicable to all of the programs of the FAO/WHO. Collectively this statement of procedures and standards is known as the Codex Alimentarius. This Commission was established in 1963 by the two organizations. There are three primary purposes of the standards and procedures: to protect the health and safety of the beneficiaries of the programs, to support the systems of fair trade that are applicable to the suppliers and obtainers of food, and to ensure that all of the activities of the programs—whether undertaken by a government or a nonprofit organization—are coordinated to work at highest efficiency.

The Codex is a broad document. It must apply in nations with very few resources and those with many resources. It covers such things as hygiene standards and procedures, the proper transport of food, and the procedures for the import or the export of food. The breadth of the Codex even includes such things as the acceptable levels of drugs in animals that will be slaughtered for food. Other matters, such as mineral supplements, have been reviewed but have not been implemented.

The FAO/WHO programs are conducted primarily in lesser developed nations where there are hygiene issues and problems with food contamination. The protocols and standards established in the Codex make the requirements for hygiene and health standards important and objective. They set procedures for aid workers and others to apply on the ground, and they also provide standards to protect the people from being sent substandard or contaminated products. The procedures also establish methodologies for the introduction of foods to avoid, problems caused by lack of technology, or differences in cultural perception.

The Codex Alimentarius Commission has 183 members. A goal of the commission is that all nations, including those lesser-developed nations, participate in the setting of the standards and procedures of the Codex. It is also recognized that many of the lesser-developed nations have not participated in the making of the Codex. This is ironic because most of the Codex is directly applicable to them. One reason for the nonparticipation is the lack of monetary resources in the lesser-developed nations. To ameliorate this, the FAO and the WHO established the Codex Trust Fund in 2003 to raise money to support the participation by lesser-developed nations in the commission and in the establishment of standards.

One strong area of concentration of the Codex is food security and food-borne disease. These are serious problems in lesser-developed nations, but in particular they affect the very young, the elderly, and those with compromised immune systems. The procedures that are discussed in the Codex start with the fields and follow the food to consumption. The rules of the Codex allow the WHO and the FAO to work with various entities within the country—the government, nongovernmental organizations, and farmers and sellers—to ensure food safety and improve food conditions.

One of the important aspects of the Codex around the globe is that all foods that are imported by FAO/WHO programs must comply with the standards set by the Codex. This protects some countries from having substandard foodstuffs or foods that are contaminated by veterinary drugs or pesticides passed off to another country. It also raises the standards of food handling in those nations where they might otherwise not be high, thus allowing the possibility that the food raised in those countries might be exported.

Compliance with the Codex affects all foods exported from developed nations and imported into developing nations, nations in distress because of a disaster, and when participating in any other FAO/WHO program. The Codex provides an inspection and certification program for import and export. Thus, complying with the Codex includes certain types of labeling (ingredients, additives, and nutrition issues), levels of pesticides, levels of veterinary chemicals, food additives, age of the food, and other important issues that affect the safety and sanitation of the food including how to apply the **Hazard Analysis Critical Control Point**. In addition to food safety, the Codex sets standards for vitamins and minerals.

The **World Trade Organization** considers the Codex a standard when it is resolving disputes regarding issues of food safety. The basis for this position is the Agreement of Sanitary and Phytosanitary Measures and Agreement on Technical Barriers to Trade established in 1995. In addition it references the Codex when resolving consumer protection disputes. The Codex is published in several official languages—English, Spanish, French, Chinese, and Arabic. The Codex has not been adopted by every nation, although it does apply to the programs of the FAO/WHO. Some nations object to the reference to the Codex by the WTO as a standard. They object because the Codex is not something adopted by each nation and to have it referenced as a standard when not all nations have even participated in establishing it can be viewed as a lack of due process. Those who support the use of the Codex argue that the reference to the Codex is not limiting. It does not forbid or preclude reference to other standards. The WTO appellate process could review the method of adopting the provisions of the Codex to determine the reasonableness of the process, which could diffuse some of the controversy and lend legitimacy to the position of the WTO.

Another controversy is over the attempts by members of the commission to have the commission include certain issues important to that member nation in the Codex. These arguments and concerns come from many different political positions. Some members of Congress have expressed concern that the Codex will be imposed within the United States. Members of the Slow Food movement complain that the Codex is too influenced by agribusiness.

See also: Appendix 15: Uruguay Round Agreement on Agriculture; Appendix 16: World Trade Organization Ministerial Conference Decision; Appendix 17: World Medical Assembly Declaration on Hunger Strikers.

Further Reading Codex Alimentarius Web site, http://www.codexalimentarius.net; The International Commission on the Future of Food and Agriculture. *Manifesto on the Future of Food.* July 15, 2003, http://www.farmingsolutions.org/pdfdb/manifestoinglese.pdf.

Elizabeth M. Williams

COMMACK SELF-SERVICE KOSHER MEATS, INC. V. RUBEN, ET AL.

Commack Self-Service Kosher Meats, Inc. v. Ruben, et al. (2002) overturned the long-standing Kosher Fraud Law in the state of New York that had been designed to prevent the intentional fraudulent misrepresentation of certain foods as kosher. The law was enforced by the New York Department of Agriculture and Markets. The basis of the court's decision was that the law violated the Establishment Clause of the First Amendment to the U.S. Constitution.

The case was brought to the district court for the Eastern District of New York by Brian and Jeffrey Yarmeisch, the owners of Commack Self-Service Kosher Meats, Inc., in Commack, Long Island. The company had been cited several times by the Department of Agriculture and Markets for improperly labeling various meats as kosher and by labeling them "soaked and salted." The law defined kosher as food that was "prepared in accordance with the orthodox Hebrew religious requirements." The company had a rabbi supervise its procedures and was not cited for unsanitary conditions or other health-related matters. Despite its requests for clarification and specific guidance, the company was repeatedly cited over the course of several years.

Finally in January 1996 the owners of the company sued the Department and the Director of Kosher Law Enforcement Division of the Department, Rabbi Luzer Weiss. The basis of the lawsuit was that the New York state law violated the clause of the First Amendment of the U.S. Constitution, known as the Establishment Clause, which states that the government will "make no law respecting an establishment of religion." In addition to this argument the plaintiffs claimed that the law deprived them of their right to freedom of religion in that they prepared food in accordance with Conservative Jewish procedures and that they and others of different faiths, such as Muslims who were eating in accordance with the halal rules, were being forced to comply with orthodox religious law.

In addition the plaintiffs argued that the law was vague in that it does not specify what the requirements are, but rather references religious rules for specifics. There were also other minor arguments such as lack of intentionality. This was especially important in light of the repeated requests by the plaintiffs for clarification from the Department.

The defendants filed a motion for summary judgment, asserting that the law was valid on its face. The plaintiffs filed a cross motion for summary judgment asserting that the law was unconstitutional on its face. The district court ruled on the summary judgment in favor of the plaintiff. The judgment stated that the New York law, specifically New York Agriculture and Markets Law sections 201–1, 201-b(1), 201-e(2-a) and (3-c), 201-h, and 26-a, violated the First Amendment to the U.S. Constitution. The court enjoined the Department from enforcing the law.

The defendants appealed the judgment to the United States Court of Appeals for the Second Circuit. The Second Circuit reviewed the record of the trial and affirmed the decision of the lower court. In its analysis, the Second Circuit stated that to enforce the law, the Department had to determine what was kosher. Similarly a company wishing to comply with the law had to determine what was kosher. The law defined kosher by a reference to orthodox religious rules of a particular religion. The specifics needed to determine whether food preparation was kosher could only be learned by reference to the religion, thus the law supported and established the orthodox Hebrew religion as an official arbiter of the law.

The Second Circuit also ruled that the New York law interfered with the free exercise of the plaintiffs' religion in violation of the equal protection clause. Although the defendants argued that there was no dispute as to what constituted kosher, the Circuit Court stated that there was indeed disagreement even without orthodox Hebrew law as to what constitutes kosher. And in addition there was disagreement between Jews who were not orthodox and those who were as to what was kosher. By forcing non-orthodox Jews to comply with orthodox rules, the state of New York was not allowing non-orthodox Jews to freely exercise their religious beliefs.

In enforcement, the Department, representing the state of New York, was required to reference religious tenants not specifically found in the law. Thus, the state was enforcing religious law, not the secular law in violation of the First Amendment.

The Second Circuit said that all parties agreed that the purpose of the law was to protect consumers from fraud, which is a valid use of the regulatory power of the state. The question was the way that the law went about this task. It did so in violation of the U.S. Constitution. The court said that existing consumer protection laws were sufficient to allow manufacturers and other food purveyors to claim that food that it labeled was kosher, and they could establish by what rules they considered it kosher. This would allow the consumer to be informed and allow the consumer to make choices without reference to religious rules in the state law. In other words, the law went too far in establishing the definition of kosher, when a less far-reaching method of protecting the consumer was available. The purposes of the law could be advanced with less entanglement with religion.

The court stated that less than 30 percent of the purchasers of kosher products are orthodox Jews. Others are Muslim or those who wish to eat in accordance with kosher principles regarding treatment of animals or for other reasons.

This case was not decided by the U.S. Supreme Court. In *Employment Div., Dept. of Human Resources of Oregon v. Smith*, 494 U.S. 872 (1990) the Supreme Court stated that while practices that impact religion can be regulated, this is allowable for secular purposes and only the secular aspects of the religion. The law must be neutral regarding the religion. This case is important in that it is a recent interpretation of the position of the law regarding the separation of religion and the state balanced against consumer rights in food labeling.

See also: Kosher and Halal Labeling; Appendix 2: *Commack Self-Service Kosher Meats, Inc. v. Weiss.*

Further Reading Commack Self-Service Kosher Meats, Inc. v. Rubin, 106 F.Supp.2d. 445 (E.D. N.Y. 2000); *Commack Self-Service Kosher Meats, Inc. v. Rubin,* 294 F3d 415 (2nd Cir. 2002).

Elizabeth M. Williams

COMMUNITY-SUPPORTED AGRICULTURE

Community Supported Agriculture (CSA) refers to a direct-to-consumer relationship between a farm operator and the consumers of the agricultural products where the consumers provide up-front support to the producers in return for a share of the products actually produced throughout the season. In a CSA, also known as subscription farming, the consumer may bear the risk of a lack of agricultural success, but many CSAs place more of the risk on the producer who owes the consumer for what has been paid for in advance, regardless of the farmer's actual production.

CSAs may be entirely owned and operated by the farmer, with only money contributed by the consumers, or in rarer situations the consumers may also provide land, capital, and/or labor to the farm operation to a varying degree. If the members contribute labor to a significant degree, they may be treated as employees for the purposes of state common law legal liability and state and/or federal occupational health and safety laws. Whatever the arrangement, a clearly structured and worded CSA membership agreement is important to spell out the rights and responsibilities of all parties to the arrangement.

The CSA concept began in Europe and CSA operations have been active in the United States since the later 1980s, with over 1,000 CSAs now operating in the United States according to the University of Massachusetts. Line Farm in Massachusetts was the first operation known as a CSA in the United States. The modern direct consumer–supported farm concept may have originated in Japan in an arrangement known as teikei. Farms may be entirely devoted to CSA or they may also sell to farmer's markets, roadside stands, restaurants, or other customers.

Some CSAs require members to come to the farm to pick up their products or they may deliver them to pick-up locations or individual residences.

Given the variety of CSA arrangements and farm operations, CSAs may be structured through a variety of business and legal arrangements. They may be sole proprietorships, partnerships, cooperatives, or incorporated businesses, and they may own their land outright or through a trust, lease their land, or otherwise gain the right to farm it. As a farm operation, many CSAs carry farm insurance, which may also include liability insurance, and specialized insurance may be necessary if members visit the farm and conduct activities like picking, driving vehicles, or visiting animals and livestock.

In 1976, Congress enacted the Farmer-to-Consumer Direct Marketing Act to promote direct marketing of agricultural commodities, including roadside stands, farmer's markets, and by house-to-house sales. The act was later amended in 2005 to explicitly include CSA programs. The act directed the **U.S. Department of Agriculture** (USDA) to work with state departments of agriculture to promote direct marketing and authorized grants to agricultural cooperatives, nonprofits, and other organizations to develop and support direct marketing of agricultural commodities and to states to provide assistance to low-income seniors to purchase direct marketed agricultural products. In 2006, 14,575 farmers served 825,000 seniors with $15 million in support from USDA.

As marketers and sellers of food products, CSAs are generally subject to state and federal food safety laws. For example, the Federal Food, Drug, and Cosmetic Act prohibits the sale of raw, unpasteurized milk in interstate commerce, and state laws may restrict or ban its sale in intrastate commerce. Cow-share programs, a subset of a few CSAs, where the consumers actually purchase the cow or share of the cow and pay the farmer to care for it, may or may not constitute the sale of raw milk, depending on the state. In addition, most states also have specific laws regulating producers of eggs, covering grading standards, sanitary conditions, and labeling.

States generally apply more regulation and inspection requirements on produce sold for resale, such as to a grocery store, than for direct-to-consumer marketing, and many have thresholds for exemptions from some regulations and inspections. But many generally applicable federal and state food safety requirements apply to CSA producers. State laws covering food vendors and involving inspections by either agricultural or health departments are common, and these will vary depending on whether the CSA produces only fruits and vegetables, or also meat, dairy, or processed food, which are generally subject to greater levels of regulation.

See also: Milk, Raw.

Andrew G. Wallace

CONTRACTS

Contracts are documents basic to the operation of almost every business—restaurants, food manufacturers, grocers, farms, vineyards—in short, the entire food and beverage industry. Each industry relies on contracts to make the business work.

Many diverse types of agreements are forms of contracts, such as leases and sales, orders, employment agreements, and construction agreements.

A contract is a mutual exchange of obligations or promises. Contracts can be oral or written. Many contracts, which make it possible to do business on a day-to-day basis, are oral. They rely on what the courts call "a meeting of the minds." This means that two or more people have agreed on a course of events, had a meeting of the minds, and have proceeded with their actions fully expecting the other parties to do what they agreed to do. The freedom to enter into contracts, often called liberty of contract, is a judicial concept. It does not mean that people may enter into any contract—minimum wage laws and other employment laws limit total freedom of contract—but people may engage in a very broad conduct under contract.

For example, when a person calls a business and makes an order, there is an agreement to deliver that item and a further promise to pay for the item—that is a contract. Pizza delivery is a good example of this type of agreement. It is not in writing. The parties generally do not know each other, but nevertheless, business is conducted successfully. Having to reduce this contract to writing would impede the flow of business.

The law recognizes several elements as necessary to form a legally enforceable contract. They are offer and acceptance, consideration, legal subject matter, and competency. The offer and acceptance represent the exchange of obligations or the mutual promises made between the parties. For example, if one orders a meal in a restaurant, the restaurant agrees to serve the meal and the diner agrees to pay for the meal. These are the mutual obligations that form the basis of the contract. Another example might be the agreement to provide fertilizer to a farmer and the farmer's agreement to pay for the fertilizer.

Acceptance can be tacit or implied—when a person prepays for an order, the deposit of the check or running of a credit card implies acceptance. The offeree (the party accepting the offer to enter into the contract) is then obligated to perform by filling the order or doing whatever has been ordered. A contract may be explicitly accepted, where the offeree says, "Yes, I'll fulfill that order." Contracts where the offer and the acceptance are explicit are known as "bilateral contracts." A "unilateral contract" is one in which the contract is accepted by simply performing the obligation.

It is essential that the subject matter of the contract be legal. If the subject matter is not legal, then the contract is not enforceable, even if there was a meeting of the minds. For example, it is illegal to kill and sell or serve endangered species as food. An otherwise legal contract to purchase that animal is based on illegal subject matter and thus is not enforceable. Therefore, a person who has placed such an order, but refuses to pay, cannot be successfully sued. The courts will not enforce an illegal contract. It is illegal to sell alcoholic beverages to people under a certain age; doing so is not only illegal, but renders the contract unenforceable.

Another important element of a contract is adequate consideration (or cause in Louisiana). Consideration is the quid pro quo that balances the mutual obligations. One type of consideration is money. Other types of consideration include anything of value, such as the goods purchased in a sale, a person's efforts or work, a trade secret, good will, and reputation built up by a company. It is possible for a one party to have an obligation that is not exactly equivalent in value to the obligation of the other party without nullifying the contract. The marketplace often is the scene of shifting values. Commodity prices can change in a period of days, rendering a costly early purchase of corn less valuable, as the market floods with corn. It is also possible that a person can knowingly overpay for something, simply because it is something desired and the value to the purchaser is higher than the normal market value. Contract law recognizes that setting value is not a precise science. However, where there is a true lack of equivalency of value, there may be inadequate consideration, causing the contract to fail.

Finally, the parties to the contract must be competent. This means they must be of the age of majority and mentally competent. Mental competency is generally assumed, unless a person is acting obviously incompetent, either by use of drugs or alcohol or because of mental illness.

A written contract represents a memorialization of the meeting of the minds. There are advantages of having a written contract. It forms a clear statement of the intent of the parties. Memories can fade over time and changes in situation may make memories shift. Putting it in writing allows the parties to define terms when the contract involves complex matters like leases and sales, where they are many factors involved. The writing allows the parties to clearly state the obligations and promises of both sides. It also allows for the statement of anticipated damages, should a breach occur.

Some types of contracts must be in writing to be enforceable. The common law support for this requirement derives from the Statute of Frauds. These types of contracts include those involving real estate transfers, contracts that cannot be performed within a year, and certain other matters regarding estates, marriage and sureties. The Uniform Commercial Code requires that the purchase of goods of a value over a certain value must be in writing, although there are exceptions.

A failure to live up to the obligations of a contract is known as a breach of the contract. When a breach occurs, the harmed party may bring an action for damages or for specific performance. Specific performance is the requirement that the breaching party must perform what was agreed to in the contract. Courts prefer to award damages rather than force even breaching parties to do something, even when they have agreed to do it in their contract. Damages are usually an award of money representing the harm done to the aggrieved party by the breach.

See also: Appendix 1: *United States v. Fior D'Italia, Inc.*; Appendix 7: *In the Matter of McCormick & Company, Inc.*

Elizabeth M. Williams

COOPERATIVES

A cooperative is a group of people who come together to engage in a particular activity to achieve a particular mutual benefit. Such a benefit is generally a mutual financial benefit. A traditional cooperative is not owned by anyone, but by all of the participants. It does not operate to make a profit. All of the financial return is shared among the members. There are large cooperatives that produce food such as Land O'Lakes and Sunkist. These coops work in concert for their mutual advantage by pooling milk to produce dairy products that the members could not afford the equipment to make alone. Similarly the citrus juice is pooled and produced under a single brand and marketed as one product.

Consumer cooperatives are not cooperatives of producers, but of consumers or buyers. They are often called buyer cooperatives (or coops). They are often made up of people who wish to combine to purchase health food, organic foods, or natural foods. By buying in bulk and reselling to members, the coop assists its members in buying natural foods at a good price. These coops have been connected with the early natural foods movement when it was often hard to find natural foods.

A buying club is usually an informal organization of friends or other like-minded people who order in bulk and share the order. A coop that is more formally organized, for example, that forms a nonprofit organization and has many members, may form a grocery store. These organizations may have a member price and a price for nonmembers who may also shop there. The coop members share the work of selecting and ordering the food, perhaps unloading the delivery truck, going to pick up the order, dividing the order, or repackaging it.

Many cooperatives operate by preordering food. This allows the coop to purchase only what it knows will sell. Cooperatives are almost always nonprofit organizations, but they are not tax-exempt. They are not eligible for 501(c)(3) status. The organization may not earn a profit if it only operates at break-even levels. Thus, if the members pay when they preorder, any necessary adjustments can be made when the members pick up their fulfilled orders. The need for accurate record keeping is essential. Some cooperatives do not allow separate orders, but rather collect the same amount for each membership share, and provide the same food for each membership share. Although the coop does not charge enough to make a profit, it will usually charge enough to cover the administrative costs of operating the coop. This means the costs of transportation, storage, packaging, bookkeeping, and so on.

Cooperatives may be incorporated as nonprofit corporations or as regular business corporations. They operate as cooperatives because of the way their by-laws are written. The by-laws should ensure that the coop will operate democratically and voluntarily. It is designed to operate for the benefit of members in proportion to their purchases or membership level. Some states, like California, have well-developed cooperative laws. The law recognizes that even those who intend to operate as a coop may decide that they prefer to incorporate as a business organization, not a coop. The rights and responsibilities of the board of directors, the officers, and the members are important components of a coop.

Subchapter T of the Internal Revenue Code recognizes patronage dividends, and doesn't tax the coop for the savings of members that are returned to the members. The members who receive the refund may have to declare the refund as income, however.

A cooperative business may subtract the amount of patronage dividends from its taxable income. In order for the patronage dividend to qualify for exclusion from the income of the cooperative, there must be a statement in the by-laws or the membership agreement that requires the coop to provide this refund to its members. This obligation is the factor that makes the payments to members excludable from coop income. A cooperative may raise capital under Subchapter T by declaring a written notice of allocation of a patronage dividend. If the coop gives the members 20 percent of the allocation, it may retain the rest for use as capital. The member must declare the entire allocated amount as personal income. If the cooperative keeps the allocation as a nonqualified investment, it may pay the patronage dividend at a later date and take the deduction in the year it pays the dividend.

Principles of the International Co-operative Alliance

1. Voluntary and Open Membership
2. Democratic Member Control
3. Member Economic Participation
4. Autonomy and Independence
5. Education, Training, and Information
6. Co-operation among Co-operatives
7. Concern for Community

Source: International Co-operative Alliance http://www.ica .coop/al-ica/.

Most cooperatives do not qualify as tax exempt organizations. However, the law allows credit union and rural utility cooperatives, both of which are highly regulated, to qualify as tax exempt entities. These special cooperatives must qualify under both state and federal law to be tax exempt.

Cooperatives are a model of business that are often used in developing countries because they pool resources, create economies of scale, and allow for social interaction and cooperation that are often culturally important to do business. The United Nations has declared that 2012 is the International Year of Cooperatives. The UN has said that cooperatives are of particular importance in helping women in developing nations have a business voice.

There are several principles that apply to a cooperative business. The first principle is that the organization is voluntary and is open to all who not only desire membership, but also are willing to participate responsibly in the cooperative. Also cooperatives are democratically controlled and members participate economically in the organization. Cooperatives are independent and provide education and training for members. They coordinate and cooperate with other cooperatives. And cooperatives operate for the good of the community.

Agricultural businesses are commonly operated as coops. Farmers can operate more efficiently in production by cooperating and can market cooperatively under one brand name and obtain better placement in grocery stores. Cooperatives must clearly state the responsibilities of members as well as their objectives to remain competitive and not act in concert in a noncompetitive manner.

See also: Anti-Trust Law and Food Manufacturing Consolidation; Anti-Trust Law and Grocery Store Consolidation; Cooperatives, Agricultural.

Further Reading International Cooperative Alliance http://www.ica.coop/al-ica/; National Cooperative Business Association http://www.ncba.coop.

Elizabeth M. Williams

COOPERATIVES, AGRICULTURAL

An agricultural cooperative, also known as a farmers' cooperative, refers to an entity organized to mutually benefit its member farmers through the marketing of their products at the maximum possible price and through obtaining farm equipment and other supplies at the minimum possible price, effectively strengthening its members' position in an economic market. Agricultural cooperatives are essentially a group of farmers pooling resources in different areas of activity, coming together as a larger and more powerful entity as they cultivate and harvest agricultural products. There are several types of cooperatives. A supply cooperative would be organized to achieve the best prices on the elements needed for agricultural production and to obtain these items for the farmers to use. These elements may include fertilizer, seeds, and **pesticides**. A marketing cooperative, such as Sunkist and Sun-Maid, is organized to market members' agricultural products. A third type of cooperative is a service cooperative, which provides various services to its members. **Cooperatives** may be a combination of these as well.

Generally, agricultural cooperatives differ from other corporations in that they are formed by their members to serve the needs of their members. Member-farmers provide the risk capital and are also the users of the services of the cooperative. They are owned and governed by their member-farmers and each member-farmer has only one vote, making a cooperative a democratic entity. They typically operate at cost and offer only a limited return on investment. The basis for the limited return on investment is the fact that cooperatives are not meant to be for-profit entities, hence the benefits they are granted at the state and federal level. The Capper-Volstead Act limits the return to a maximum of 8 percent to the members. Additionally, members participate in the net margins based on the quantity or value of the business conducted with and for them. Examples of agricultural cooperatives include Blue Diamond Growers (almonds), Humboldt Creamery (dairy), Dairy Farmers of America, and Ocean Spray (cranberries and citrus). Most cooperatives begin as small businesses, but may grow to generate billions of dollars in revenue. Ocean Spray, a marketing cooperative, was created in 1930 by three growers who wanted to expand the market share of cranberry products. Now one of the largest juice producers, it represents the success a cooperative can achieve for its members. According to the **U.S. Department of Agriculture** (USDA), agricultural cooperatives account for a significant amount of economic activity in the agricultural industry.

Benjamin Franklin began the first successful cooperative, a mutual fire insurance company, in Philadelphia in 1752. By 1804, a group of dairy farmers in Connecticut organized a marketing cooperative. The first permanent, recorded cooperative in England was founded in 1844. Known as the Rochdale Society, this cooperative developed a list of 11 principles that became the basic tenants of cooperative societies. Though the principles have evolved, their basic ideas remain. Agricultural cooperatives enjoy benefits at both the state and federal level. The favorable attitude toward cooperatives is apparent in the availability of special incorporation statutes, certain federal income tax deductions, partial antitrust exemptions, and judicial recognition of the unique nature of the cooperative.

State Statutes

A cooperative is a corporation, rather than a club. State statutes vary in their incorporation statutes for cooperatives. Some states incorporate cooperatives as a special type of business corporation or a type of nonprofit. The nonprofit status is derived from the idea that cooperatives are generally not organized to be for-profit ventures. They are organized to benefit their members.

For tax purposes, state statutes usually follow federal statutes when dealing with cooperatives. State statutes vary in their treatment of cooperatives, but they generally prohibit interference with cooperatives. They impose penalties for interference such as civil fines, criminal penalties, and treble damages. They may also authorize injunctions.

Taxes

Cooperatives may pay property, sales, and employment taxes. Additionally, they pay a single tax on earnings at the membership level. However, cooperatives may take certain federal income tax deductions. Net income on business conducted with and for patrons (those members and nonmembers who use the cooperative services on a cooperative basis) is not taxable. Patrons pay tax on net income refunded to them, while the cooperative does not pay taxes on that. This deduction is granted under Subchapter T of the Internal Revenue Code. The main point of debate is whether cooperative income is from patronage or nonpatronage business as this determines the cooperative's tax liability. Courts tend to rule that income is patronage based if it facilitates the service activities of a cooperative rather than only making it more profitable.

Some cooperatives may qualify for further tax deductions of they are considered "exempt" under section 521 of the Internal Revenue Code. This deduction is also allowed under Subchapter T of the Internal Revenue Code.

Partial Antitrust Exemptions

Under the Capper-Volstead Act (1922), cooperatives receive partial antitrust exemptions. Some theorists have questioned whether the exemption continues to be necessary in light of the size of many modern cooperatives. They particularly question the need for antitrust exemptions in the dairy industry. The Government Accountability Office (GAO) supports the relevance of the Capper-Volstead exemption, even for large cooperatives like the dairy farmers cooperatives, claiming that they are small compared with the distributing and processing firms that purchase their products. Although the **Federal Trade Commission** (FTC) assumes the role of antitrust enforcement for other corporations, the USDA is charged with antitrust enforcement for agricultural cooperatives. Although the cooperatives enjoy this exemption, the USDA is supposed to ensure that they do not abuse it. The USDA is regularly criticized for not overseeing antitrust enforcement in cooperatives, especially in pricing activities.

Securities

Membership stock, equity, and debt instruments of cooperatives are not generally considered securities at the state or federal level. If they were considered securities, the legal requirements of the cooperative would engender registration and disclosure requirements.

Agricultural cooperatives are increasingly common in the developing world. For example, South Africa passed a Cooperatives Act in 2005. The act embraced the internationally recognized and adopted principles of cooperation, originally based on the Rochdale principles.

Further Reading Chaddad, Fabio R., and Michael L. Cook. "Understanding the New Cooperative Models: An Ownership-Control Rights Typology." *Review of Agricultural Economics* 26, no. 3 (September 2004): 348–60; Hawke, Stephen D. "Antitrust Implications of Agricultural Cooperatives." *Kentucky Law Journal*. 73 Ky. L.J. 1033 (1984–1985); Matthews, Marry Beth. "Recent Developments in the Law Regarding Agricultural Cooperatives." *North Dakota Law Review*. 68 N.D.L. Rev. 273 (1992); Ulmer, Al. *Cooperatives and Poor People in the South*. Atlanta, GA: Southern Regional Council, 1969.

Stephanie Jane Carter

COPYRIGHT OF RECIPES AND DISHES

The Copyright Law of the United States generally does not protect recipes or dishes made from them. Cookbooks have received some copyright protection, but not against copying of individual recipes.

Copyright protects original works of authorship, such as literary works, that are fixed in a tangible medium of expression. It does not extend to mere facts or to any idea, procedure, or process, regardless of the form in which it might be embodied in a literary work, such as a cookbook.

Recipes have been variously defined in dictionaries as a process for making something, a set of rules to be followed when duplicating foods and particular dishes, and a list of ingredients appearing with the steps to be followed for creating an item prepared for eating or drinking.

As such, recipes are considered under copyright law to be ideas and factual statements of ingredients and are not protected. Also, at least under copyright law, recipes are not considered to have sufficient originality for protection. Individual dishes prepared from recipes have never been covered by copyright law, but they might be protectable under other legal theories. Cookbooks, being compilations of elements that are not copyrightable, are only eligible for copyright to the extent they feature original selection and arrangement of recipes or material beyond the recipes themselves. For example, original artwork or photographs used in the presentation of a recipe in a cookbook would be protected by copyright. Also, a recipe would have some measure of copyright protection if included in a creative narrative how the dish might be prepared. Such narrative might include anything from musings about the spiritual nature of cooking to suggestions for music and place settings. What would be important and protectable in such cases would be the way in which the ideas and facts were expressed, and not the facts or ideas themselves.

Over the years, there have been numerous cases in which chefs and authors of cookbooks have attempted to convince courts that recipes should be protected under copyright law.

Folklore places the first confrontation in 1638 under what was then France's equivalent of copyright law. A chef sought protection for his "fragrant sauce" for vegetables and, not succeeding in court, stormed a competitor's restaurant kitchen, thrusting handfuls of hair into the pots in which his sauce was being prepared.

In modern times, at least in reported U.S. cases, more moderate approaches have been taken and disputes have been of a more scholarly nature. In 1892, for example, the U.S. Supreme Court affirmed a lower court's ruling in favor of a woman who had written a book of "receipts" that were copied by a publisher who added and subtracted copy and substituted another name for that of the author. The Court dealt with many legal theories, but had nothing whatsoever to say about the threshold questions of whether recipes could be copyrighted. Apparently, the question was never raised.

In a North Dakota case in 1924, another court simply assumed that recipes could be copyrighted to the extent that they served to advance the culinary art. This case, however, seems to have never been accepted as a precedent.

In 1991, the issue of copyrighting recipes was squarely addressed in court and resolved. The publisher of a book of yogurt recipes sued the publisher of another book of yogurt recipes, and a ruling against the publisher who sued spelled out in detail the law as it exists today.

See also: Trademarks.

Further Reading 17 U.S.C. 101 et seq; *Belford Clark & Co. v. Schribner*, 144 U.S. 488 (1892); *Fargo Mercantile Co. v. Brechtel and Richter Co.*, 295 F. 823 (8th Cir 1924); *Feist Publications, Inc. v. Rural Tel. Service, Inc.*, 499 U.S. 340 (1991); Levenson, Barry M. *Habeas Codfish*. Madison: University of Wisconsin Press, 2001; *Marcus v. Rowley*, 695 F2d 1171 (9th Cir. 1983); Nimmer, Melville B., and David Nimmer. *Nimmer on Copyright*. Albany, NY: Matthew Bender, 1997; *Publications International, Ltd. v. Meredith Corp.*, 88 F3d 473 (7th Cir. 1996); *Superfine Products, Inc. v. Denny*, 54 F. Supp 148 (N.D. Ga. 1943).

William T. Abbott

CORKS

A cork is a type of bottle closure made from the outer bark of the cork oak tree (*Quercus suber*), which is an evergreen oak that grows best in the Mediterranean regions of Western Europe and North Africa and places with similar climates. The cork bottle closures are most commonly used with wine bottles, though non-cork closures such as rubber or plastic stoppers or metal screw-off caps are growing in usage and popularity.

Corks have been used to seal bottles and other containers for food and beverages for thousands of years. Dom Pérignon helped popularize the use of cork for sealing wine bottles in the 1600s. The cork oak forests are also useful. The cork oak trees create rich forests that support mammal, bird, insect, and plant species. The trees protect the coast from erosion. Additionally, the cork industry provides employment opportunities for many people, notably in North Africa. Since cork used for closures comes from the outer bark of the cork tree, the trees do not have to be cut down to be harvested for this product.

Still, to be a positive enterprise, the cork forests must be sustainably and responsibly managed. In May 2008, Congress amended the Lacey Act of 1900 to ban the import, export, purchase, or sale of illegally harvested plants or plants products. This is relevant to cork production and import. There are also nongovernmental groups that help ensure that these products are responsibly grown and harvested. The Forest Stewardship Council (FSC) is an organization with the goal of promoting responsible forestry. The FSC offers a certification for responsible forestry and the products from those forests. The certification is a nongovernmental way of regulating forestry and promoting responsible, sustainable practices. Recognized in more than 50 countries, the FSC accreditation allows consumers to easily identify cork and other forest products that have been responsibly grown and harvested. The FSC certification can also be applied to wineries that use sustainably harvested corks. In 2007, Willamette Valley Vineyards in Oregon became the first winery to earn the FSC distinction.

The FSC has been criticized for certifying large monoculture plantations. However, organizations such as the World Wildlife Fund pledge support to the FSC. Governmental regulation is often characterized as government involvement in issues it may not know enough about. In fact, some forestry organizations fight government intervention because many of their regulations work against what their goals are because of a deficit of knowledge. Another issue in the cork industry is that the use of other closures for wine bottles is growing in use and popularity. Many companies have begun using synthetic corks and screw-off caps as an alternative to traditional cork. Since the cork industry and these forests are largely dependent on the wine industry, the use of other closures can be detrimental to the industry, the forests, and the people who work with them. Many publications report that the new stoppers prevent leakage and "moldy cork" and do not harm the aging process in wine. The new stoppers are perceived as a superior product, and there is evidence that the use of these will continue to grow.

See also: Beverage Closures and Containers, Alternative.

Stephanie Jane Carter

COUPONS

A coupon refers to a document in print or digital form that is offered in exchange for something of value, such as an item or a reduction in price when the item is purchased. They are often used as a type of marketing incentive. They are typically issued by manufacturers or retailers for use and are commonly found in print media such as magazines or newspapers, or online. When a coupon is issued through a manufacturer, it is usually redeemed at a retail outlet. The retailer then sends the coupons to a clearing house that ensures the validity of the coupon. The manufacturer then issues a refund to the retailer. A newer form of coupon is through GPS technology. When consumers pass a coupon-offering establishment, the coupon will appear on their smart phone.

Coupons were first used by Georgia tycoon Asa Griggs Candler, who bought the formula for Coca-Cola in 1887. To promote his product, he issued handwritten coupons for free Coca-Cola. He gave soda fountains free syrup to use for the free sodas. Shortly after that, cereal manufacturer C.W. Post used coupons to market Grape Nuts, offering one cent off purchase. Coupons became enormously popular during the Great Depression, when families had less money to spend on groceries and used coupons to save money. As chain supermarkets grew in the 1940s, so did the use of coupons. With such a large number of coupons being distributed and redeemed, the Nielson Coupon Clearing House was created in 1957 to validate coupon redemptions. In the 1990s, digital coupons that consumers could print were introduced. Coupon codes were also introduced. In 2008, cell phone coupons that could be scanned debuted. Coupons soared in popularity again in 2009, with the onset of the recession. The offer and redemption of physical coupons has been declining since 1992, while the use of online coupons continues to increase.

Coupons offer value in a variety of ways. They may be in the form of rebates gained by mailing proof of purchase to a manufacturer. They may be in the form of a discount that is taken when an item is purchased. Generally, the merchant gives the discount and is reimbursed by the manufacturer. Often, the merchant is required to supply the manufacturer with proof, usually in the form of a sales receipt, which demonstrates that the sale was made.

Depending on its terms, a coupon can legally represent a promise and, consequently, a legal obligation known as a unilateral contract. A contract is created between the manufacturer who distributes the coupon and the merchant who accepts the coupon. A contract is also created between the manufacturer who distributes the coupon and the customer who decides to take advantage of the offer. As soon as the offer is accepted, the unilateral contract is enforceable. Therefore, unilateral contracts created by coupon promises are enforceable under contract law. For this reason, language on coupons must be very explicit. Coupons usually offer clear expiration dates and language that disallows transferring the coupons or redeeming them for actual money.

Misuse of coupons, usually in the form of coupon fraud, can entail criminal penalties. Merchant have committed coupon fraud when they return coupons to the manufacturer and accept the refund for items that were never actually purchased. Creating fake coupons and redeeming them for items of value is another action that constitutes coupon fraud. According to 2010 estimates, coupon fraud cost manufacturers and retailers about $500 million each year. In the past, coupons have been protected against counterfeit reproduction through the use of holograms and watermarks. In fact, some print coupons were printed with watermarks that stated void. Coupon fraud has grown as technology has made it easier to create counterfeit coupons and as consumers get more of their coupons from online sources. According to NCH Marketing Services, Inc., the redemption of fraudulent coupons increased 14 percent between 2008 and 2009. Coupon Information Corporation is a nonprofit group that monitors coupon fraud for food companies. The criminal penalty for coupon fraud varies from state to state.

Coupons may or may not reduce the amount of sales tax on an item. If the retailer offers the coupon, the item does not incur the full sales tax amount because the item was not offered at full price. If the manufacturer offers the coupon, full price is still considered to be paid, but the manufacturer refunds part of it to the store.

A recent issue regarding coupons has been their resale on online auction sites such as eBay. The Grocery Manufacturers Association (GMA) and the Food Marketing Institute asked that eBay ban copyrighted, nontransferable coupons on the site. They claimed that the sale of the coupons in most cases is unlawful because most coupons explicitly state that they are not transferable. They also claimed that the sale of the coupons violated intellectual property rights. They worked together with eBay to develop policies regarding the sale of coupons on the site and the GMA occasionally monitors the sale of coupons on the sites that are in violation of the policies. The policies include a ban on selling expired coupons, except where they are collectible, a ban on selling electronic coupons, a ban on selling coupons in bulk, and limiting the number of coupons that offer a free product without requirement of purchase.

There are other classes of coupons in addition to coupons meant to market a product. For example, **food stamps** are basically coupons for food. In times when goods must be rationed, coupons are often used to control the amount of a product a person can purchase. The World Food Program, which is a type of international **food bank**, has used coupons in emergency areas to control the distribution of food. These coupons still follow the basic definition of a coupon—a document that can be used in exchange for something of value. These types of coupons often entail the same issues of fraud as manufacturer and retail coupons.

See also: Groceries, Taxes on; Internet Sales.

Stephanie Jane Carter

COURT SYSTEM
The court system is part of the judiciary. It is a mechanism that allows for resolution of controversies, whether civil, criminal, or governmental. The court system is established in the U.S. Constitution and in the constitutions of the various states. Controversies of all varieties can be resolved in the court system.

Civil controversies refer to disputes or other matters involving private persons and businesses. These matters can include, for example, divorce, contractual disputes, real estate controversies, **tort** controversies, estate administration, name changes, and adoption.

Criminal matters that may be resolved in the courts may include traffic violations, common law crimes such as murder or theft, and crimes defined by law such as violating noise levels, polluting, and intentionally adulterating food. A civil matter can include an action, known as a "private attorney general" matter, in which legislation allows a private party to bring an action to enforce the law, when an appropriate governmental agency has not.

Governmental controversies are those controversies that involve an action by a citizen or a business against the government for one or more of several reasons. These reasons can be to force the government to enforce a law, to challenge the interpretation of a law as either being unconstitutional or not properly interpreted or applied, and to resolve controversies within the government or between governments.

State and federal court systems are designed to allow parties to present matters of controversy to be decided by a jury or judge at a trial. After that decision is made it is subject to review by an appellate system. The appellate system may have one or two tiers.

The beginning of the process is the trial. At the trial the parties present the facts and the evidence that supports the facts to the judge or jury. They define their positions. They ask for redress. After considering the evidence and deliberating, redress is either granted or not. At trial both the law and facts are interpreted. And all parties who may have an interest in the controversy are allowed to present evidence and argument. The facts as they are established in the record made of the trial are very important. This is the opportunity to build the foundation for an appeal.

In building the record during the trial, it is also important for the parties to point out to the judge errors in the decisions of the court as the trial proceeds. Objections should be noted with reasons to support the objections. Exception should be taken when objections are overruled. All issues that are decided incorrectly for a particular side should be preserved for the record.

The appellate process is based on errors of law or errors of fact that are tantamount to an error of law. Because there is no retrial and no new evidence taken, the entire review of the proceedings is based on the trial record. The person who brings the appeal, that is, the party who is dissatisfied with the decision of the trial court, is called the "appellant." The appellant files a brief with the appellate court. The brief is a document that outlines, with specific references to the transcript and the evidence and the errors made by the judge and the jury. The other party, responding to the appeal, is called the "appellee" or "respondent." The appellee files an answer brief that points out to the court the false arguments made by the appellant.

Because the finder of fact has firsthand experience observing the evidence being given, seeing the reactions of the witnesses, watching the demeanor of the parties, the appellate process is based on the principle that the trier of facts decisions about the facts is correct. When the trier of fact is the judge, the standard to overturn the decisions about the facts is not as high, and may be attacked as an abuse of discretion. The appellate court merely has the record to go by. So it is legal error that forms the basis of the appeal. The error rises to the level of reversible error. Occasionally when the facts are wrong, the court can find that the error in fact is equivalent to an error of law.

In addition to pointing to errors of law and citing specific references to errors in the transcript of the trial, the briefs establish the legal error by pointing to precedent. "Precedent" is a term that refers to decisions made in other cases. Precedent is persuasive when it comes from a court of an equivalent level, such as another federal court of appeals, or from another jurisdiction. Often states will look to decisions of other states for guidance when there is no precedent in that state. However, when a superior court has made a decision, that decision is binding precedent. By citing precedent in a brief, the parties establish what the law is and what the interpretation of the law should have been in the trial.

Some parties may have an interest in the outcome of a matter but may not be a party to the action. With leave of the appellate court these parties may file a brief with the court, known as a brief *amicus curie*, often called an amicus brief or a friend of the court brief. Often these briefs expand the scope of consideration by the appellate court, because they explain to the court how the decision may affect others beyond just the parties in the case. In addition the amicus brief may argue matters beyond the errors that are argued in the briefs of the parties.

Sometimes the appellate court will affirm the judgment of the lower court. This means that the appellant has failed to establish error sufficient to overturn the lower court decision. The appellate court may reverse the decision of the lower court. In such action, the appellate court is convinced that sufficient error occurred to overturn the decision of the lower court. The appellate court may affirm in part and reverse in part, as when they affirm that wrongdoing occurred, but lower the damage award.

When the appellate court needs more information, as when the judge in the lower court may have not allowed certain testimony to come into evidence, it can remand the case back to the lower court with an order to admit that evidence. Only the trial court can take evidence, so after the evidence is taken, the case may either be reconsidered by the lower court or returned to the appellate court for decision. This can be a difficult procedural process, if the court had been decided by a jury. It may actually be necessary to recall the jury or retry the matter.

Another form of error is an error in procedure. This is called a "denial of due process." When an appellate court reviews the decision of the court which is related to the resolution of a dispute between two private parties, the review is called appellate review. When the appellate court reviews a judgment in its capacity to interpret a law or regulation for constitutional sufficiency, the appropriate term is "judicial review."

Federal System

The federal courts are a three-tiered system consisting of trial courts, appellate courts, and the Supreme Court. The trial courts are divided into two types of courts. The constitutional courts are the courts created by Article III, Section 1 of the U.S. Constitution. These are the various District Courts, the Circuit Courts of Appeal, and the Supreme Court. Legislative courts are created by Congress by virtue of the power of the government to regulate and monitor. Such courts as the Bankruptcy Court, the Court of Military Appeals, and the Court of Federal Claims are examples of legislative courts. These are not courts of general jurisdiction, rather they have limited jurisdiction. Appeal from most special courts is through the Court of Appeals and the United States Supreme Court.

The court system is divided into 94 districts by state or region and further identified by the geographic region within the district. For example, California is divided into the Northern District, the Central District, the Southern District, the Western District, and the Eastern District. In the federal system the District Courts are the trial courts. It is here that evidence is taken and testimony heard. District courts are courts of general jurisdiction. It is not uncommon for a district court to hear criminal matters as well as civil matters.

An appeal of a judgment or verdict from the district court within the circuit is to the appropriate Circuit Court of Appeals. There was a time when judges actually traveled from town to town hearing cases. They were said to be riding a circuit. It is from this that the name Circuit Court of Appeals comes. In some circuits, the Fifth, for example, the judges travel to more than one city within the circuit so that not all hearings must take place in one particular city. There are 11 numbered circuits, the District of Columbia Circuit, and the Federal Circuit.

The Court of Appeals for the Federal Circuit hears those appeals from the specialized courts like the Court of International Trade. The jurisdiction of this circuit is nationwide, as some district courts may sit as a specialized court for purposes of convenience. For example, a case that has many witnesses that is far from Washington, D.C., may be heard by the district court sitting as a specialized court. Any appeal from the judgment would be to the Court of Appeals for the Federal Circuit, not the geographical circuit court. But it is easier for the parties not to have to transport all witnesses to Washington, D.C.

After review by the Court of Appeals the losing party may wish to bring yet another appeal. The court of last resort in the United States is the Supreme Court. There are two ways to bring a matter before the Supreme Court. One is by direct appeal and the other is by writs of certiorari. Although there are a few instances of a right of appeal to the Supreme Court, most review is a discretionary decision by the high court to hear a case. The appealing party petitions the Supreme Court to issue a writ of certiorari. A "writ of cert," as they are known, is an order from the Supreme Court to the lower circuit court to send the record of the case to the higher court. The Supreme Court can either grant the petition for cert, which is consenting to review the lower court judgment, or deny the petition for cert, which is refusing the review.

The Circuit Courts of Appeal generally sit in panels of three judges. A majority of judges is sufficient for a decision. But sometimes the court will sit *en banc*. This means that the entire court will hear a matter. Again a majority of judges is sufficient for a decision. But this action ensures that the entire circuit will consistently decide similar cases. Thus a resolution by the appellate court would not be based on the random selection of judges on a panel.

States

Most states today have a three-tiered system that parallels the federal system; however, there are exceptions with some states having only two tiers. At common law, there were equity courts and law courts. Law courts were required to follow precedent. Courts of equity were more flexible, and acted as a sort of appeal, when the application of the law was harsh or unfair.

States have different names for the various levels of courts such as superior court or appeals court. For example, the trial court in New York is called the

> **From the U.S. Constitution, Article III—Judicial Branch**
>
> Section 1—Judicial Powers
> The judicial Power of the United States, shall be vested in one supreme Court, and in such inferior Courts as the Congress may from time to time ordain and establish. The Judges, both of the supreme and inferior Courts, shall hold their Offices during good Behavior, and shall, at stated Times, receive for their Services a Compensation which shall not be diminished during their Continuance in Office.

Supreme Court. It is important when reading cases from the various states that you ascertain the names of the various levels of courts in that state so that one knows where in the hierarchy the decision was made.

On rare occasions involving issues that derive from the constitutionality of law or state conduct, decisions from state courts can be appealed to the Supreme Court.

See also: Appendix 1: *United States v. Fior D'Italia, Inc.*; Appendix 2: *Commack Self-Service Kosher Meats, Inc. v. Weiss*; Appendix 3A: *Pelman, et al. v. McDonald's Corporation*; Appendix 3B: *Pelman, et al. v. McDonald's Corporation*, Amended Complaint; Appendix 3C: *Pelman, et al. v. McDonald's Corporation*; Appendix 4: *Arnett, et al. v. Snyder*; Appendix 5: *North American Cold Storage Co. v. City of Chicago*; Appendix 6: *United States v. Park*.

Elizabeth M. Williams

CPR FOOD INDUSTRY DISPUTE RESOLUTION COMMITMENT

The CPR Food Industry Resolution Commitment is a voluntary agreement, among organizations that have signed the commitment, to try alternative dispute resolutions such as mediation or arbitration before resorting to litigation. CPR is an acronym that refers to the International Institute for Conflict Prevention and Resolution. The purpose of the CPR Food Industry Dispute Resolution Commitment and other commitments formed under CPR is to mitigate the costs, time, and burdens of litigation, most of which are unpredictable.

In 2010, Best Foods, Borden Chemical, Inc., ConAgra Foods, Inc., Eric A. Taussig, General Mills, Inc., Gerber Products Company, Hershey Foods Corp., International Multi Foods Corp., Kellog Company, Kettle Foods, Inc., Nestlé, PepsiCo, Inc., Pillsbury, Ralston Purina Company, Reckitt and Coleman Inc., and Universal Foods Corp. were members of the CPR Food Industry Dispute Resolution Commitment.

The commitment states that claims of false advertising, disputes regarding company-owned trademark, trade names, and service marks, trade dress disputes, disputes claiming unfair trade practices, patent disputes, trade secret disputes, disputes involving the hiring of those employed by the competitor, and contract disputes will all proceed according to the CPR Food Industry Resolution Commitment when disputes arise between organizations that have signed the agreement. Procedures include negotiation, mediation, submission of claims of false advertising to the National Advertising Division of the Better Business Bureau (when they fall in the jurisdiction of that division), and adjudication.

The CPR has resolution agreements for other food entities as well. The CPR Franchise Mediation Program was established in 1993. It represents a commitment to follow CPR procedures in the case of franchise disputes. While this agreement involves many food franchise companies, it is not limited to food organizations. It encompasses franchise organizations, including these signatories in 2010: Church's, Popeyes, Arby's, Baskin Robbins, Burger King, The Coffee Beanery, Subway Sandwich Shops, Dunkin Donuts, East Side Mario's Restaurants, Jack in the Box, KFC, Hardee's Food System, Little Caesar Enterprises, McDonald's, Pizza Hut, Shoney's, Taco Bell, and Wendy's.

Alternative dispute resolution is often favored by corporations and by the courts. It reduces the burden on the court system and reduces the amount of publicity a corporation may receive in litigation.

Stephanie Jane Carter

CREDIT CARDS AND THE RESTAURANT INDUSTRY

As credit cards have proliferated throughout the restaurant industry, they have wrought a gradual change in the reporting and recently in the taxation of the business. Today, even fast food restaurants accept payment by credit card. What was once a cash business that depended on the memory of the wait staff, cryptic handwritten notes, and a cash box has been transformed into a business where almost all transactions can be traced. The use of cash has been greatly reduced. Orders are entered into a computer and paid for through a computer.

Restaurants

Today the restaurant is required to report tips paid to its wait staff. The Internal Revenue Service (IRS) has taken the position, supported by the Supreme Court, that the percentage of tips reflected on the credit card slips of a restaurant represents the percentage to be applied to all tips, even cash tips, received by the wait staff. The restaurant, which must pay its contribution to taxes on the wait staff tips, must calculate them then and cannot use under-reported taxes as stated by the wait staff as the basis for their calculations. When the case was first decided, there was concern that many waiters who had relied on under-reporting to increase their income would leave the profession.

In addition, the restaurant has the fiduciary responsibility to protect the patrons from credit card theft by restaurant employees. When cash was the primary method of payment, a different sort of diligence was required. Swipe devices called skimmers that capture and store information from credit cards before the card is swiped for payment have been used in restaurants, when the wait staff takes the credit card out of view of the patron. New wireless readers that can be brought to the table are a way to reassure patrons that such theft cannot take place. Restaurants are the primary business where a credit card is taken away from the patron to complete the transaction. Most new devices mask the credit card number on the receipt to protect patrons from theft.

Another form of misunderstanding if not actual fraud is the inclusion of the tip or gratuity in the credit card total given to the patron, but where there is still a blank line that looks like a tip line on the check. Unknowing patrons may add a tip without realizing that they had already been charged. This also takes the decision of how much to tip away from the patron. A dishonest server could also increase the tip amount written in by the patron and enter the new amount into the system after it is signed by the patron. If the tip amount is increased, it merely appears that the patron has made an addition error on the signed credit card slip.

Some states, Massachusetts for example, have considered legislation that would require retailers and restaurants to take responsibility for theft of credit card information from their machines.

There are now some restaurants that are working with credit card companies to provide special offers to consumers who use particular cards, earning rewards or special incentives for use.

An area of conflict regarding credit cards and the payment of tips is the cost of commission and transaction fees that may be withheld from tips when paid to the wait staff. The restaurant must clearly deal with this when setting its policies for paying tips to the wait staff. The Internal Revenue Service has not based its computations on the discounted amount of tips. But the restaurant could be absorbing the cost of the commission if they paid the face amount to the wait staff. The chain, Bonefish Grill, for example, has made it a company policy not to withhold the commissions from the tips paid to its wait staff. This is a company-by-company policy.

Patrons

As more people use credit cards to pay at restaurants, either because they want the record of their expenditures or because of the convenience of not needing cash, the decision of a restaurant not to accept credit cards is becoming a serious business decision. Small, inexpensive restaurants might not be able to survive if they had to pay the commission and transaction fees to credit card companies, because the restaurant margin is too small. Other restaurants may have to be very good or have very loyal customers to not accept payment by credit card.

One consumer complaint is the restaurant that does not clearly inform patrons before they begin to order that it does not accept credit cards. The embarrassment of not having cash is a strong motivator not to return, especially if there is no convenient ATM nearby. Especially at high-end restaurants, the need to carry several hundred dollars in cash makes not accepting a credit cards extremely non-customer–friendly. Many restaurant blogs include comments about this problem in their reviews.

Restaurants have advocated for the passage of the Credit Card Fair Fee Act, which would permit restaurants to band together to negotiate a favorable credit card fee. This would require amendments to the **antitrust laws**. The National Restaurant Association has supported this bill.

Those restaurants that provide special incentives in cooperation with credit card companies may find that they engender both loyalty in customers and also attract new customers who wish to try a new place without great risk. These incentives could mean special two-for-one offers or a free course, such as dessert, with a special card.

Most credit card companies do not allow a retailer to offer a discount for paying cash. The practice also makes customers believe that they are not paying the appropriate price for their meal, especially when the discount is greater than the commission and transaction fees would be. The practice may be counterproductive for the restaurant, which could lose a favorable credit card relationship and could confuse or irritate a patron.

See also: Fior D'Italia v United States; Appendix 1: United States v. Fior D'Italia, Inc.

Elizabeth M. Williams

CULINARY SCHOOLS, REGULATION OF

The number of culinary schools in the United States and the number of chefs who have attended culinary school has grown significantly since the late 1990s. Although culinary school is not a necessary step to becoming a chef, the competition for higher paying positions has made it an attractive option. The U.S. Bureau of Labor Statistics reported that chefs and head cooks made up only 12 percent of the 941,600 jobs held by chefs, head cooks, food preparation and serving supervisors in 2008. The Bureau of Labor Statistics also reported that the highest earnings for these jobs are in upscale restaurants and hotels. Many of these positions are more easily obtainable with a culinary school degree. Accredited schools ensure the employer, the student, and the public that a school adheres to a set of standards.

There are several types of culinary schools, including two- and four-year colleges, community colleges, private institutions, and technical schools. The American Culinary Federation Foundation Accrediting Commission (ACFFAC) is the largest accrediting agency for culinary schools and culinary education programs. In 2010, the ACFFAC accredited more than 200 formal training programs and also sponsors apprenticeship programs. The ACFFAC is recognized by the Council for Higher Education. The ACFFAC also operates as a third-party endorser for federal funding. Other accrediting bodies include the Western Association of Schools and Colleges, the Middle State Association of Schools and Colleges, the Southern Association of Colleges and Schools, the Northwest Association of Schools and Colleges, the North Central Association of Colleges and Schools, and the New England Association of Schools and Colleges.

Some large hotels and restaurants offer apprenticeship and other training programs as an addition or an alternative to culinary school. The Office of Apprenticeships under the U.S. Department of Labor's Employment and Training Administration keeps a list of registered apprenticeships. Several regulations apply to registered culinary apprenticeships. For example, Equal Employment Opportunity in Apprenticeship (Title 29, C.F.R., Part 30) is a network of policies that promotes equal opportunities in registered apprenticeship programs. Registration incentives include tax benefits for employers and workforce development grants in some states. The Department of Labor also provides printed rules that update the National Apprenticeship System. These regulations were updated in 2008 (Title 29 C.F.R., part 29).

The median wage-and-salary earnings for chefs and head cooks in 2008 was $38,770, according to the U.S. Department of Labor Statistics. The middle 50 percent of those earned between $29,050 and 51,540, with the bottom 10 percent earning less than $29,050 and the top 10 percent earning more than $66,680. Many culinary school graduates will not be in the top 10 percent of that group. Some argue that the cult of the celebrity chef has glamorized the culinary profession in the eyes of young people, creating beliefs that the field is lucrative and that chefs generally become celebrities. On May 7, 2007, *The New York Times* reported that two-year culinary programs, including tuition and supplies, can reach $48,000, with the maximum of $14,125 covered by federal low-interest loans. For students who only want to cook, the amount they pay for culinary school can be financially crippling to pay back on meager salaries. Several lobbying groups, such as Student Loan Justice, have tried to change regulations applying to culinary school student loans. Many professional chefs who work with young people advise them that culinary school is expensive, that the profession in not as glamorous as it appears on television, and that for people who just want to cook, less expensive culinary programs or apprenticeship programs may be the more financially prudent choice.

Regulation of a restaurant associated with a culinary school where students prepare food for sale to customers is governed by the same rules that are applicable to commercial restaurants in that locale. This means that food handling and storage rules, **Americans with Disabilities Act** requirements, and **Hazard Analysis Critical Control Point** rules are applicable. The school is a place for students to learn what these regulations are.

See also: Americans with Disabilities Act and Restaurants.

Stephanie Jane Carter

D

DEPARTMENT OF HEALTH AND HUMAN SERVICES

A relatively new cabinet department founded in 1979, the Department of Health and Human Services (HHS) was created by splitting what was formerly the Department of Health, Education, and Welfare (created in 1953 during the term of President Dwight D. Eisenhower) into Health and Human Services and the Department of Education. The portfolio of HHS contains the public health of the United States and maintaining the welfare of the citizenry. Although the Social Security Administration was originally a part of HHS, that function was transformed into an independent agency in 1995. Today, HHS has the administration of the U.S. Public Health Service and the Family Support Administration.

The HHS is responsible for many health-related programs. It also is responsible, along with the **Food and Drug Administration** and the **U.S. Department of Agriculture** (USDA), for food safety. The Food Safety Working Group, which advises the president and the **executive branch** on matters of food safety, is made up the representatives from the USDA and the HHS. This group has recommended, for example, that the Office of Homeland Security (HS), which has jurisdiction over imports into the United States, put into place food security and safety measures that will ensure the importation of healthy and safe food. This resulted in the creation of the Commercial Targeting and Analysis Center for Import Safety by HS. Although it is administered by HS, the Center is run in cooperation with the USDA's Food Safety and Inspection Service, the **Environmental Protection Agency**, the **Food and Drug Administration**, and others agencies, whose experts are available when needed.

The HHS is responsible for all aspects of public health, which includes diseases. But it also includes illness caused by food-borne pathogens, lifestyle diseases like obesity, mental and emotional conditions that are related to food such as anorexia nervosa and bulimia nervosa, as well as such public health problems as Type II diabetes, gout, and alcoholism.

A part of HHS is the U.S. Public Health Service Commissioned Corps. This is the uniformed branch of the Public Health Service headed by the Surgeon General. The Corps is made up of only commissioned officers who are generally considered noncombatants. They can be assigned to the armed forces, however, by the president. The Corps members wear a uniform that is like the Navy uniform with the special Public Health Service insignia. The Corps began its existence as first the Marine Hospital Fund and then the Marine Hospital Service in 1871. Corps members originally help with the health of merchant marines, but came to enforce other public health-related matters such as quarantines.

Since 2000, the Surgeons General have addressed the public health issue of obesity. In 2001 the Surgeon General issued a Call to Action, calling attention to the public health problem that obesity represented and asking for the government to act toward preventing the condition. The call to action listed a number of recommendations for lifestyle changes and activities that could be adopted by schools. Having the Surgeon General identify a public health problem gives that problem a high priority in the eyes of the public, as well as the public health community.

In 2010 the Secretary of HHS, the Surgeon General, and First Lady Michelle Obama announced an initiative to combat obesity in both adults and children. There is a role for HHS and the Surgeon General in advising other agencies of government as to how those agencies can support the initiative, as well as producing guidelines and recommendations for schools, parents, and all citizens; collecting statistical information regarding obesity and its complications; and disseminating that information to citizens.

The **Centers for Disease Control and Prevention** (CDC) is another agency that operates under the aegis of HHS. Despite the public position of HHS and the Surgeon General, the CDC has stated that while obesity continues to be high and a public health problem, it appears to have leveled off in 2003 to 2004. The CDC has yet not determined the reason that the incidences of obesity did not continue to grow. The CDC has also conducted studies of the health costs attributed to obesity. They estimated that in 1998, when the study was conducted, that $78.5 billion of health costs could be attributed to obesity-related illnesses. About half of those costs were borne by the Medicare and Medicaid systems.

The CDC has published a number of studies that indicate that obesity is a larger problem for those in poverty or those at risk for poverty. This circumstance was recognized by Michelle Obama in her initiative against obesity. This is important not only as a public health issue, but also a social welfare issue. Social welfare issues are also administered by HHS.

The Centers for Medicare & Medicaid Services (CMS) are administered under HHS. The Social Security Administration, however, determines eligibility for Medicare and produces the checks for payment of Medicare-covered expenses. Similarly the CMS administers the Medicaid program. Unlike Medicare, which operates as a federal system, each state administers its own Medicaid program. These programs are not all identical and can reflect the cultural and political differences of each state. It is the responsibility of CMS to ensure that the states comply with federal Medicaid regulations and requirements. Both of these programs are enabled by the Social Security Act of 1965. The HHS through its Office of the Inspector General (OIG) investigates Medicare fraud. It has a large enforcement branch that investigates criminal activity. Besides regular training as criminal investigators and officers, the OIG officers receive training in forensic accounting and other special training to uncover fraud and abuse in both the Medicare and Medicaid systems. The OIG operates in cooperation with state law enforcement in investigating Medicaid fraud and abuse. HHS through the OIG also is tasked under the Child Support Recovery Act with investigating the intentional avoidance of paying child support in all states and the District of Columbia.

See also: Obesity Lawsuits.

Further Reading Department of Health and Human Services. http://www.hhs.gov.

Elizabeth M. Williams

DIET FOODS

Diet foods are foods that have been modified to fit a body modification diet. Body modification could include building muscle or gaining weight. Most diet products are targeted to accommodate the national preoccupation with losing weight. They include prepackaged foods such as Lean Cuisine. They also include foods with "diet" labels like "low-fat," "lite," "sugar-free," "fat-free," and "reduced calorie." "Low-fat" is legally defined as less than three grams of fat per serving. "Fat-free" is defined by the government as less than half a gram of fat per serving. They also include foods that contain imitation fats and sugar substitutes. There are also diet foods sold under diet programs, such as Jenny Craig, Slim-Fast, and Nutri-System. The diet food industry has been increasing over the last few years because Americans are obese and overweight, while living in a society that favors thinness. Adults with a body mass index (BMI) between 25 and 29.9 are considered overweight, while adults with a body mass index of 30 or over are considered obese. A national survey headed by Youfa Wang, an associate professor at Bloomberg School's Center for Human Nutrition, predicts that 86 percent of American adults will be overweight or obese by 2030. Ninety-six percent of non-Hispanic black women are predicted to be overweight or obese and 91 percent of Mexican American men will be overweight or obese. The study also projects that health care spending related to these weight issues will be as much as $956.9 billion.

There are several reasons the diet food industry is such a lucrative industry. A society in which the majority of the citizens are overweight favors thinness. Models and actors represent the extreme of this aesthetic. Rather than simply being slim and healthy, the actors and models are typically emaciated. This is, as stated, in stark contrast to the rest of the population. This fact, along with the health issues, has caused the diet food industry to grow. According to the U.S. **Food and Drug Administration**, Americans spend more than $40 billion yearly on weight-loss reduction products, such as diet foods and drinks. The health issues associated with being overweight or obese and the actual cost of these medical procedures adds to the national preoccupation with losing weight. The call to decrease waistlines comes from popular culture with its preference for an aesthetic of thinness, from medical professionals concerned with health, and from officials who are concerned with the cost of this health care. Weight concerns boost the sale of diet foods and drinks.

Nutritionist and author **Marion Nestle** believes that the food industry promotes an "eat more" culture. Indeed, with so many foods on the market and only a limited number of people to purchase them, it would be beneficial to the food industry if everyone could eat a little more. Whether or not the food industry promotes this in an intentional or irresponsible way, the fact is that people are eating more. As incomes rose over the last few decades, people began performing less manual labor. People could afford things like cars and the gas to fuel them. Computers made life even easier. People began leading more sedentary lives. Sedentary lives often lead to snacking, which leads to weight gain. Time constraints have also aided the diet food industry in diet food sales. Instead of cooking something healthy from scratch, it is much easier and at times faster to put an item labeled "diet" into the microwave. Moreover, studies show that consumers are confused about diet and health. Ultimately, consumers feel less conflicted when buying a product that is labeled with low-fat, diet, low-calorie, or other diet term. Confused about diet and short on time, consumers can simply buy a ready-made product that boasts the thing that consumers want, using labels that consumers perceive as healthy. Whether these products are actually healthy is a source of contention.

There are several issues with diet foods. Firstly, most nutritionists believe that many diet foods can actually cause overeating. A reason for this is that consumers think they can eat more of something because it is labelled diet OR has a "diet" label. In the end, they often consume more than they would have if they had eaten the full-calorie, full-fat version. Some people refer to this as the "Snackwell's Syndrome." Snackwell's is a brand of snack food that gained popularity in the 1990s. Marketed as diet foods, they are usually a fat-free version of something that was normally high in fat. However, the products still had a large number of calories. "Snackwell's Syndrome" became uniquely associated with the act of over-consumption of a product that boasts of lower amounts of a product the consumer is trying to avoid. The term has actually moved from the food industry into the energy industry. With so many energy-saving products on the market, experts warn consumers about over-consuming energy and driving utility bills up as a result of using more of these "low-energy" items. Basically, low-fat does not mean low-calorie. Studies have shown that consumers are less likely to read nutritional information because of the large number of health claim labels in the marketplace. They understand diet food labels such as "fat-free" to mean healthy, and that it is okay to eat more of them. In fact, the health or diet claim on the package makes consumers feel less guilty. A 2006 study by Cornell University showed that people, especially overweight people, were eating more of the low-fat snacks than if they were just eating regular snacks, resulting in more calorie intake.

Some nutritionists believe that diet foods may help people develop tastes for junk foods. Instead of substituting unprocessed vegetables, seafood, or meat for the food deemed unhealthy, people simply substitute the "healthy" version of the unhealthy food. For example, potato chips are considered junk food. The companies that make potato chips now market baked chips that are low-fat. Regardless of their fat content, they are still low-nutrient. Potato chip companies also began to market fried, fat-free versions of their chips. They are fat-free because they are fried in Olestra, a non-absorbable, energy-free fat substitute. Consumers who would never have eaten potato chips started eating the baked and fat-free version. Consumers compensated for the fat deficit in the chips by eating more. Instead of eating a healthy diet, these foods allow consumers to eat more top-of-the-pyramid foods. By doing that, nutritionists believe the consumer develops a taste for junk food.

Diet foods often cost more. An unaltered piece of food, such as celery or an apple, is inexpensive and healthy. Diet foods are typically value-added products that cost more because of the "added value." Recently, food companies have started to market the "100-calorie pack." They have split their products into smaller portions and packaged them. However, these cost more than the versions that have not been split up into the packs. Consumers would save money by splitting their food into portions themselves.

At times, food companies have used synthetic compounds to replicate, substitute, or replace naturally occurring ingredients that have been deemed unhealthy. Because of this, diet foods may contain more artificial flavors and preservatives to make up for the things that they lack. Potato chips fried in Olestra were foods with a large amount of an artificial additive. The FDA originally required Olestra products to carry a label warning consumers that the product could cause loose stools and prevent the absorption of some vitamins. It is questionable whether such diet foods are worth the harm they cause. There is a group of people known as "junk-food dieters" who eat the diet forms of processed foods to lose weight instead of cutting portion sizes or eating a healthy food. Nutritionists think that "lite" foods send the message that it is acceptable to continue to eat junk food instead of switching to healthful food. Even if the products are low-fat or low-calorie does not mean that they have the nutrients necessary to maintain a healthy diet.

Many critics say that instead of eating junk foods, consumers should simply eat "real food." Author **Michael Pollan** has recommended that if one's grandmother would not recognize it as food, then it should not be eaten. He goes further to recommend that consumers eat real food with a diet of many vegetables and keep **portion sizes** small.

Diet foods may do more harm than good. However, they do show that people want to improve their diets. Although consumers perceive diet foods as healthier, it is worth reading the nutrition information on the back of the package. It is noteworthy that, despite the increase in spending on diet foods, the weight of most Americans has been increasing as well.

See also: Additives and Preservatives; Dietary Supplements; Labeling Definitions; Lite Labeling; Trans-Fats.

Further Reading Finkelstein, Eric A., and Zuckerman, Laurie. *The Fattening of America.* New York: John Wiley & Sons, 2008; Goldstein, Mark A., and Myrna Chandler Goldstein. *Controversies in Food and Nutrition.* Westport, CT: Greenwood Press, 2002; Nestle, Marion. *Food Politics: How the Food Industry Influences Nutrition and Health* Berkeley: University of California Press, 2007; Wansink, Brian. *Mindless Eating: Why We Eat More Than We Think.* New York: Bantam, 2006.

Stephanie Jane Carter

DIET FOODS, SPECIAL

There is no U.S. regulatory definition of **diet foods,** per se, but there are certainly foods that are considered diet foods of all types. These are foods that are either naturally low in calories, such as vegetables, or that are modified in some way to reduce calories, such as sugar-free sodas. But also included in the diet food category are foods modified by the reduction or removal of another component, such as fat. An example is fat-free mayonnaise. The legal rules and regulations that apply to all foods still apply to "diet" foods.

Diet food may also include food intended to be eaten by people who are on special diets for reasons of health, for example, diabetes, high cholesterol, or renal disease. As different diet fads, such as a high-carbohydrate diet and a raw food diet, arise, diet food reflects the fashion of the moment through a change in **labeling**. Today, beers are labeled with carbohydrate counts as well as calories, so that this beverage addresses fat and weight loss concerns. The law, through its regulations, changes to support the changes in societal attitudes and needs, as well as to protect the consumers as they follow these new fashions.

Words generally associated with diet foods include light or **lite** or low, as in low salt, and various "free" foods, as in sugar-free and fat-free. Other terms associated with diet foods include low-fat and high-fiber. To be able to use these terms on a label or make health claims about the foods, a food producer must comply with the regulations promulgated by the **Food and Drug Administration** and the **U.S. Department of Agriculture**. These regulations also cover the comparisons with non-diet or unaltered foods that may be claimed by the producers.

Diet foods can also mean foods that people avoid because of an allergy or intolerance. For example, people who are lactose intolerant may drink soy milk as a substitute for cow's milk. Those with allergies, such as an allergy to peanuts, will seek out food that does not contain peanuts. Those with renal disease will avoid proteins. Those with celiac disease avoid food products with gluten. Once again, the label is key to informing the consumer of the contents of the product.

The term "diet food" can now also be claimed by restaurants. With increased regulation requiring **labeling** for food in restaurants, the nutritional components including calories, fats, and carbohydrates are used by restaurants to promote weight loss. It is a classic example of using what could be a burden and turning it into an advantage. That is what the Subway chain has done with its claims that eating its sandwiches results in weight loss, as represented by its spokesman, Jared Fogel. Subway markets some of its sandwiches by advertising and posting their fat content. Subway also recommends exercise. It is an example of embracing the labeling, which other fast food restaurants are reluctant to do.

Other special diet foods could be considered: kosher foods, foods for vegans, and food eaten on diets to promote longevity. As well, special diet foods are created to be eaten on a special plan for weight loss and calorie restriction, such as Weight Watchers, South Beach, or Jenny Craig. These brand-name special diets must conform to the labeling laws in their diet claims and nutritional labeling.

See also: Labeling Definitions; Labeling, Nutrition; Lite Labeling; "Natural" Labeling.

Further Reading Title 21 *Code of Federal Regulations* Part 105; Willett, Walter C., and P. J. Skerrett. *Eat, Drink, and Be Healthy: The Harvard Medical School Guide to Healthy Eating.* New York: Free Press, 2005.

Elizabeth M. Williams

DIET ORGANIZATIONS, REGULATION OF

The weight loss industry is actively mining the fears of obesity and the desire for weight loss that so many people have. Diet organizations such as Weight Watchers, Overeaters Anonymous, Jenny Craig, Atkins, and Nutrisystem offer counseling and some also offer products such as food. These organizations are businesses that collect monthly fees or other payments for their services. The breadth of diet programs is large and varied. Some gyms offer weight loss programs in conjunction with gym memberships.

Congress has not established specific regulations regarding these weight loss organizations. They may contain components that are regulated by already existing regulations, however. For example, if the organization and its system include food, the food component is regulated by all of the applicable food regulations of the **Food and Drug Administration** (FDA), the **U.S. Department of Agriculture** (USDA), the **Federal Trade Commission** (FTC), and anything else that might be applicable. However, there is no set of regulations that monitors and controls all the components of the organization.

There are legal difficulties associated with some regulation of these organizations. The freedom of people to associate with other like-minded people is protected by the First Amendment of the United States Constitution. Merely providing a place where people wish to congregate to engage in legal behavior is not regulated. As well, proposing methodologies for losing weight, giving people encouragement for this activity, and discussing plans of action are all protected speech, also under the First Amendment.

Jody Gorran, a Florida businessman, filed suit against Atkins Nutritionals, Inc., in 2004 (*Gorran v. Atkins Nutritionals, Inc.*, No. 2004-CC-006591-MB [Fla. Palm Beach County Ct. May 26, 2004]), claiming that after following the Atkins plan he developed high cholesterol and other physical ailments that were alleged to be related to following the diet. The plaintiff learned that the American Heart Association and the American Dietetic Association considered the diet dangerous, although the Web site of Atkins Nutritionals asserted the efficacy of the diet. The complaint claimed that Gorran had relied to his detriment on the negligent misrepresentation of the healthiness of the diet and claimed damages under the Deceptive and Unfair Trade Practices Act in the state of Florida. After the filing of Gorran's suit, Atkins Nutritionals filed for protection of the bankruptcy court, which stalled further proceedings. When the company came out of bankruptcy, the matter was removed to the District Court for the Southern District of New York.

The question before the court was whether the Web site and book were simply speech protected by the First Amendment, discussing diets and weight loss. If the Web site and book were found to be commercial speech, there would be limits on their freedoms, and the accuracy of the speech and reliance on it would be actionable. The plaintiff argued that as the Web site existed only to sell products of Atkins Nutritionals, it did not exist as a forum for discussion and comment, and it was clearly marketing to sell a product, that is, commercial speech. However, the court dismissed the case, ruling that the book and Web site were guides to eating a low carbohydrate diet, thus protecting the defendant from **liability**.

Since 1990, the FTC has pursued enforcement actions for more than 100 weight loss claims that were false or deceptive weight. Most claims are defended as being mere puffery, but the courts have defined puffery as being the sort of claim that cannot be objectively measured and that when made most people would not rely on it. The FDA, which regulates food labeling, could also assert itself, if the claims made by the product are found on the label.

As there is no specific regulation of diet organizations, the mission, so to speak, has fallen on the FTC on the basis of advertising claims. There are no standards and few actual studies, other than those conducted by the diet companies, comparing the different methodologies of the different diet organizations. The FTC monitors advertising claims based on the truthfulness of the claim or whether it is misleading and whether there is objective substantiation of the claim. The review of truthfulness is a review of the claims in advertising. Advertising can be found in many media, and the FTC monitors it all.

Weight loss products that are marketed with a claim of efficacy, but that contain a disclaimer in fine print that they work as a part of an overall diet and exercise program, are the types of advertisements targeted as misleading by the FTC. The thrust of the advertisement—use this product to lose weight—is misleading, because the real cause of the weight loss is the overall diet and exercise program. Moreover, without a showing that the product itself contributes to weight loss, the FTC may find the advertisement deceptive.

If the advertiser has sufficient objective evidence that shows that it can support its claim, then it is safe from the FTC, which requires scientific tests, research, or studies as the basis of the claim. The tests cannot be done by the company, but by professionals in the field. The anecdotal stories of individuals are insufficient evidence of the claims of weight loss due to the use of the product. Clinical human trials conducted in accordance with accepted scientific protocols are required as support for claims.

Since 1997, the FTC has been monitoring weight loss claims under its own program known as "Operation Waistline." This program is a concerted effort by the FTC to expose deceptive claims and to discourage them by the imposition of fines, making examples of diet claims that are the most egregious. The FTC has stated that as many as half of the claims of the diet products and organizations are misleading, if not deceptive. Because the FTC has no standards in place that describe minimum requirements of diet organizations, there is only the case by case review of claims, which is an increasing burden on the FTC as the weight loss industry grows.

See also: Advertising of Food; Court System, Torts.

Further Reading Cleland, Richard L., et al. *Federal Trade Commission Weight-Loss U.S. Advertising: An Analysis of Current Trends.* Washington, DC, Department of Health and Human Services, Federal Trade Commission Staff Report, September 2002.

Elizabeth M. Williams

DIETARY SUPPLEMENTS

According to the Dietary Supplement and Health Education Act (DSHEA) of 1994, a dietary supplement is something ingested that contains a "dietary ingredient." A "dietary ingredient" may be a single ingredient or a combination of ingredients such as vitamins and minerals. These ingredients may be any dietary substance, like an amino acid or an herb, to supplement the diet. The U.S. **Food and Drug Administration** (FDA) is the agency that regulates dietary supplements. But dietary supplements are monitored and controlled under their own set of regulations. They are neither food nor drugs. They are monitored separately from prescription drugs and over-the-counter drugs.

The FDA regulates three types of claims that may be found on labels of dietary supplements. These are the same three groups that apply to conventional foods. First, health claims, defined by a specific substance and a disease or a condition that is related to health, may be used on labels of dietary supplements. A health claim has been made when a specific substance is named in reference to the disease or health-related condition. Claims made about the level of nutrients are a second category of claims. The final category is structure/function claims. According to the FDA, these claims "address a role of a specific substance in maintaining normal healthy structures or functions of the body." Health claims are subject to FDA review and authorization while structure/function claims are not. FDA regulations allow two types of health claims to be asserted on the dietary supplement labels. The first is a Nutrition Labeling and Education Act (NLEA) Authorized Health Claim. This type of health claim establishes a connection between the dietary supplement and a possibility of contracting a disease. Health claims are regulated by the NLEA of 1990, the Dietary Supplement Act of 1992, and the DSHEA. The second type of health claim for dietary supplements is a Qualified Health Claim. For this type, there is not enough scientific evidence for the FDA to issue regulations. So, phrases that temper the claim are added to indicate that the scientific evidence supporting the claim is limited. The FDA's "Consumer Health Information for Better Nutrition Initiative" creates a mechanism to make these limited claims.

The second category of claims on dietary supplement labels is a Nutrient Content Claim. This type of claim provides for a description of percentage level of a dietary ingredient even when no Daily Value has been established. The third category of claims is a Structure/Function Claim. Since the FDA does not pre-approve these claims, it is required that the claim must actually state that the FDA has not evaluated the claim. Dietary supplements are different from drugs, so they must include a statement that the supplement is not designed to "diagnose, treat, cure, or prevent any disease." The DSHEA has established some regulations for making such claims. If the supplement label did make this claim, it would immediately change the classification to a drug and would then have completely different regulations.

There were several landmark decisions, acts, and amendments that led to the current nutritional supplement industry. Over the last few decades, the regulations that governed the supplement industry have become unraveled because of a successful lobbying campaign by the supplement industry. In the 1970s, the FDA classified vitamins A and D as drugs because they cause toxicity symptoms at high levels. The supplement industry sued and the FDA was prohibited from classifying high-potency supplements as drugs for "irrelevant" reasons such as lack of nutritional need or toxicity. In 1976, Congress introduced the Proxmire Amendment, an amendment to the Food, Drug, and Cosmetic Act. The Proxmire Amendment said that the FDA may not set maximums on the amounts of vitamins or minerals allowed in a supplement, classify the supplement as a drug if its dose exceeds what the FDA considers nutritionally rational, or restrict the combinations of vitamins and minerals in a supplement. This was a major step forward for the dietary supplement industry. If supplements had been classified as drugs, they would be subject to much more regulation. Later that year, the FDA proposed that supplements be treated as over-the-counter drugs and carry a label that said that they should only be used when their need has been determined by a physician. The FDA withdrew this proposal but maintained that if dietary supplements claimed that they treated, cured, mitigated, or prevented any diseases, then they were marketing themselves as drugs, and they would be treated as drugs by the FDA.

The next set of landmarks in dietary supplement regulation came in the 1990s. The NLEA forced the FDA to start authorizing health claims for foods as well as dietary supplements. Before this, health claims were forbidden. The claims had to be substantiated by significant scientific evidence. The FDA also had to develop separate authorization process for supplement health claims and had to decide whether to authorize 10 specific health claims. A major controversy in the supplement regulation debate was whether they should be subject to regulation as food or as drugs. The supplement industry preferred to be considered food so they would be subject to less regulation.

Senator Orrin Hatch (Rep-Utah) introduced the Health Freedom Act of 1992, which was to block the FDA from using health claims as an excuse to regulate dietary supplements as drugs. Hatch was reportedly concerned that the FDA could put anyone out of business through overregulation. The act did not pass, but Congress did pass the Dietary Supplement Act of 1992, which barred the FDA from applying the forthcoming food labeling rules to dietary supplements for a year, giving the dietary supplement industry time to organize an opposition. This led to a major advance for the supplement industry, the DSHEA.

The DSHEA broadened the definition of supplements to vitamins, minerals, amino acids, botanicals, metabolites, and diet products. It makes the FDA responsible for proving that a product is harmful, rather than making the manufacturer prove it is safe. Given the budget constraints in the FDA, this charge proved difficult. The DSHEA ended the FDA's authority to remove harmful products from market. It allowed for products to remain on the market even while court proceedings against the manufacturers are under way or while approvals are obtained. It also authorized the structure/function claims when a disclaimer is included that says that the statement has not been evaluated by the FDA and that the product is not intended to diagnose, treat, cure, or prevent any disease. It allowed supplements a place in the food category, but not identical to foods. Under the DSHEA, the burden of ensuring that the supplement is safe before it is marketed is on the manufacturer of the supplement. In most instances, the manu-facturers have no requirement to register their products with the FDA or get FDA approval before selling dietary supplements. There is no minimum standard set by the FDA. It is the also the manufacturers' responsibility to ensure that information on the product's label is truthful and not misleading. The FDA's role does not begin until after the product has reached the market. Only when a product is found to be unsafe does the FDA have an obligation to do something. After the product has been marketed, the FDA is responsible for monitoring safety and product information. Dietary supplement advertising falls under the jurisdiction of the **Federal Trade Commission** (FTC). The **Food and Drug Administration Modernization Act of 1997** (FDAMA) required the FDA to permit nutrient content and to monitor claims of health-giving properties of regular foods when the claims are substantiated by published, authoritative statements by the federal public health agencies or the National Academy of Sciences. These criteria apply to supplements as well. In 1998, *Pearson v Shalala* took more regulatory authority away from the FDA. Congress had given the authority to the FDA in NLEA to give prior approval to health claims of foods, but the FDA created a very difficult standard to approve such claims. After 10 years, only 10 claims had been approved. Durk Pearson and Sandy Shaw were manufacturers of supplements who wished to assert four specific health claims on the labels of their supplements that were backed by scientific information. The scientific data were also widely accepted and commonly touted in the media. The FDA denied the use of the claims, so Pearson and Shaw brought suit. The D.C. Court of Appeals ruled that the labels of dietary supplements may make medical claims on the condition that they also carry a disclaimer that the FDA has not granted approval of the claims. In 2007, the government implemented a serious adverse event reporting law and gave final rule on good manufacturing practices.

In May 2009, the FDA warned General Mills about cholesterol-reducing claims the company made for its Cheerios cereal. The press gave the warning more coverage than it may have in the past, signaling that the FDA and the public may consider a stricter treatment of this industry.

Major issues in the supplement debate include how restrictive the FDA should be in its regulations. Also, through the history of the supplement regulation battle, the FDA has lost some of its power to regulate food and drugs as well. The increased number of health claims on products undeniably help sell more of a product (Supplement sales were $4 billion in 1997. Directly after the DSHEA was enacted, they rose to $15 billion. By 2007, sales were reportedly $23.7 billion.) However, they have also left the public confused about health and the validity of the claims. Studies show that many people believe the health claims because they are in print or because they believe that the government authorized them. In fact, many of the supplements, other than vitamins and minerals, have not been tested in a controlled clinical setting and many health professionals are unclear on the effects of them. The relaxed rules on health claims for dietary supplements, coupled with the fact that health claims sell, mean that more conventional food and over-the-counter drug companies are adding supplements, and their health claims, to their products.

See also: Labeling, Nutrition; Neutraceuticals.

Further Reading Nestle, Marion. *Food Politics: How the Food Industry Influences Nutrition and Health* Berkeley: University of California Press, 2007.

Stephanie Jane Carter

DISTILLERIES

Home Distilling

Although federal law allows the making of wine and the making of beer at home for personal use without a license, it does not allow for any non-licensed home distilling of spirits for home consumption. This means that home distilling may not be engaged in for purposes other than home consumption. Stills may be sold and purchased, for example, for other types of distilling, such as for making distilled water or the distilling of essential oils. Even for home consumption, federal law requires distillers to obtain a license. The licensing fees and the taxes are high enough to discourage home distillers from applying. In addition there are other requirements that make home distillation impractical.

Unregulated commercial distilling and home distilling was practiced in the early United States. In 1791 the first tax on whiskey was initiated in the form of the Whiskey Act. In 1794 a protest known as the Whiskey Rebellion, an uprising in rural Pennsylvania, was suppressed by the National Guard and negotiators. The tax was enacted in an attempt by Secretary of the Treasury, Alexander Hamilton, to reduce the national debt. During Prohibition (1919 to 1933) the practice of making moonshine—unregulated and illegal spirits—flourished. Moonshine has a reputation for being full of impurities, such as methanol, and is associated even today with rebellion against federal regulation.

On the repeal of Prohibition the federal government began to license and regulate distilleries. No home consumption exception has been successfully enacted. In 2001, Congressman Bart Stupak of Michigan introduced a bill into the House of Representatives to allow home distilling, but the bill did not pass.

The policing and enforcement of the laws applicable to distilling fall under the Alcohol and Tobacco Tax and Trade Bureau (TTB; formerly the Bureau of Alcohol, Tobacco and Firearms) of the U.S. Treasury Department. This office is responsible for enforcement of all laws covering the production of liquor. Prosecution of home distillers who operate without the requisite license can result in a criminal penalty of 10 years' imprisonment. The illegal distiller's house can be civilly seized if it is the site of the distilling (see 26 U.S.C. 5601 and 5602 for penalties that can be imposed on such illegal operations).

Micro-Distilleries

Many states are reducing the licensing fees and changing the distribution requirements of micro-distilleries, making it possible for small commercial operations to sell their product directly to the public. Oregon, for example, has created a marketplace for micro-distilling by reducing annual license fees, allowing for direct sales to the public and liberalizing the laws of giving away samples. These laws often parallel the laws allowing wineries to make direct sales to the public at the winery.

In contrast, the state of Washington required all spirits to be distributed through the state liquor control board for distribution. This makes the cost of small-batch liquor cost-prohibitive. State and federal taxes can represent as much as 32 percent of the purchase price of a bottle of liquor. A new law, a "craft distillery bill" with limitations on size of production, was introduced by Senator Chris Marr of Spokane in 2010. It passed through the Washington legislature with only one dissenting vote and took effect in July 2010. The new law is applicable to distilleries that produce less than 20,000 gallons of spirits per year. Their license fee is $100 per year instead of the $2,000 per year paid by larger distilleries.

There are still differences in liberality between the Washington and Oregon type laws. Oregon allows for micro-distilleries to obtain ingredients from anywhere around the world. Washington requires that half of the ingredients must come from the state of Washington.

Micro-distillery laws have been passed in states such as Michigan, and other states are considering similar changes in the law.

Commercial Distilleries

Since Prohibition the federal government has regulated distilleries. Bourbon and other liquors are defined by the Federal Standards of Identity for Distilled Spirits, found in the **Code of Federal Regulations** at 27 C.F.R. 5.22. It is regulated as to content of the mash as well as aging requirements, location of production, and other factors such as **alcohol content**. Part 19 of 27 C.F.R. provides the details of the application for a distillery license. These requirements include the payment of an excise tax, the filing of a bond with an application, a location and equipment that comply with the requirements stated in the law, the maintenance of prescribed records and documentation, and the submission of regular reports. The tax is not required for forms of alcohol produced for purposes other than human consumption, such as **ethanol** produced as fuel, but other requirements apply.

The TTB is responsible for alcohol production licensing, the collection of excise taxes, the regulation of alcohol labels, and alcohol advertising. To produce alcohol, the distillery must obtain a basic permit from the TTB. Production may not begin until this permit has been obtained. Each distillery must be separately registered. The application process may include fingerprinting, background investigations within the United States as well as Interpol, and physical inspection of the distilling site. This process can take months.

In addition to the federal requirements, there are state requirements. A company that has distilleries in more than one state must comply with the requirements in each state where a distillery exists. Having a basic permit from the TTB does not exempt a distillery from complying with state requirements. Many states have other restrictive requirements that will not allow licenses for owners of certain other types of businesses, such as liquor distribution businesses. It may be that the state licensing process cannot begin until after the federal licensing or permitting has

Definitions of Whisky in the Code of Federal Regulations (27 CFR 5.22 [b])

(b) *Class 2; whisky.* "Whisky" is an alcoholic distillate from a fermented mash of grain produced at less than 190° proof in such manner that the distillate possesses the taste, aroma, and characteristics generally attributed to whisky, stored in oak containers (except that corn whisky need not be so stored), and bottled at not less than 80° proof, and also includes mixtures of such distillates for which no specific standards of identity are prescribed.

(1) (i) "Bourbon whisky," "rye whisky," "wheat whisky," "malt whisky," or "rye malt whisky" is whisky produced at not exceeding 160° proof from a fermented mash of not less than 51 percent corn, rye, wheat, malted barley, or malted rye grain, respectively, and stored at not more than 125° proof in charred new oak containers; and also includes mixtures of such whiskies of the same type.

(ii) "Corn whisky" is whisky produced at not exceeding 160° proof from a fermented mash of not less than 80 percent corn grain, and if stored in oak containers stored at not more than 125° proof in used or uncharred new oak containers and not subjected in any manner to treatment with charred wood; and also includes mixtures of such whisky.

(iii) Whiskies conforming to the standards prescribed in paragraphs (b)(1)(i) and (ii) of this section, which have been stored in the type of oak containers prescribed, for a period of two years or more shall be further designated as "straight"; for example, "straight bourbon whisky," "straight corn whisky," and whisky conforming to the standards prescribed in paragraph (b)(1)(i) of this section, except that it was produced from a fermented mash of less than 51 percent of any one type of grain, and stored for a period of two years or more in charred new oak containers shall be designated merely as "straight whisky." No other whiskies may be designated "straight." "Straight whisky" includes mixtures of straight whiskies of the same type produced in the same State.

(2) "Whisky distilled from bourbon (rye, wheat, malt, or rye malt) mash" is whisky produced in the United States at not exceeding 160° proof from a fermented mash of not less than 51 percent corn, rye, wheat, malted barley, or malted rye grain, respectively, and stored in used oak containers; and also includes mixtures of such whiskies of the same type. Whisky conforming to the standard of identity for corn whisky must be designated corn whisky.

(3) "Light whisky" is whisky produced in the United States at more than 160° proof, on or after January 26, 1968, and stored in used or uncharred new oak containers; and also includes mixtures of such whiskies. If "light whisky" is mixed with less than 20 percent of straight whisky on a proof gallon basis, the mixture shall be designated "blended light whisky" (light whisky—a blend).

(4) "Blended whisky" (whisky—a blend) is a mixture which contains straight whisky or a blend of straight whiskies at not less than 20 percent on a proof gallon basis, excluding alcohol derived from added harmless coloring, flavoring or blending materials, and, separately, or in combination, whisky or

neutral spirits. A blended whisky containing not less than 51 percent on a proof gallon basis of one of the types of straight whisky shall be further designated by that specific type of straight whisky; for example, "blended rye whisky" (rye whisky—a blend).

(5) (i) "A blend of straight whiskies" (blended straight whiskies) is a mixture of straight whiskies which does not conform to the standard of identify for "straight whisky." Products so designated may contain harmless coloring, flavoring, or blending materials as set forth in 27 CFR 5.23(a).

  (ii) "A blend of straight whiskies" (blended straight whiskies) consisting entirely of one of the types of straight whisky, and not conforming to the standard for straight whisky, shall be further designated by that specific type of straight whisky; for example, "a blend of straight rye whiskies" (blended straight rye whiskies). "A blend of straight whiskies" consisting entirely of one of the types of straight whisky shall include straight whisky of the same type which was produced in the same State or by the same proprietor within the same State, provided that such whisky contains harmless coloring, flavoring, or blending materials as stated in 27 CFR 5.23(a).

  (iii) The harmless coloring, flavoring, or blending materials allowed under this section shall not include neutral spirits or alcohol in their original state. Neutral spirits or alcohol may only appear in a "blend of straight whiskies" or in a "blend of straight whiskies consisting entirely of one of the types of straight whisky" as a vehicle for recognized flavoring of blending material.

(6) "Spirit whisky" is a mixture of neutral spirits and not less than 5 percent on a proof gallon basis of whisky, or straight whisky, or straight whisky and whisky, if the straight whisky component is less than 20 percent on a proof gallon basis.

(7) "Scotch whisky" is whisky which is a distinctive product of Scotland, manufactured in Scotland in compliance with the laws of the United Kingdom regulating the manufacture of Scotch whisky for consumption in the United Kingdom: *Provided,* That if such product is a mixture of whiskies, such mixture is "blended Scotch whisky" (Scotch whisky—a blend).

(8) "Irish whisky" is whisky which is a distinctive product of Ireland, manufactured either in the Republic of Ireland or in Northern Ireland, in compliance with their laws regulating the manufacture of Irish whisky for home consumption: *Provided,* That if such product is a mixture of whiskies, such mixture is "blended Irish whisky" (Irish whisky—a blend).

(9) "Canadian whisky" is whisky which is a distinctive product of Canada, manufactured in Canada in compliance with the laws of Canada regulating the manufacture of Canadian whisky for consumption in Canada: *Provided,* That if such product is a mixture of whiskies, such mixture is "blended Canadian whisky" (Canadian whisky—a blend).

been obtained. This need for serial applications can cause the entire process to take many months.

In addition to licensing and permits that are directly related to the manufacture of liquor, distilleries must comply with other requirements such as zoning laws, parking and other general business requirements, all of which add cost and time to the establishment of the legal business.

See also: Alcoholic Beverage Control Stores.

Further Reading Alcohol and Tobacco Tax and Trade Bureau. www.ttb.gov.

Elizabeth M. Williams

DISTRIBUTION OF FOOD

The distribution of safe and nutritious food throughout the country is a complex yet absolutely important task. Access to good food is the basis for good health and is an important mission of the government. But this mission relies on the private and the public sectors for its successful operation.

Mechanisms govern national and international distribution of food, such as various modes of transportation, storage, import and export customs laws, and the laws of private contracts. These mechanisms may be private but regulated by government, like transportation on interstate highways, or they can be totally governmental and reflect governmental priorities and policies, like **food stamps** and school lunch programs. But all affect the distribution of food and affect its pricing and its availability.

Transportation

The laws affecting interstate transportation are applicable to the transportation of food. There is the additional overlay of food safety over the normal transportation regulations. The Sanitary Food Transportation Act as variously amended describes the food requirements and the powers of the Secretary of Transportation. The **U.S. Department of Agriculture** (USDA) issued the *Guide for Security Practices in Transporting Agricultural Food Commodities in October 2004*. In addition the U.S. Department of Homeland Security (U.S. Customs and Border Protection) adopted the Customs-Trade Partnership Against Terrorism (C-TPAT) and Container Security Initiative, which ensures the safety and security of containers, including those containing food. The **Food and Drug Administration** (FDA) adopted the Bulk over the Road Food Tanker Transport Safety and Security Guidelines in 2003. Finally the Department of Transportation and its divisions—the Federal Highway Administration, the Federal Motor Carrier Safety Administration, the Federal Aviation Administration, the Federal Railroad Administration, and the Maritime Administration—all work together to create an infrastructure for intermodal transport of food to various locations around the country.

Customs

If foods must be brought into the United States from another country, they must first pass through customs. U.S. Customs and Border Protection (CBP), under Homeland Security, secures the integrity of the food coming into the United States, protects agriculture by limiting certain products, plant diseases and pests, and makes it possible for Americans to enjoy the products of other nations. Customs operates whether the food enters the country by land, sea, or air. The Harmonized Tariff Schedule of the United States contains a list of the foods and agricultural products that may be ordinarily imported into the United States. The list includes live farm animals, bulk agricultural commodities and products, and prepared foods. The CBP enforces the food and beverage regulations of other agencies at the point of entry.

Distributors

Food in the United States can be sold directly to consumers or be transported and sold to retailers who resell to consumers. When the goods are sold across state lines they are subject to the safety rules of the FDA and the USDA and other agencies, such as state departments of agriculture. But the method of sale—direct to consumer, sale to distributors with resale to retailers and then to consumers—is also subject to the private law of contracts. Contract law is one of the matters traditionally reserved to the states for oversight. Many states have unique contract laws, but to facilitate interstate sales, most states have adopted a form of the Uniform Commercial Code. This means that the seller and buyer, from different states, can operate as though the laws of contracts and commerce were the same in their respective states, thus making interstate sales easier. Thus, a contract between a supplier in one state who is distributing to five other states through a supplier in yet a sixth state can do business without investigating each state or hiring legal counsel from each state.

Alcohol distributors have been mandated by law since the repeal of Prohibition in 1933, and they create a three-tiered system of distribution of alcoholic beverages. However, food is not so limited. Thus, it is generally unnecessary to find a food distributor to sell food products. A manufacturer of granola, for example, could go from grocery to grocery to sell its product directly and not use a distributor. However, for convenience, a manufacturer might desire to be represented by a distributor to increase the number of retailers where the product could potentially be sold.

Farmers markets and even sales at and from farms and roadside stands are a form of direct sales that allow farmers to sell directly to consumers and restaurants without the mark-up caused by the distributor's layer in the chain of distribution. There has been concern recently that small and family-owned farms might disappear and the current movement to distribute food through green markets and the popularity of **community-supported agriculture** (CSA) is one more positive step in the food distribution chain, which may also help family farms.

Food Stamps and Commodities

The USDA has a number of programs that allow for distribution of foods to the needy. One program encourages states and certain agencies, like school districts, to directly contract with commercial entities to process bulk commodities into food that can be used for such distribution as school lunch programs. It is the mission of the Commodity Supplemental Food Program to ensure the nutrition of pregnant women, nursing mothers, children up to the age of six, and the elderly (over age 60) by distributing to them USDA commodity foods. Funds are provided to the states for the administration of this program. The Department of

Defense Fresh Produce Program makes fresh fruits and vegetables available to the USDA for distribution. Schools and states have been the beneficiaries of this program as well as military installations and Indian reservations.

See also: Alcohol, In-State Distribution of; School Breakfast and Lunch Programs; Subsidies.

Elizabeth M. Williams

DRINKING AGE

Drinking age refers to the legal drinking age, that is, the minimum age at which a person may legally drink alcoholic beverages. With the repeal of Prohibition in 1933, the states were able to set their own rules regarding the minimum drinking age under the authority established by the Twenty-first Amendment to the Constitution. Most states set a legal drinking age at 21, which was the generally recognized age of majority. A minority of the states had lower drinking ages between 18 and 20. In the 1970s, the states began to lower the legal drinking age to 18. The reason for this action was an attempt to give young people all of the rights of majority in light of the passage of the Twenty-sixth Amendment, which gave the right to vote to those who reached the age of 18.

Before 1984, this issue was considered within the purview of matters reserved for state action by the Tenth Amendment. At that time, the drinking age varied from state to state. Some states allowed 18-year-olds to drink beer but not spirits. In some states people had to wait until they were age 21 to drink spirits. Other states, like Louisiana, allowed 18-year-olds to drink legally.

In an effort to control the abuse of alcohol, the federal government entered into the arena of minimum drinking age. But it was prohibited by the Tenth Amendment from enacting a federal minimum drinking age that would supersede state law. Thus, the federal government enacted a law that allowed it to influence the laws of the various states by the use of the enticement or threat of the reduction or loss of federal highway funds for noncompliance with the desires of Congress.

The Federal Uniform Drinking Age Act of 1984, 23 U.S.C. 158, mandated that states change the minimum legal purchase or possession age for all alcohol to age 21 or the state would lose or suffer a reduction its federal highway funds under the Federal Highway Aid Act. This law does not have the effect of wholesale prohibition of "possession" by those under the age of 21. There are exceptions. Those exceptions include possession in private clubs or other private establishments, which include homes; for medical or dental purposes in a hospital or other medical establishment; when the person is selling for a licensed retailer, manufacturer, or wholesaler—such as a clerk in a store where liquor is sold; and for religious purposes when the person is accompanied by a parent or spouse or legal guardian, when that person is over the age of 21.

In light of the room given by the federal law, the states have not uniformly enacted laws that prohibit the consumption of alcohol by those under the age of

21. Some states allow 18-year-olds to be present in a place where alcohol is consumed, even if they are not allowed to consume it, including serving it as a bar-
tender. In other states, those under age 21 may consume liquor on private
property when in the presence of their parents, legal guardian, or spouse when
that person is over age 21. Other states actually use the vague term "family member" without defining who a family member is.

A number of states have not changed the drinking age in spite of the federal
law. Thirty states allow parents to allow their children under the age of 21 to drink
within their homes with their consent. Some states tied the continuation of their
change in the drinking age to the federal law with an automatic repeal if the federal
law is repealed. These states had mixed reasons for resisting the changes required
by the federal legislation, not the least of which was financial. For example, those
states who enjoyed "spring break" tourism were hit hard financially by the increase
in the minimum drinking age. The federal law was challenged as an unconstitutional usurpation of the rights reserved to the states under the Tenth Amendment
in *North Dakota v. Dole* (483 U.S. 203 (1987)). The case proceeded all the way to
the U.S. Supreme Court, which upheld the federal law. The high court held that
this Act was in conformance with the U.S. Constitution under the Taxation and
Spending Clause. With the decision by the Supreme Court, the states that might
have held out had little incentive to not comply with the federal law.

There has been recently an argument that the legal minimum drinking age
should be reduced to allow people to begin drinking earlier so that they learn
about responsible drinking. Some groups of college educators, such as the Ame-
thyst Initiative, have advocated the reduction in the drinking age. Others, such as
the National Institute on Alcohol Abuse and Alcoholism College Drinking Task
Force and Mothers Against Drunk Driving urged college administrators to rigorously enforce the minimum drinking age laws on campus to reduce alcohol-
related traffic accidents and deaths and to also reduce alcohol-related sexual
assaults. The statistics regarding traffic accidents and fatalities related to alcohol
have been used by both sides to bolster their arguments. In recent years, the
move to revisit these laws has been increasing.

Another common argument advanced in support of lowering the minimum
drinking age is that people in the United States become majors or adults at the
age of 18. At this age they serve in the armed forces and may marry, enter into
contracts, and vote, yet they are not legally allowed to drink. Still another argument is that in those states where the community culturally supports a higher
drinking age the statistics show that the higher drinking age does reduce traffic
fatalities. In those areas where the drinking age was "forced" on the states and
thus not supported by the local culture, the number of fatalities has not been
affected. This argument is that the actual age is arbitrary and that it is culture that
creates any benefit of minimum drinking age.

See also: Advertising of Alcohol Products, Alcohol; State and Federal Law, Conflicts
between; In-State Distribution of Alcohol; National Distribution of Alcohol.

Elizabeth M. Williams

DUMPING

Dumping is a trade practice that is predatory and involves attempts to acquire market share and destroy the competition. It may refer to actions regardless of location, but is most often used in the context of international trade. Specifically dumping refers to the practice of selling a product in a rival market either at less than the cost of producing it or at less than the price for which it sells in its own market.

Free market advocates do not consider dumping a negative act. They consider it advantageous to consumers, because it lowers prices for consumers. On the other hand, advocates for workers and for preserving certain ways of life argue that dumping is a threat. The net cost of dumping is up for debate. There is a cost in either the payment of higher prices or in the loss of certain ways of life.

Dumping, as it is defined by treaty, is a permissible basis for protectionist duties levied against the products of the dumping nation. The **World Trade Organization** (WTO) regulates dumping and protectionist duties. To prove a case of dumping, three points must be made. First, there must be evidence that a large amount of product from the offending nation has been introduced into the attacked nation at a very low price. Then the attacked nation must prove that its industry has actually been harmed and is threatened. Finally the attacked nation must establish a causal connection between the dumping and the harm.

Once dumping has been established there are several options available to the threatened nation. One option is to create safeguards to protect the market share of the domestic industry. Both U.S. crawfish farmers and tilapia growers have claimed a loss of market share due to dumping by various Asian seafood producers. A safeguard can be a measure that limits the amount of an import of a particular product without actually naming a particular nation as an offender. Thus once the maximum allowable amount of the product has been introduced in a given period, no more is allowed to be imported. This amount would be based on the previous market share enjoyed by the domestic product.

The most severe action that a nation might take is to levy protective duties on the products imported from the nation identified as the dumping offender. This obviously is the most targeted and the most charged action that a nation might take. Protective tariffs are the most extreme and scrutinized form of protectionism in the international community, often resulting in retaliatory levies based on the other countries claims of dumping. It must be considered whether saving or protecting the tilapia market is worth the risk of other retaliation.

Within an individual nation the political power of the harmed industry must be balanced against the other trade activities of that nation and the possible economic consequences over all.

See also: Importation of Food, Tariffs, World Trade Organization.

Elizabeth M. Williams

E

EGG PRODUCTS INSPECTION ACT

The Egg Product Inspection Act (EPIA) was passed in 1970 to ensure that the marketplace has access to healthy shell eggs and egg products. The goal of the EPIA is to prevent undesirable shell eggs from reaching consumers either directly or incorporated into processed foods. This act is an example of regulation to protect the consumer when food is processed, and the intermediate product is not within the control of the consumer and cannot be evaluated by the consumer.

The phrase "egg products" means eggs that are taken from their shells at plants called "breaker plants" where they are processed. There are several egg products. There are whole eggs, separated yolks, separated whites, and various blends that are processed. Egg products come in several forms—liquid, frozen, and dried. Egg products are used by restaurants, hospitals, schools, and many other types of facilities selling fresh food for consumption, as well as by bakeries and food manufacturing facilities. Egg products can be found in dry mixes, such as pancake mix or instant pudding, pasta, frozen desserts, mayonnaise, candies, and baked products.

The EPIA requires mandatory pasteurization of all egg products, whether ultimately refrigerated, frozen, or dried. Pasteurization is achieved when eggs or egg products are heated rapidly and maintained at a minimum required temperature for a stated length of time. The heat kills salmonella bacteria but is not intended to boil the eggs or to change its characteristics such as texture, appearance, flavor, nutrition, or use.

The act also requires that breakage plants that manufacture egg products in any of its forms—liquid, dry, or frozen must be inspected continuously by the **U.S. Department of Agriculture** (USDA). The law is applicable to all such facilities. Applicability is independent of size and applies to all egg-breaking facilities. Likewise, it applies to facilities whether products are sold in a limited local market, across state lines, or internationally. Companies that carry, truck, and take in shell eggs and egg products also are subject to being inspected regularly.

Eggs delivered to breaking plants are placed into cooling rooms for holding. They are cleaned in water that must be at least 20 degrees warmer than that of the egg as well as sprayed with a sanitizer before breaking. They cannot be broken if they are wet, and must wait until they are merely moist. Shell eggs and egg products generally are placed into three categories.

1. *Refrigerated liquid products*: To create these products, eggs are broken and separated; liquid eggs are placed into covered containers. These products are ready for transportation to bakeries or other facilities for immediate use or are ready for additional processing at appropriate facilities.

2. *Frozen egg products*: Any part of the processed egg can be frozen. This may include whole eggs, whites, yolks, predetermined blends of whole eggs and yolks, or whole eggs and milk, and blends that include other products such as sugar, corn syrup, or salt.

3. *Dried or dehydrated egg products:* Dried eggs are also called egg solids. Dehydrated egg products have been manufactured and available in the United States since 1930, though quality in the early days was considered poor. Improved dehydrated egg products are used in numerous convenience foods and in the food service industry.

The provisions of the EPIA are carried out by the USDA. The act is enforced by the USDA and the **Food and Drug Administration**.

See also: Appendix 11: Bill AB 1437 Introduced into the California Legislature Dealing with Shelled Eggs.

Further Reading Egg Products Inspection Act. http://www.fsis.usda.gov/regulations_&_policies/EPIA/index.asp; Food Safety. http://www.usda.gov/factbook/chapter9.pdf.

William C. Smith and Elizabeth M. Williams

EMBARGOES

The strict definition of "embargo" is an action by a government that prevents the free movement of merchant ships in and out of the country's ports. The limitations may be limited to ships traveling to and from a particular port that the government wishes to block. The government that imposes an embargo is trying to limit trade with a particular country or countries to maintain neutrality, affect that country's economy, and/or keep the other country from obtaining necessary goods. The broader modern use of the word is a trade prohibition against either another country or a certain product. Embargoes can involve any commodity or product, but often involve food—water, corn, rice or other essential commodities.

The Embargo Act of 1807 was a law passed at the behest of Thomas Jefferson that prohibited ships from coming and going through U.S. ports and prohibited trade with all nations. The purpose of the law was to limit or eliminate trade with England and France to maintain the neutrality of the United States during the Napoleonic Wars. There was also an incident in which an English ship impressed several American seamen into service. This action angered the country and influenced the cause of the embargo. The law was very unpopular. Most historians believe that the embargo failed. The embargoes were all effectively lifted by 1809.

The Office of Foreign Assets Control (OFAC), part of the Department of Treasury and the federal enforcement arm of embargoes and other sanctions, first derived its authority from the Trading with the Enemy Act of 1917. It currently publishes a list of embargoed countries. They are Iran, Cuba, Syria, North Korea, Myanmar, and Sudan. The OFAC controls the need for and issuance of export licenses. The decision is based on what is being exported and to where. The OFAC has a list of countries that are under sanctions, which is a lesser control than a full embargo. In addition there is a Specially Designated Nationals and Blocked Persons List and a Denied Persons list, maintained by the Department of Commerce.

Embargoes are an age-old governmental practice. They are an attempt by one country to pressure or control another country. Embargoes are considered a tool in the foreign policy array, in contrast with blockades, which are forced stopping of foreign vessels. Blockades are considered acts of aggression.

The United States has laws that make participating in a secondary embargo illegal. This means that if a foreign government imposes an embargo on another country, citizens of the United States cannot support the embargo of the embargoed country. That law is designed to keep the U.S. citizens from being controlled by the governments of other countries.

The Cuban Embargo is a long-standing embargo of the United States. It has been in effect since 1960. In 1997 the American Association for World Health issued a report that analyzed the embargo and determined that the health and nutrition of the people of Cuba had been adversely affected by it. The report indicates that caloric intake in Cuba has been greatly restricted by the embargo, causing babies with low birth weight and other nutritional problems. In addition, water purification chemicals are not making it through the embargo, causing an increase in water-borne illnesses. The embargo has affected the lives of the ordinary citizens of Cuba. U.S. embargoes imposed on other countries do not usually include bans on the sale of food or essential medicines.

In 2000, the U.S. farm industry complained that it was being adversely affected by the Cuban Embargo. The Trade Sanctions Reform and Export Enhancement Act was enacted, which softened the restrictions of the embargo and allowed food and essential medicine to be traded with Cuba for humanitarian purposes. At first Cuba refused trade, but after Hurricane Michelle in late 2002, Cuba relented and began to trade with the United States. Trade has continued to grow. Today the United States is a major food supplier to Cuba.

Many people criticize this embargo as being unsuccessful in changing the actions of the Cuban government; however, it is has made Cuban people poor, hungry, and less healthy; has restricted the freedom of the people of the United States to travel to Cuba; and farmers and others from trading with the country. Some argue that the maintenance of the embargo is a bargain to attract votes from the staunch anti-Castro community of Florida.

During World War I the United States suffered a food shortage. Production was limited by a number of factors, including bad weather, and at the same time European demand for U.S. food was high. This demand reduced the food supply alarmingly. The price of food was rising by huge percentages. The reaction of the government was to enact an embargo to keep food within the country.

After World War II, the United States used embargoes during the Cold War. The United States emerged without the damage to agricultural land and urban areas that left Europe in need of help to recover. The United States began a number of economic sanctions against the Soviet Union that included embargoes. The Export Control Act of 1949 was the formal expression of those sanctions. Initially the embargo against the Soviet Union was very strict. The embargoes imposed on the Eastern European countries were much looser in an attempt to cause unrest between those countries and the Soviet Union. As relations with the Soviet Union improved, trade increased, including food sales.

An embargo of U.S. ships going to England, France, and Israel during the Suez Canal crisis in 1956 stopped those powers from taking military action against Egypt. This was an embargo against allies, yet it worked to avoid a military invasion.

The United States imposed embargoes against North Korea, North Vietnam, and China. These proved unsuccessful and caused U.S. allies to object, especially after the end of the Korean War. President Richard M. Nixon famously lifted most of the Chinese Embargo for strategic reasons, that is, to increase U.S. trade with China. Today, embargoes are most likely to be imposed for human rights violations.

See also: Boycotts; Executive Branch and Executive Orders; Appendix 15: Uruguay Round Agreement on Agriculture; Appendix 16: World Trade Organization Ministerial Conference Decision.

Elizabeth M. Williams

ENVIRONMENTAL PROTECTION AGENCY

The Environmental Protection Agency (EPA), headquartered in Washington, D.C., is one of the independent agencies of the **executive branch**, reporting directly to the president of the United States. Because several programs were assigned to different agencies and lacked coordination, Congress created the new agency in 1970 under President Richard M. Nixon to place all of the programs under one umbrella.

The EPA's mission is to protect the environment and, thus, the health of U.S. citizens. It establishes minimum standards, monitors the environment, and enforces regulations. The various programs brought together include the elimination of air pollution and water pollution, controlling noise pollution, and limiting radiation exposure. As toxic waste disposal became more of a problem, the regulation of toxic waste was placed under the purview of the EPA, which now sets standards for its disposal.

The EPA was established as the political reaction to the clamor for a cleanup of the environment, which the government had previously assumed could clean itself. Before the EPA had been created, there was no governmental mechanism for the type of action necessary to take control of the environmental degradation and its deleterious effects on the health and the quality of life of the citizenry.

One of the EPA's programs derives from the Environmental Response, Compensation, and Liability Act of 1980, also called the "Superfund." The act was passed to create a framework for the restoration of toxic waste sites. This act requires that those parties who caused the problem, that is, dumped toxic waste, finance the cost of the clean up. Importantly, the EPA also monitors the activities of other federal agencies and reports on the impact of their activities on the environment. Furthermore, the EPA coordinates and assists state and local governments in their attempts at maintaining a clean environment within their geographic boundaries.

The EPA also works with private organizations, working to keep the environment clean.

The EPA employs 17,000 people in Washington, D.C. It has 10 regional offices and laboratories around the country. Employees include the gamut of specialties necessary to run any agency like media and computer employees, but it also employs engineers and scientists who specialize in the environment.

The EPA administers all of the environmental laws: the Clean Air Act; the **Clean Water Act**; the Comprehensive Environmental Response, Compensation, and Liability Act and the Superfund Amendments and Reauthorization Act; the Emergency Planning and Community Right-to-Know Act; the Federal Insecticide, Fungicide, and Rodenticide Act; the Federal Food, Drug, and Cosmetic Act; the National Environmental Policy Act; the Oil Pollution Act of 1990; the Safe Drinking Water Act; the Solid Waste Disposal Act; Resource Conservation and Recovery Act; and the Toxic Substances Control Act.

The EPA conducts many programs (some of which are described in the following discussions) that safeguard the food supply of the United States.

AgSTAR Program
The AgSTAR program promotes the installation of bio-gas recovery systems in confined animal feedlots. The goal of the program is to reduce methane emissions.

Pesticide Environmental Stewardship Program
The goal of the Pesticide Environmental Stewardship program is to encourage the stewardship of the soil and the environment by voluntary means and by not merely following the standards but exceeding the standards.

The National Clean Diesel Campaign
The National Clean Diesel Campaign (NCDC) includes these campaigns: Clean Construction USA, Clean Ports USA, Clean School Bus USA, and Diesel Retrofit. The NCDC is part of a plan to make diesel engines cleaner. This effort has been partly regulatory and partly voluntary. This program has the cooperation of national, state, and local agencies, such as school districts, as well as nongovernmental partners.

Coal Combustion Products Partnership
The Coal Combustion Products Partnership (C2P2) is a program that combines the efforts of industry and the government to encourage efficient energy production through the use of coal, reduce the overall consumption of energy, reduce the level of greenhouse gases emitted into the atmosphere, and reduce the amount of solid waste by encouraging the industry to recycle. For example, one goal of the C2P2 program is to replace Portland cement with coal ash in concrete. The goal is to go from the 12.6 million tons used in 2002 to 20 million tons of coal ash in 2010. It is predicted that reaching this goal will result in the reduction of greenhouse gases by at least 6.5 million tons each year. It will also increase the reuse of coal combustion products from 35 percent to more than 45 percent.

Combined Heat and Power Partnership

Combined Heat and Power (CHP) is known by another term, "cogeneration." The CHP is a methodology that allows for power and thermal energy to be generated from one source. The CHP Partnership (CHPP) operates on a voluntary basis. It is designed to encourage the use of regeneration and, thereby, reduce the impact of the generation of power on the environment. Each participating facility installs a CHP system. The system is tailored to satisfy both heat and energy requirements of the participating facility. This retrofitting with CHP makes the facility more efficient—both decreasing the costs of energy generation and production of heat. The CHPP works when members of the cogeneration industry, the EPA, appropriate state and local agencies, energy consumers, citizens, and environmental groups join together to keep making improvements to the systems, let others know about the benefits of cogeneration, and facilitate the joining of the program by new participants, including food industry participants.

Community-Based Childhood Asthma Programs

The connection between environmental pollution and the incidence and control of asthma is the motivation behind the creation of the Community-Based Childhood Asthma Program. This voluntary program is conducted in conjunction with public health officials at the federal and local levels in an attempt to reduce the incidence of attacks by reducing environmental triggers. This program identifies best practices and allows families who have children with asthma to help reduce triggers in the home, in schools, in day care centers, and other public and private places. Most families have an asthma management plan and this program is intended to be part of that plan, which also may include medical treatment and drug and other therapies.

EnergyStar

The EnergyStar program is designed to help citizens make intelligent choices when purchasing products, such as appliances, that use energy. This program is applicable to both business and private investment in energy-efficient appliances. The program is administered jointly by the EPA and the U.S. Department of Energy. In addition to using less energy, citizens and businesses can save money by using energy-efficient products and promote a cleaner environment. To make it easier to participate, the EnergyStar program has created a rating system that quantifies the energy efficiency of the product. The EPA has worked with producers in all of the sectors of appliance production to support the use of the EnergyStar label on all products. In addition, all the it encourages producers to create more efficient products to achieve a better rating, create better practices for new construction and retrofitting to achieve higher ratings, and inform consumers in all markets of the benefits of these efficiencies.

Great American Woodstove Changeout Campaign

Woodstoves manufactured before 1988 are generally inefficient. To encourage the transition to more efficient models, the EPA and environmental organizations and industry have joined together to form the Great American Woodstove Changeout Campaign. The campaign encourages the installation of more efficient clean-burning stoves that are EPA-certified. One of the goals of the program is to reduce air toxicity both inside and outside, reduce solids in the air, reduce the potential hazards for fire, and improve overall efficiency.

Green Power Partnership

More and more sources of green power are being identified. The Green Power Partnership encourages the use of green power sources instead of conventional sources, which may be inefficient and have a great environmental impact. This program is voluntary. Those renewable sources of energy, such as solar and wind power, allow commercial and other entities to reduce their environmental impact. The EPA educates, puts groups together, creates resources, and has a program of publicizing partners. Many organic food producers include green production in their practices.

Labs 21

Labs 21 is a joint program of the EPA and the U.S. Department of Energy. It encourages laboratories on a voluntary basis to participate in the reduction of energy and reduction of pollution by laboratories. Laboratories are high energy users as well as major polluters in all areas—water, air, and soil. The EPA and the U.S. Department of Energy are working together to help with best practices in new construction and retrofitted laboratories to reduce energy costs and diminish environmental damage. The EPA has set a goal to make all EPA laboratories energy self-sufficient so that other laboratories in the country can use their practices as a model.

Outdoor Wood-Fired Hydronic Heaters Program

Old outdoor wood-fired hydronic heaters are one more example of inefficient appliances that may still be in use. The Outdoor Wood-Fired Hydronic Heaters program addresses this inefficiency by helping producers create and sell more efficient outdoor hydronic heaters.

Radon Risk Reduction

Exposure to radon has been identified as the second leading cause of lung cancer. The Radon Risk Reduction (RRR) program has a goal of eliminating and minimizing this hazard. As real estate changes hands, radon problems in a home can be identified and remediated, if necessary. New home construction is also a part of the program. The RRR program is intended to increase radon reducing features in new home construction.

Responsible Appliance Disposal Partnership

Many of the chemicals found in old appliances deplete the ozone. When appliances are not disposed of properly these chemicals from old freezers, computers, refrigerators, air conditioners, and humidifiers can leach into the environment and do damage. The Responsible Appliance Disposal (RAD) program supports those who recover the ozone-depleting chemicals like foam insulation and refrigerant from old appliances and see that they are properly disposed of. RAD partners are varied and include universities and utility companies. They ensure that those components like metal, plastic, and glass that can be recycled are recycled. The polychlorinated biphenyls (PCBs), mercury, and used oil are recovered and properly disposed. The EPA collects and distributes data on the proper collection, disposal, and recycling of the components recovered from disposed appliances. In addition the EPA collects statistics about disposal and recovery so as to properly review the program. These benefits, when properly marketed, can help encourage others to participate and help Congress understand the benefit of continuing the program. The RAD partnership also operates an awards program to further encourage participation.

SmartWay Transport Partnership

The SmartWay Transport Partnership educates consumers to the benefits of choosing truck and rail companies that operate in the most green energy-efficient manner and apply other green practices. Retailers and other consumers are encouraged either to select an environmentally efficient carrier or to buy products from those manufacturers who use efficient carriers.

Greenhill

The Greenhill Advanced Refrigeration Partnership is a voluntary program composed of the EPA, the chemical industry that produces refrigerant, the refrigeration manufacturers, and the grocery industry. It is designed to encourage the protection of the ozone layer around the earth by the use of green technologies, environmental support plans, and methodologies. The implementation of the Partnership should additionally reduce greenhouse gases and result in significant efficiencies and monetary savings. Because it is a voluntary program, partners do not limit themselves to complying with minimums, but rather pledge to do all that they can to affect the goals of the program. They agree to measure their current impact, including current refrigerant emissions, and then create a plan for the reduction of the emission complete with target goals and dates. In addition the partners agree that they will use nonozone depleting products and efficient refrigeration techniques as they improve their facilities or build new ones. The EPA hopes that through this program there will be significant improvement in the thinning of the ozone layer.

WasteWise

WasteWise is a recycling program of the EPA. It shows the public how recycling and reuse can help save money and be more efficient. It encourages and promotes the use of recycling to reduce the production of waste materials and the purchase of products made of recycled materials. It encourages the manufacture of products with recycled materials. This program has a recognition component to further encourage participation.

The Environmental Protection Agency's budget was $7.8 billion in 2009. Almost half of its budget is used for state-operated programs which regrant to programs and projects within their respective states.

See also: Carson, Rachel; Clean Water Act; Dumping, Ethanol, Pesticides; Runoff, Agricultural; Solid Waste.

Further Reading Environmental Protection Agency Web site, http://www.epa.gov/

Willliam C. Smith and Elizabeth M. Williams

EQUAL EMPLOYMENT OPPORTUNITY COMMISSION AND RESTAURANTS

The Equal Employment Opportunity Commission (EEOC) is the federal agency that protects citizens from violations of the various civil rights laws that apply at work. These laws include the **Americans with Disabilities Act** (ADA) and the Equal Rights Act. Today, the protected classes include race, religion, national origin, age, gender, disability, whistle blowing about any discrimination, or standing up to discrimination. The EEOC can investigate claims for discrimination levied against federal agencies. In addition it can bring a suit for discrimination against an employer. The EEOC derives its authority from the Civil Rights Act of 1964. The agency is specifically mentioned in several additional statues: the Age Discrimination in Employment Act of 1967, the Rehabilitation Act of 1973, the ADA and its amendments.

The EEOC has been at the center of controversy for many years. One of the biggest complaints is its backlog. For political reasons, it is often underfunded and unable to respond in a timely manner to all of the complaints that are filed. From 2006 to 2008 the EEOC saw complaints rise by about 25 percent. This happened while the agency was experiencing a reduction in staff because of budget cuts.

In 2009 the EEOC was found to have violated the National Labor Standards Act (NLSA) in the manner that it handled overtime. According to the arbitrator who made the determination, the EEOC was requiring its employees who worked overtime to take compensatory time. The agency was not paying overtime. The arbitrator determined that the agency has a clear requirement under the law to time and one-half for overtime worked in a given week. The workers who were working overtime were not exempt employees under the NLSA. Many labor advocates are hopeful that this ruling will result in an increase in the budget of the EEOC.

The Civil Rights Act of 1964 prohibited, among other things, racial discrimination in public accommodations and employment. The law was deemed constitutional by the Supreme Court despite initial claims that it was delving into areas traditionally reserved to the states. The Fourteenth Amendment and the Fifteenth Amendment to the constitution and the Commerce Clause were the basis for supporting the law. The meaning of public accommodations has been determined to include restaurants and hotels, as well as theaters and stores. This part of the law is applicable in the food industry but is not enforced by the EEOC. This enforcement is the role of the Justice Department. The employment discrimination provisions of the Civil Rights Act are enforced by the EEOC, however.

In 1963 the Equal Pay Act passed. This bill required that those working in the same job doing similar work, whether male or female, had to be paid the same amount. The inclusion of sex in the antidiscrimination provision was intended to defeat the bill, because of its absurdity. That was a miscalculation, and sex discrimination was also monitored by the EEOC. The law applies both in hiring and in the course of employment.

The process of filing a complaint with the EEOC can be done in writing—in person or by mail—or by telephone. Under the Civil Rights Act and other civil rights laws, the complainant is required to file the complaint within 180 days of the occurrence of the discrimination. In those areas where there is a state agency charged with protecting the state's citizens against discrimination, the initial complaint must be filed with the state agency. Then a complaint can be filed with the EEOC within 300 days of the occurrence or 30 days after the determination by the state agency that it will not pursue the complaint, whichever is earlier. Missing the deadlines can make EEOC unable to pursue a complaint.

There is a requirement to file a complaint with the EEOC before bringing a private lawsuit for discrimination. However, a case based on the Equal Pay Act can be brought without an EEOC filing. But if the pay discrimination is also a violation of the Equal Rights Act, there may be an EEOC filing requirement.

After a complaint or charge is filed, the EEOC may either schedule a priority investigation when there appears to be discrimination or a due-course investigation where the facts are less clear. During the investigation, the EEOC may request documents and interview people. It may attempt to settle with an employer. The EEOC may recommend the case for the Mediation Program, to which both parties must consent. This may shortcut the resolution of the issues. If the mediation does not work, then the investigation can continue. If the agency does not find a violation the charge can be dismissed. If the agency dismisses the charge, the complainant has 90 days in which to bring a private action. This dismissal is called a "right to sue" notice. Under some laws, the right to sue notices can be requested without investigation.

Restaurants can be highly emotional environments because of the pressure of performing quickly. Besides sex and racial discrimination, an area of prohibited discrimination is retaliation. When a person is punished or fired in retaliation for an action taken by an employee, the restaurant can face an action even when the underlying cause of the retaliation is found to be groundless. Hostile environment and sexual harassment are problems that the restaurant industry has to face. Even religious discrimination, which has increased in recent years, is an area that restaurateurs must watch. Most religious discrimination complaints are based on a failure to make adequate accommodations for religious needs. These can include letting people off early or allowing them to not work on certain religious days. Dress code accommodation is also an area of concern.

According to the law, the restaurant is responsible for the improper conduct of its employees. Thus, a hostile work environment, sexual harassment, or other types of discrimination that may be perpetrated by employees may cost the restaurant, even when the actions are not the approved policy of the business.

See also: Administrative Procedures Act; Litigation; Minimum Wage Law and Restaurant Workers.

Further Reading The Equal Employment Opportunity Commission Web site http://www.eeoc.gov/

Elizabeth M. Williams

ESPIONAGE, FOOD

Industrial espionage is the use of dirty tricks, undercover employees, and theft of information to learn about the activities of competitors and manipulate the marketplace. The food and beverage industry can be just as involved in these activities as other industries. Some of the activities are illegal.

In 2001 there was a worldwide health concern about beef and foot-and-mouth disease. Cattle around the world were destroyed to avoid the spread of the disease. It has been theorized that rather than being an actual health threat, that this major health concern and the subsequent reaction to it were really acts of corporate sabotage. Two things can happen in the middle of these health crises: the stock of an affected company can plummet in value making it cheaper to acquire and those companies found to be clean and safe during the crisis can garner larger market share. Similar claims of manipulation of the marketplace have been made about reported but unsubstantiated claims of E. coli contamination. The stock of Hudson Beef Company fell in 1997 and Tyson Foods Corporation was able to purchase the company and eliminate a competitor.

In 1997 it was reported that a person who died in China was a suspected victim of bird flu. Immediately after this report, the United States stopped imports of chicken from China. Within a few days, more than 1 million chickens were killed in China to curb any spread of the disease. The Chinese government was under great pressure to limit exports of chickens. Some followers of the world marketplace and the Central Intelligence Agency (CIA) claim that the CIA caused the outbreak of bird flu so as to shore up domestic chicken companies and allow U.S. chicken interests to more easily obtain a place in the Chinese market while the market was vulnerable.

The situations described are a form of dirty tricks, misinformation, and disinformation being used to manipulate markets. But other forms of espionage, while using spy tactics, are not based on fraud. For example, when there was serious flooding in Iowa that threatened the corn crops, corn futures prices were soaring and had been for two weeks. There was concern that the entire corn crop would be lost. The **U.S. Department of Agriculture** (USDA) was on the ground interviewing farmers to determine the extent of the actual and potential losses. But the hedge funds were using satellites to observe the extent of the flooding. They learned, before the USDA, that the flooding was not as devastating as was being reported, and invested accordingly. When the USDA reported that the flooding was not going to destroy the harvest, the hedge funds had already invested, knowing that the prices would begin to fall. The hedge funds' advance knowledge allowed them to profit.

In 2008 Burger King hired private investigators to engage in surveillance of a group of young people, the Student/Farmworker Alliance, trying to improve the conditions of farm workers in Florida. The college students were working in partnership with a group of farm workers in Florida called the Coalition of Immokalee Workers. This group had been urging fast-food companies to look into the conditions of the tomato workers. The tomatoes were being supplied to the fast food industry. Burger King responded to the request for consideration by hiring an investigator who was accused of being unlicensed.

In the 1930s during periods of labor unrest, corporations used investigators to infiltrate labor unions. After a series of congressional investigations this practice was held to be an unfair labor practice. There have not been investigations of corporate espionage in recent years.

Rumor is part of the corporate espionage arsenal. Snapple was accused of being racist in 2009 and McDonald's has been accused of grinding worms into its burgers. Even when the rumors are not successful in scuttling the company, they can cost the company millions in marketing countermeasures. Just that expenditure of money can be a threat to smaller companies.

Another form of espionage is product tampering. Gerber experienced this phenomenon when there were accusations of glass in its baby juices in 1986. Gerber considered itself in a no-win situation. Consumers who had concerns did not contact the company but rather the media, which fed the publicity machine, while selling newspapers and magazines. Gerber was criticized for the way that it responded to the situation. Instead of assuaging the public, the company attempted to quiet the media, and this caused widespread mistrust in consumers. This illustrates the tricky nature of espionage. Proper handling by the accused company could make the company a winner. In 1993 Pepsi Cola successfully survived a claim that needles and syringes were being found in Pepsi cans.

Attempts to manipulate the market have included kidnapping of corporate executives, threats of extortion, and other illegal activities. These can be handled by law enforcement through normal channels. Breaking into corporate files to steal proprietary information is also an illegal action that can be prosecuted when proven. But there are less obvious forms of theft, for example, the enticing of an employee of one company to take a job at a competitor company. Although the new employee may not actually share secrets, which belong to the original employer, it is impossible for ideas and concepts not to pass between the competitors. Knowledge of products in development, marketing plans, launch of product dates, and strategies are all examples of the types of information an employee may reveal, sometimes without even realizing it.

Computer hacking and the planting of viruses are examples of using the computer to access files. Companies that have trade secrets that are formulas, recipes, and strategic plans often keep only hard copies of this type of information, kept in a safe with limited access, instead of keeping it on a computer. Even non-networked computers and those without Internet access can be vulnerable.

See also: Trade Secrets.

Further Reading Javers, Eamon. *Broker, Trader, Lawyer, Spy: The Secret World of Corporate Espionage.* New York: HarperCollins, 2010.

Elizabeth M. Williams

ETHANOL

Ethanol is the type of alcohol that is created by the distillation of fermented materials such as grain mash or fruit. Ethanol is the alcohol in the spirits such as brandy, whiskey or other liquor. In addition to being an alcoholic beverage, this ethyl alcohol is a biofuel that has been used as an additive to petroleum-based fuels. In some states, the use of up to 10% biofuel as an additive in gasoline is mandated by law. Most cars manufactured today can run on a blend of gasoline and ethanol.

Although it is a renewable resource, ethanol as a fuel is controversial as it is currently produced. One basis for the controversy is that agricultural land and resources that could be growing food crops have been diverted to growing crops that will be converted to ethanol fuel. Another controversy is that the federal government is subsidizing the growing of crops for conversion to ethanol fuel, when it is arguable that the cost of fertilizing the soil that grows the crops grown for fuel costs more than the savings that are realized using the biofuel. There is further argument that the production of ethanol fuel is not "clean," because it requires the use of petroleum-based fertilizer. Much ethanol in the United States is produced from corn. Sugar cane is considered a more efficient source of ethanol, but it receives fewer federal subsidies.

The Small Ethanol Producer Tax Credit is a special federal tax credit that is designed to level the playing field to allow small farmers and ethanol producers to compete with larger ethanol producers. The credit is a production income tax credit of $.10 per gallon with an annual cap at 15 million gallons. This same gallon limit is the definition of the production limits to qualify for the credit, with an additional production capacity limitation of 30 million gallons. This credit is authorized by the American Recovery and Reinvestment Act of 2009.

In 2007, Portland, Oregon's City Council was the first to require that gasoline sold within the city must be a blend of at least 10 percent ethanol. Several other states require ethanol blends for environmental reasons. Others require it because of the need to meet federal emission standards within the city.

The California Air Resources Board (CARB) has adopted rules and standards effective January 2011 that are known as the California Low Carbon Fuel Standard. This ruling includes the consideration of the carbon load and other costs in producing ethanol from corn and other products in determining the standards. Corn ethanol producers objected to this move by the CARB, arguing that the final product of the ethanol is the only thing that should be considered in setting standards. Unless the rules are amended, corn-based ethanol produced in the Midwest will not qualify under the standard, thus will not be able to be sold in California.

The U.S. **Environmental Protection Agency** (EPA) promulgated in 2009 a notice that it was going to make new rules, that is, the Renewable Fuel Standard. Proposed regulations were published for 60 days under the provisions of the

Administrative Procedures Act. These proposed rules also referenced indirect carbon loads in the determining of the values of the standard.

A new organization, the Biofuels Interagency Working Group, was established by Presidential Directive by President Barack Obama. The Group consists of the **U.S. Department of Agriculture**, the EPA, and the Department of Energy. The purpose of this group is to encourage and improve the use and production of biofuel, including the crops used to produce the fuel and the development of the technology to produce biofuel from cellulose. This working group is exploring the blurred line between the production of food and the production of fuel.

There is growing controversy that the continued world deforestation, world poverty, and hunger, as well as other sociopolitical problems are aggravated by growing crops for biofuel, instead of growing crops for food. The development of technology that could use other renewable biological sources for the production of ethanol could solve those controversies, collectively known as fuel versus food.

There is discussion that the blend mix of ethanol and gasoline will rise from 10 to 15 percent. Current U.S. law mandates that 12 billion gallons of ethanol be incorporated into gasoline during 2010. This goal is widely known as E15 – a fuel that contains a ration of 15% ethanol and 85% gasoline. Reaching this goal or even exceeding it has implications for agriculture and the production of corn. Production of the corn hybrids most suitable to the production of ethanol will take that acreage out of food production. Even if E15 is maintained, it is anticipated that there will be several waves of litigation attempting to control or change E15. Some of the **litigation** will center on the carbon load of growing corn to produce ethanol. Other litigation will center on the reduction of food acreage. Still other litigation will deal with questions of equal protection and the subsidies for corn as opposed to other potential ethanol crops, such as sugar cane.

It is also anticipated that car manufacturers, already economically threatened, will bring protective litigation seeking to ensure that they will not be held liable for potential damage to old cars. There is concern that the engines of older cars will not be able to safely run on the ethanol blend.

Currently, the support of biofuels, once considered a clean source of renewable energy, has been tarnished by concerns that the growth of the raw materials to produce these fuels is less clean than the production of petroleum products. The agricultural toll of growing corn as the raw material for biofuel means reducing acreage dedicated to food production, which raises the cost of food. It also means that the need for fuel encourages deforestation in favor of farmland, impacting those who do not have sufficient agricultural land and also negatively impacting the earth. The fuel versus food controversy is integrally bound into the agricultural laws and regulations of the United States, as well as the rules of the EPA and Department of Energy. These rules have not always been coordinated toward the same end.

See also: Environmental Protection Agency; Farm Bill.

Further Reading Farm Policy.com http://www.farmpolicy.com/?p=1089

William C. Smith and Elizabeth M. Williams

EUROPEAN UNION REGULATIONS

The European Union is both a political and economic organization of 27 European countries. The European Union has developed a standardized system of laws so that people, goods, services, and capital can move freely from one state to the next. In addition, the European Union has a common currency, the Euro. Members also have common policies on matters that affect all members such as agriculture, fisheries, and area development. Members of the European Union currently include Austria, Belgium, Bulgaria, Cyprus, the Czech Republic, Denmark, Estonia, Finland, France, Germany, Greece, Hungary, Ireland, Italy, Latvia, Lithuania. Luxembourg, Malta, the Netherlands, Poland, Portugal, Romania, Slovakia, Slovenia, Spain, Sweden, and the United Kingdom. To become part of the European Union, a state must conform to the Copenhagen Criteria, which were defined at the 1993 Copenhagen European Council. These criteria include requiring a stable democratic government that respects human rights and the rule of law, a healthy market-based economy, and acceptance of all the aspects of membership. The European Commission acknowledged the importance of the agro-food sector to the larger economy in its "White Paper of Food Safety 2000." In 2002, the European Union established the European Food Safety Authority (EFSA). This is a separate and autonomous food law branch. It is responsible for assessing the safety of foods and communicating with the public regarding food safety issues.

There were several important cases in the history of the European Union's food policy. At its inception, European Union food policy dealt with the free movement of goods. Although food law encompasses much more now, there were several important decisions in shaping food law in respect to the free movement of goods. *Dassonville* involved Scottish whiskey being imported to Belgium from France. It had been purchased by French distributors. Belgian legislation required a certificate of origin to be made out in the name of the Belgian importer. This particular whiskey lacked the certificate. The final decision in 1974 in the case was that the Belgian legislation hindered trade among European Union member states. The case of *Cassis de Dijon* is also widely recognized as a landmark in the development of European Union food law. Cassis de Dijon, a French liqueur, contained less than the required amount of alcohol to be marketed in Germany. The courts found that the German restriction had no reason to exist. The only thing it did was restrict French liqueurs from entering the German market. French liqueurs usually have a lower alcohol percentage than their German equivalents. The court decided that as long as the product had been lawfully produced and marketed in a Member State, then it should be free to move throughout the European Union. Moreover, if Germany were permitted the restriction, then German products could move freely while French products could not. This case dealt with the concept of "mutual recognition." More restrictive states would benefit if this were allowed. The *Fietje* case ruled that a "provision which prohibits the sale of certain alcoholic beverages under a description other than one prescribed by national law to beverages imported from other Member states, making it necessary to change the label . . ." is overly restrictive. The *Kelderman* case dealt with brioches imported from France to the Netherlands and the Bread Act. The brioches did not have the amount of dry matter required by the Dutch Bread Act. The court found that where the national rules applied to "the importation of bread lawfully produced and marketed in another member state they were restrictive and incompatible with Article 28 EC." The *Rau* case questioned whether a Belgian law, which required that margarine sold at retail be cube-shaped, was compatible under European Commission law. A German company was trying to sell cone-shaped margarine in Belgium. The Belgian government claimed that the law was not overly restrictive to trade because margarine can easily be adapted to cube shapes. The Belgian government also claimed that the cube-shaped margarine protected the consumer from confusing butter and margarine, two different products. The European Commission ruled that the cube-shaped requirement was overly restrictive because it would cost a great deal to change the shape of the margarine and alter its packaging. The European Commission also found that the cost of changing the shape and packaging of margarine was greater than the benefit it awarded consumers, the benefit of preventing confusion. Moreover, the prevention of confusing butter with margarine could equally be accomplished with clear labeling. *Commission v. Germany* found that Germany was being overly restrictive by not allowing beer with **additives** to be marketed in Germany. The *Drei Glocken* case regarding Italian pasta rules was decided in a similar way. There were several more cases dealing with the movement of goods; however, all reflect a similar mindset of increasing the ease of trade among Member states.

"The Green Paper," published in 1997, recognized the importance of the international dimension on trade and economic welfare. It recognized that food legislation must be seen in the context of the international market. It also continued to recognize consumer safety as top priority. It recognized that food labeling can be a problem. It sought to both give the consumer information through proper food labeling, while avoiding unnecessary "detail provisions." In fact, this continues to be a major issue. In the 2009 European Union elections, voters were urged to consider, "How much labeling do we need?" The "White Paper on Food Safety" (2000) set a new approach to food law and policy, the "farm-to-fork" concept. This concept is also known as the "stable-to-table" concept. This concept recognizes the nature of food production as cohesive with each aspect dependent on others for success. The White Paper focused on the role of the European Union on food policy, but it also noted the importance of enforcement at national, regional, and local levels. The White Paper also noted that confidence on the part of consumers and trading partners was waning in the areas of food science, food law, and food controls. The European Union has said that greater transparency and openness are the tools to restore consumer confidence. Most notably, the White Paper established an independent European Food Authority. The food authority would be charged with issuing scientific advice on food safety, operating the Rapid Alert System for Food and Feed (RASFF), communicating food safety issues to consumers, and networking with national agencies and scientific bodies. In 2002, the European Union defined overarching principles of food law and established the EFSA. The European Union defines food as "any substance or product, whether processed, partially processed, or unprocessed, intended to be, or reasonably expected to be, ingested by humans. It includes drink, and any substance intentionally incorporated into the food during its manufacture." Medicinal products and feed are defined as different from food. Originally, food law in the European Union was based on the free movement of goods. Over time, it began to encompass much more. The food laws are created to serve the consumer and the consumer's best interest. Food laws are intended to support fair trade, to protect human life and heath, and to protect animal health and welfare, plant health, and the health of the environment.

Traceability is the ability of food to be traced from the farm, or origin, to the table, or final destination. It ensures that when there is a food safety issue, it can be traced and stopped at its source.

One of the main aspects of the European Union is the Common Agricultural Policy (CAP). Its goals are to increase production of farms, establish a stable food supply, ensure that farmers have a decent quality of life, stabilize markets, protect animal health and welfare, and ensure reasonable prices for consumers. The European Union attempts to accomplish these goals in a variety of ways. The "farm-to-fork" approach is considered a general principle in food safety for the European Union. It ensures a high level of protection of

Precursor to the European Union

The treaty that established the European Economic Community (EEC) was signed in Rome, on March 25, 1957. The countries of Europe determined that they could not survive another European war. With an eye toward peace and cooperation, the EEC, the precursor to the European Union, was begun with these simple words:

His Majesty the King of the Belgians, the President of the Federal Republic of Germany, the President of the French Republic, the President of the Italian Republic, Her Royal Highness the Grand Duchess of Luxembourg, Her Majesty the Queen of The Netherlands,
DETERMINED to establish the foundations of an ever closer union among the European peoples,
DECIDED to ensure the economic and social progress of their countries by common action in eliminating the barriers which divide Europe,
DIRECTING their efforts to the essential purpose of constantly improving the living and working conditions of their peoples,
RECOGNIZING that the removal of existing obstacles calls for concerted action in order to guarantee a steady expansion, a balanced trade, and fair competition,
ANXIOUS to strengthen the unity of their economies and to ensure their harmonious development by reducing the differences existing between the various regions and by mitigating the backwardness of the less favored,
DESIROUS of contributing by means of a common commercial policy to the progressive abolition of restrictions on international trade,
INTENDING to confirm the solidarity which binds Europe and overseas countries, and desiring to ensure the development of their prosperity, in accordance with the principles of the Charter of the United Nations,
RESOLVED to strengthen the safeguards of peace and liberty by establishing this combination of resources, and calling upon the other peoples of Europe who share their ideal to join in their efforts,
HAVE DECIDED to create a European Economic Community. . . .

Preamble to the Treaty of Rome (1957)

human life and also takes into account animal health and welfare, plant health, and the environment.

Genetic engineering has gained consumer attention across the globe in recent years. The debate is often seen as the United States supporting genetic engineering because the largest genetic engineering companies are American. The European Union takes a different approach to genetic engineering. Eight genetically engineered crops are authorized in the European Union for "feedstuffs." The approved organisms are four maize varieties, three grape varieties, and one soy variety. In general, the European Union's policy on genetic engineering reflects a more cautious approach. Although many in United States consider genetically engineered foods as safe and wholesome, the European Union believes these foods should be proven safe before they are put on the market. In 1998, the European Union imposed a moratorium on new approvals of genetically modified organisms. They cited a fear of long-term health and environmental impacts.

See also: Appendix 15: Uruguay Round Agreement on Agriculture.

Further Reading Holland, Debra, and Helen Pope. *EU Food Law and Policy*. The Hague: Kluwer Law International, 2004.

Stephanie Jane Carter

EXECUTIVE BRANCH AND EXECUTIVE ORDERS

The executive branch of the federal government is led by the president of the United States. The U.S. government is made up of three branches—legislative, executive, and judicial—that are established in their authority by the U.S. Constitution. These three branches of government each have powers and roles that are defined by the Constitution. And each has the ability to limit and check the actions of the two other branches under a system known as checks and balances. The purpose of checks and balances is to ensure that no one branch has an unbalanced amount of power.

The president, as leader of the executive branch, oversees the various agencies that are legislatively created by Congress. The executive implements the **legislation** passed by Congress. These agencies make and promulgate rules and regulations that are a form of law. These agencies also have authority to inspect and enforce the rules and regulations. Although the agencies must follow the mandates of the law and their mission is established by law, because the agencies are a part of the executive branch, they are also influenced by the executive. Thus the general mandate of the enabling legislation can be influenced by an interpretation made by the executive.

This can also work in reverse. If Congress is not satisfied with the rules and regulations of the agency, it can pass new legislation eliminating loopholes or establishing the proper interpretation of the regulation; for example, in 2005 when Congress amended the law to clarify the details of the promulgated regulations. A court case brought by Arthur Harvey challenging the regulations on ten different counts was not successful at the trial level. However, three of his counts were found to be supportable by the First Circuit Court of Appeals in Maine. The three counts overturned by the appellate court were addressed by Congress in the 2005 amendments.

In addition to the duty to see to the day-to-day operation of the country, the chief executive is also the commander-in-chief of the U.S. Armed Forces.

The vice-president and the heads of administrative agencies form a part of the executive branch. Should the president die or otherwise be unable to serve, the vice-president would succeed the president. The vice-president is elected. Votes are actually cast by the electoral college, thus an elected official succeeds the president in the official succession of power. The vice-president serves as president of the Senate, another interlocking aspect of the three branches of government. The vice-president does not vote unless required to break a tie in the Senate. The appointment of agency heads is a very important and policy-influencing role of the executive. Thus the secretary of agriculture, the head of the **Food and Drug Administration**, and the head of other government agencies are examples of the type of power held by the executive.

The cabinet is the group of advisors to the president who are agency heads. The secretary of agriculture is the first cabinet member in the line of succession to the presidency after the vice-president, the Speaker of the House, and the Senate President pro tempore. There are currently 15 members of the cabinet.

Presidents have been issuing Executive Orders from the beginning of the presidency. The first recognized Executive Order was issued in 1789. Executive Power is established in the U.S. Constitution in Article II, Section 1. Executive Orders are directed at executive agencies.

Executive Orders have been used to advance important issues in the history of the United States. The Emancipation Proclamation, for example, in which President Abraham Lincoln freed slaves, was an executive order. Many people have criticized the use of the Executive Order, claiming that Presidents use the technique to legislate—clearly the power given to Congress. But without the Executive Order the ability of the president to carry out the law would be compromised.

Governors have the authority to issue Executive Orders. These Orders have authority over the agencies that form the executive branch. States of emergency after a disaster, for example, are issued by Executive Order. The consequences of a state of emergency are defined by state law, depending on the nature of the emergency. But it will usually entail the calling out of the state national guard under the authority of the governor. A state of emergency can also allow a governor to contract for and distribute food to those in need during and after an emergency. Mayors also have the power to issue Executive Orders. Curfews issued after the declaration of a state of emergency after a local disaster can be a result of such an order.

Michelle Obama and the Organic Garden at the White House

Michelle Obama, First Lady of the United States, has begun an organic garden at the White House. In addition to starting the garden and sharing its bounty with school children, she has made comments about healthy eating and food security and food justice. The role of the First Lady, not officially a part of the Executive Branch, but certainly influential, is a constantly changing one. But if she continues to discuss the importance of healthy eating and influences young people to eat well, she may do more than any legislation can to change eating in the United States.

All Executive Orders can be criticized as an assertion of legislation by the executive, regardless of level of government. But without them the executive has no way to direct the agencies under his or her leadership. Ultimately it is a matter of balance and transparency. These will keep the executive in check, but should it be necessary, either the courts or the legislature can block an executive order under the appropriate circumstances.

See also: Administrative Procedures Act; Code of Federal Regulations; Court System; Food and Drug Administration; Organic Foods Production Act.

Further Reading Congressional Research Service Report, "*Harvey v. Veneman* and the National Organic Program: A Legal Analysis" http://www.nationalaglawcenter.org/assets/ crs/RS22318.pdf; Federal Register–executive orders http://www.archives.gov/federal -register/executive-orders/

Elizabeth M. Williams

F

FAIR PACKAGING AND LABELING ACT

The Fair Packaging and Labeling Act (FPLA) of 1966 sets requirements for product labeling and packaging. One of the goals of the act is to provide consumers with sufficient information to make intelligent and informed comparisons of brands. The FPLA requires that all processed foods be labeled to qualify for distribution. The law requires that the label have specific information, including the common name of the product. The name and place of business of the manufacturer, packer, or distributor must also appear. A content statement of the net quantity must appear. An ingredient list with the common or usual name of each item, beginning with the most primary ingredient and listed in descending order, is also required.

The law requires that all of this information must be placed so that it is noticeable, readable, and understandable with ordinary use and under usual conditions. Generally if part of the label is printed in a language other than English, the information must also appear in English.

Part of the rationale of the act is to give the consumer sufficient information to know the origin of the food. This means that the manufacturer must be identified with the name, street address, city, state, and zip code, all printed in English. Sometimes food is packaged or distributed, but not manufactured. In those cases the same information, name, street address, city, state, and zip code of the packager or distributor must be printed in English on the label. In those instances where the food is not manufactured by the entity on the label, the label must contain that information in the form of phrases such as "manufactured for" or "distributed for."

It is essential that the label reflect the net quantity of the food contained in the package. This information is not only required by the Fair Packaging and Labeling Act, but also by the Federal Food, Drug, and Cosmetic Act. The proper form of that quantity label depends on the type of food. The law requires that the quantity be accurate, and that it be either weight, count, or other measure such as volume. When appropriate the quantity of the food item should be given as drained weight, in those instances where the food is packaged in or with a liquid that is not considered part of the food, such as pickles packed in liquid.

It may be a good marketing principle, but the law requires that the common or ordinary name by which the food is known be prominently placed on the label. This name must be boldly presented parallel to the package when seen in the regular display format. If the food is further processed, for example, shredded, sliced, or pitted, then a word that describes this form of the food must also appear on the label, unless a picture of the processed food appears on the label or if the food is visible through the container.

The ingredients list should reflect the descending order of the ingredients by weight. They must be listed by their ordinary names, not by chemical names or other biological name. Each of the foods that form components of the processed food must be listed. Chemical ingredients like colorants or preservatives or other additives must also be listed as ingredients and with the same rules.

Some foods are characterized by a predominant and defining ingredient, such as shrimp cocktail. If the amount of shrimp is insufficient in relation to its other ingredients, the manufacturer may not be able to label it by its common name. Many foods are so defined in the **Code of Federal Regulations** (CFR).

Although preservatives and other food additives and colorants may be required to be included in the ingredients list, butter, cheese and ice cream do not have to list their colorants, except for FD&C Yellow No. 5, which must always be listed. Spices do not have to be individually identified, but can be listed merely as "spices." The CFR requires that certain specific flavorings and colorants must be identified, particularly those that are artificial. But others do not have to be listed by name, but only generically as colors or flavorings

The CFR specifies the nutritional information that must be listed on food labels. Just like other labeling requirements, this is intended to inform consumers so that they can make intelligent choices. Health claims, the various ways in which nutrients are listed, and other types of labeling regulations can be found in the CFR.

In 1982, as an additional requirement, metric units were required to be added to labels. This requirement does not eliminate the need to also give quantity in U.S. customary units, such as ounces, cups, and quarts.

See also: Code of Federal Regulations, Food Allergen Labeling and Consumer Protection Act of 2004, Labeling Definitions.

William C. Smith and Elizabeth M. Williams

FAIR TRADE

Fair Trade is the special logo that has been developed by the Fair Trade Labeling Organizations International (FLO). This international organization is a consortium of 24 other organizations with headquarters in Bonn, Germany. The organization is designed to promote the economic development of the people in countries that have been traditionally exploited by large agribusiness producers in developed nations. These countries produce agricultural products such as coffee and chocolate, which are sold internationally, but traditionally have benefitted the large producers over the farmers.

To achieve its goals, the FLO sets what it calls Fair Trade Standards. These standards try to ensure that the actual farmers and producers make a living wage and have sustainable methods that will allow them to continue to produce the product. The FLO tries to establish partnerships with those who will further develop and market the products to ensure that a premium is paid to the producers so that they can improve their lives beyond the subsistence level. The FLO has worked to produce a market for Fair Trade produced foods through traditional marketing and through appealing to the goodwill of consumers.

International Standards

The International Social and Environmental Accreditation and Labelling Alliance.

ISEAL voluntary standards setting code applies to "Fair Trade":

The Code focuses on the standards development process and on the structure and content of the standard. Key steps in standards development include:

- Defining the objectives of the standard and justifying the need for its development.
- Identifying affected stakeholders and providing them with information about the Code development process and how they can participate.
- Having public consultations and ensuring that there is a balance of interests participating.
- Providing a variety of opportunities and tools (i.e., teleconferences, meetings, webinars) for stakeholders to participate.
- Ensuring a variety of opinions are given equal weight and providing for balanced decision-making.
- Making the standard and supporting documents publicly available and reviewing the standard on a regular basis.

Requirements on the structure and content of the standard include:

- Having clearly defined objectives and ensuring that the requirements in the standard contribute directly to achieving those objectives.
- Ensuring the content of the standard is clear and unambiguous, and that it is relevant to the market and builds on regulatory requirements.
- Balancing the need to adapt the standard so that it is locally applicable with the desire for global consistency in its interpretation.
- Working to harmonize standards where their content or scope overlaps.

Source: ISEAL Alliance. *Codes of Good Practice.* http://www.isealalliance.org/code.

The Fair Trade Standards are both general and specific. They are general in that they apply to all agricultural producers and partners. However, because the products that are covered by the standards are so diverse, standards are set that are specific to each product. These products include flowers, honey, cocoa, bananas, coffee, rice, sugar, tea, wine, and spices and herbs. When a product is composed of a fair trade-covered product, there are rules that allow the use of the mark. For example chocolate, which includes cocoa and sugar, must use both fair trade cocoa and sugar to use the mark. Rice, on the other hand, is a single product and thus must be 100 percent fair trade to use the mark.

In addition to the positive requirements set by the FLO, there are prohibitions. The FLO prohibits certain types of herbicides and **pesticides** that are considered harmful to the growers, to consumers, and to environmental sustainability. Not only are the standards related to wages but also to the safety of workers and the use of child labor.

To be able to use the logo, Fair Trade auditors must certify that the fair trade standards are being complied with. The audit is conducted periodically in subsequent years to maintain the certification.

Those partners who buy and market in accordance with all of the standards set by the FLO are allowed to use the FLO Fair Trade logo on their packaging, label, and their advertising. The logo is a marketing tool for the seller and distributor of the product in that it allows the consumer who is interested in the philosophical and ethical standards set by the FLO know that a product is in compliance with these standards. The Fair Trade mark is used in countries other than Canada and the United States. In the United States and Canada, labels read "Fair Trade Certified."

See also: Food Aid to Foreign Countries, Tariffs, World Trade Organization.

Elizabeth M. Williams

FAMILY FARM IN BANKRUPTCY, REORGANIZATION OF

Family Farmer Reorganization, a type of federal court **bankruptcy** proceeding, is found under Chapter 12 of the U.S. Bankruptcy Code. Chapter 12 provides for the reorganizing of debts of a small family farm or family fishing business. It aids small family farms in reducing debts and restructuring payments. It can allow a family farming or family fishing business to continue its activities, even with excessive debt.

The Bankruptcy Act of 1898 was the first permanent act that provided companies protection from creditors. It contained no special provisions for farmers, except for involuntary bankruptcy proceedings. Section 75 of the Bankruptcy Act of 1933 provided some temporary special treatment for farmers, although it was limited in scope. In 1934, the Frazier-Lemke Act provided even stronger protections for farmers, allowing federal courts to reduce the amount of a farmer's debt to a level equal to the value of the property. This act expired in 1949. The Bankruptcy Act was amended in 1938 by the Chandler Act, which added the foundation for Chapter 11 bankruptcy and Chapter 13 bankruptcy. Created in response to the large number of bankruptcies filed during the Great Depression, it reorganized the nonexempt assets of financially distressed debtors. These amendments applied to farming, as well as a number of other types of organizations. The Bankruptcy Act of 1978 completely revised the Bankruptcy Act of 1898. It also created Chapter 11 and Chapter 13, neither of which was ideal for family farmers and fisherman. Chapter 12 of the U.S. Bankruptcy Code was created as a temporary measure in October 1986, following the farm crisis of the 1980s. The first bankruptcy measure that treated farmers differently, it was made permanent by the Abuse Prevention and Consumer Protection Act of 2005, also known as the 2005 Bankruptcy Act. This act also extended Chapter 12 protection to family fishermen. Fishing operations include aquaculture, catching and harvesting fish and seafood, and cultivation or catching aquatic plants such as seaweed.

Chapter 12 is often heralded as a positive measure for family farmers and fishermen. It is simpler and less expensive than Chapter 12. Chapter 13 was better suited for those with less debt than farmers and fishermen, particularly wage-earners.

Chapter 12 requires that the person filing be a small family farmer or fisherman. To be considered as such, the government has created certain tests and lists of criteria. For example, for an individual or married couple to qualify as small family farmers or fishermen, their income must not exceed an amount prescribed by the Consumer Price Index. Seventy-five percent of the debt must come from the farmer. Their gross income must come from farming and there is a test to decide whether it does. For corporations or partnerships filing, more than half of the stock, if any, must be held by the family. The family and/or relatives must administer the farming operation, and the farming operation must make up more than 80 percent of the value of the organization. The stock must not be traded publicly and there are restrictions on debt. Besides a continuing stringent list of requirements an individual or entity must meet before being considered a family farmer and eligible for bankruptcy under Chapter 12, there is also a requirement that applies to all those filing under Chapter 12—they must have a regular annual income so that they can make regular payments on the debt. That regular annual income need not come from farming and there are some exceptions made for seasonal farming or fishing.

Major issues in family farming include what is known as the Death Tax, which taxes the value of the farm after the death of the owner and requires the descendents to pay taxes that exceed what they make off the land in a farming operation. If the farm is worth more sold as a development property, the taxes are based on that use of the land. This often forces family farmers to sell the family farm or go into so much debt that they file for bankruptcy. Many theorists also argue that family farms suffer because of a farm policy that favors large, corporate farming operations and only offers subsidies for a limited number of crops. Although Chapter 12 makes it easier to file for bankruptcy, many theorists claim that other government operations make it necessary for farmers to file for bankruptcy.

See also: Agriculture and Livestock, Urban.

Stephanie Jane Carter

FARM BILL

The Farm Bill is an omnibus bill that deals with major issues of the **U. S. Department of Agriculture** and is passed approximately every three years. The Farm Bill affects almost all areas of agricultural administration including farm subsidies, international matters, the environment, and the way of life of agricultural communities. The massive Farm Bill passed in 2008 is valid for five years.

The current Farm Bill encourages a "green attitude." There are rules and regulations that provide standards and suggestions for the implementation of programs to encourage this attitude. This is a new addition to the policy making of the Farm Bill, but it also continues past policies. One of the great controversies surrounding the Farm Bill is that, once instituted, certain programs have become a way of doing business in agriculture. Terminating these programs, when business practices have been built on them, would have a devastating economic effect on agri-business.

Crop insurance, milk loss guarantees, and other guaranteed loan programs are examples of older programs. Critics claim that the reasons that some of these programs no longer exist, or if they do, the small farmers who may need them are too small to qualify for them. Yet the economic impact of revamping the Farm Bill in a massive way is also of tremendous concern, as it will likely adversely affect prices as well as supply.

The current Farm Bill includes funds for food nutrition programs, like **food stamps**, rural development, and soil conservation. It also extends federal **subsidies**. Federal subsidies are criticized by many within and without the United States. Subsidies are given to encourage the production of certain foods, such as grains. Congress, in setting food policy, determines that to properly control food prices and have an adequate supply, farmers should be encouraged to produce certain foods by being given a direct monetary incentive—a subsidy. It is recognized that supply and demand alone cannot ensure that there is enough food. And people must eat even when farmers find it cheaper to have their land sit idle than to grow food.

Today the Farm Bill authorizes spending of about six times more money in nutrition programs like food stamps than it does in food commodities. However, the money invested in food stamps ensures that federal dollars will be used to buy food, and therefore this spending represents an important economic component of the bill. That is, not only do food stamps feed the hungry, but they cause more dollars to be invested in the food industry. When commodity prices rise, there is generally an argument against the need for subsidies. That is balanced by the need to distribute money in the form of food stamps and in government-purchased food distribution, because the high commodity prices translate into higher food prices at the grocery store.

Advocates of the soil argue the necessity for a farm bill that addresses more than the economic issues of feeding those in need and ensures international grain sales. They advocate a longer-term bill than five years. They argue that subsidies encourage the development of practices by industrial agricultural concerns to grow for the maximum money, which includes subsidies. These soil advocates claim that by eliminating natural practices (such as crop rotation) and growing the same lucrative crop year after year, the soil is being destroyed. To compensate for loss of nutrients in the soil, these same businesses add petroleum-based fertilizers, which further damage the soil. Because of the desire to save money, inadequate tilling is practiced, further degrading the soil.

To repair this damage, advocates see that a long-range plan with monetary incentives that reflect a policy designed to protect the soil should be adopted through the Farm Bill. Agricultural run-off can be reduced by the appropriate policies as well as the reduction of soil erosion.

Another controversy that is embodied in the Farm Bill is the conflict between corporate and family farms. It is not clear what the policy of the Farm Bill might be—protecting farming as a way of life, maintaining an adequate food supply, maintaining an affordable food supply, or ensuring that those in need have adequate food to eat. The method of giving subsidies is currently beneficial to commercial farms, which are willing to do what makes them the most money in the short run. Family farmers, worried about the value of their soil, may not be able to qualify for subsidies if they rotate crops or raise the wrong crops. Current attempts to revisit the Farm Bill would limit subsidies sharply to those farms with sales of at or under $500,000. This is an attempt to allow subsidies only to small family farms and not corporate farms.

Other current issues are limitations in crop insurance and certain storage regulations on commodities. Cuts in subsidies to certain farmers are one change, but in addition the actual commodities that receive subsidies are under question. When there is a change in a farm bill during

---

Commodity Credit Corporation

The original Farm Bill was passed in 1949. This law established the permanent commodity programs. Each subsequent farm bill may amend those programs, but the effect of the change expires with each bill. If the bill is allowed to expire, there is a reversion to the permanent programs. The original bill established the nonrecourse loan, administered by the Commodity Credit Corporation (CCC). The nonrecourse loan works in the following way: a threshold amount is set for a commodity. If the market price of the commodity drops below that threshold price, the farmer can choose to surrender the commodity to the CCC and not have to repay the loan. Essentially the farmer can opt to force the CCC to purchase the commodity. This mechanism has helped stabilize commodity prices and has been extended to livestock and dairy products.

---

the period of its validity, farmers who have made plans for their planting based on the provisions of the bill can feel cheated. Had the bill not been passed they might have made different planting decisions. But once the plants are in the ground, it is too late to change plans.

One component under consideration is additional funds to the children's nutrition program. This program would add money to the Farm Bill for the specific purpose of purchasing additional fruits and vegetables for children's lunch programs. This would have the two-fold effect of increasing the amount of fruits and vegetables children eat, but cause a policy shift by creating demand instead of subsidizing supply. If this policy is adopted into the Farm Bill, farmers will know that the government will be providing money to purchase fruits and vegetables. With the anticipated demand, it is likely that this will encourage farmers to grow them.

See also: Farms, Corporate; Farms, Family; Runoff, Agricultural.

Elizabeth M. Williams

FARM LABOR LAWS AND REGULATIONS

All farms that operate as businesses must comply with employment laws and regulations as mandated by various acts of legislation, including the Fair Labor Standard Act of 1938 and the National Labor Relations Act, as well as regulations enforced by the Internal Revenue Service, the Occupational Safety and Health Administration (OSHA), and the **Environmental Protection Agency**. A few laws and regulations have limited application to only a small portion of agricultural employers and employees, but others are applicable to every agricultural worker. Labor laws and other protections for workers may apply to all employees, but there are special attributes of agricultural work that require specific laws. For example, agricultural work can be seasonal. It can occur in areas that are remote for food and lodging. It may be performed by noncitizen workers who migrate from farm to farm during the season. But the basic U.S. civil rights laws prohibiting discrimination based on the recognized protected categories of gender, age, race, national origin, and religion are applicable to all. The Americans with Disabilities Act also provides legal protection for people with disabilities. Although some of these laws apply to all workers, they have particular relevance to farm labor.

Immigration and Nationality Act

The Immigration and Nationality Act (INA) prohibits the hiring of undocumented aliens. Unlike some laws, the INA is applicable to all employers and is not based on a minimum number of people employed by the farm. Employees must fill out an Immigration and Naturalization Service Form I-9 for their employers to establish their legal status. Employers are required to maintain the Form I-9 for whatever period is later, either three years after the date the person was hired or one year after employment ended.

Federal Minimum Wage

Currently the minimum wage for all workers is $6.55 per hour. The requirement to pay minimum wage does not apply to all employers, however. It is only applicable on those farms where in any quarter during the previous calendar year the farm used more than 500 man-days of labor. A "man-day" is defined as a day when an agricultural employee does agricultural labor for one hour or more. When the farmer/employer is the sole proprietor, the 500 man-day test is not applicable to the immediate family of the farmer/ employer and the minimum wage rule does not apply. When the farmer/employer is incorporated or a partner or such, the law is fully applicable, to family members as well.

Workers' Compensation

Workers' compensation is designed to pay for injuries and occupational diseases that are incurred by employees while on the job. Compensation includes medical coverage. It is applicable even when the injury is due to the negligence of the employee. Workers' compensation grants payment to the employee for time when the employee is unable to work due to injury or disease. It provides for dependents when there is a permanent disability or death. Farm owners and operators are required to provide workers' compensation for all employees. Part-time workers, juvenile farm workers, full-time farm workers and seasonal farm labor are all covered by workers' compensation. Even family members who are employed by the farm are included under the workers' compensation umbrella.

Workplace Safety

The purpose of OSHA is to ensure the safety of the worker in the workplace. OSHA has established standards for the agricultural environment, including those for slow-moving vehicles, use of fertilizers such as anhydrous ammonia, and rollover protective structures designed for farm tractors. OSHA has established minimum standards of employee training. Machinery must be properly marked and there are standards for guarding and shielding machinery. The OSHA rules do not apply when the farmer is self-employed. These rules are also not applicable when only immediate family work on the farm. If other safety laws are applicable, they may supersede OSHA regulations.

Social Security

Social Security laws and regulations apply to farm workers. This is true of all farm workers including the spouse and parents of the farmer and children who are 18 years or older, as well as nonrelative farm-worker employees. Employees are subject to Social Security withholdings. Only the self-employed farmer and children under the age of 18 are exempt from Social Security.

Federal and State Income Tax Withholding and Tax Deposits

These same farm workers are also subject to federal income tax withholding. Farm employers must use an employer identification number. The Agricultural Employer's Tax Guide contains the withholding tables for use by the employer. Agricultural employers must maintain W-4s filled out by each employee. When they deposit payroll taxes, tax deposit **coupons** are necessary. The payroll taxes, which include Social Security taxes and withheld income taxes, can be deposited only once annually when they are up to $500. Where annual taxes are between $500 and $50,000, withholdings and taxes must be deposited every month. When taxes owed are more than $50,000, payroll taxes must be deposited twice per month. Agricultural employers must file the Agricultural Employer's Tax Return each year. Employers are required to furnish employees with a W-2 wage and tax statement by January 31 of the next tax year.

Unemployment Insurance

Because farm employment is seasonal, the rules for which agricultural employers must provide unemployment insurance are specifically defined. Unemployment insurance is a factor when an employer employs 10 or more individuals in each of the 20 or more weeks during the previous quarter or the employee earned at least $20,000 in cash wages in any quarter of the current year or the previous year. Any employment, even for only a part of the day, counts in determining whether 10 workers were employed in a given week.

   When the farmer/employer is a sole proprietor, parents, spouse, and children under age 18 do not have to be covered by unemployment insurance. When the employees' weeks' test or quarterly payroll tests are applicable, then employees of partnerships and corporations must be covered by unemployment insurance. The partners of a general partnership are ruled to be self-employed and not employees for unemployment purposes. Minors are also covered, except when they are children of a sole proprietor.

Employment of Minors

Many farm workers are under the age of 18; however, various state and federal laws are applicable to minors. In some states the rules are rigorous when the employer is unrelated to the minor. However, when the employee is the minor child of the farmer/parent, the rules do not apply. Where a job is hazardous, children under the age of 16 may not be employed. The rules of the U.S. Department of Labor are used to determine the list of hazardous occupations or jobs. Some states have also promulgated lists of hazardous occupations. The lists often include such jobs as driving a tractor or operating or assisting in the use of harvesting equipment. Other hazardous jobs include working around bulls, boars, stud horses, and cows and pigs with sucklings and newborns. Working with timber or scaffolding or using certain fertilizers or other chemicals is considered hazardous as well.

Independent Contractor and Employee

Employers must define the type of relationships they have with workers, either as employees or independent contractors. The Internal Revenue Service has 20 different determinants in making this decision.

Factors to determine whether a person is an employee or an independent contractor can include how much control the employer exercises over the person performing the work, where the employer controls the work and the way that the work will be done and the time and the provision of the means to perform the work, whether the worker is enrolled in benefit programs, and whether the worker is paid regularly or paid by the job.

Withholdings are the responsibility of the employer. Where the relationship is one of an independent contractor, the contractor must pay all taxes and is not covered by workers' compensation or unemployment insurance. In the agricultural setting, lawyers, accountants, veterinarians, and construction workers are usually considered independent contractors. More traditional farm workers are employees.

See also: Boycotts, Farm Bill, Strikes and the Food Industry.

William C. Smith and Elizabeth M. Williams

FARM-TO-TABLE PRICING

Farm-to-table pricing refers to the cost of a product once it reaches the consumer. The price often depends on the activities involved with the raw product between the time it leaves the farm and arrives at a consumer's table. This price can be drastically higher than the cost of the product at the farm. One reason for the increase in price is the concept of a value-added product. Value-added refers to the additional value of a product over the amount it was worth at its previous stage of production. Value-added costs include packaging, labor, advertising, and additional ingredients. Most of the money for a product is made in the value-added phase, which can be as simple as freezing, chopping, washing, and/or packaging a product or as complex as turning corn into corn syrup and then into a popsicle or soda. Typically, the farmer receives an average of 20 percent of the amount that the consumers pay for a product. This figure is even lower for producers of fruit and vegetables, who make as little as 5 to 6 percent of the amount the consumer pays.

Critics complain that food companies are more likely to focus on the value-added activities in food production, rather than promoting the consumption of fresh fruits and vegetables. What happens at each stage of adding value is more processing, which normally compromises the nutritional value of a food. It can be argued that not all value-added activities compromise nutritional value. Adding value could be adding **dietary supplements** to a product. Adding value can be as simple as cutting the fruit or vegetables, which arguably could make fruits and vegetables more marketable. However, the consumer cannot tell how fresh a product is when it is not whole. Moreover, once a vegetable is chopped, it requires extra packaging, which causes unnecessary waste. While pre-cut vegetables and pre-washed salad may be convenient, they cost more than the uncut vegetable and the unwashed salad. Most consumers cannot afford to pay someone to wash and cut their vegetables regularly, especially when these tasks are so easy to do on one's own. Critics of this type of value-added product also complain that pre-cut vegetables leave nothing for the cook to work with. Cut beets are missing beet greens, which can be sautéed and eaten. Pre-cut carrots may not be the size one wants to use. In the case of pre-washed salad, the salad needs to be washed again by the consumer. Adding value means additional handling, which can cause contamination.

A movement that seeks to skip value-enhancing activities is called the "farm-to-table" movement. The farm-to-table movement seeks to reintroduce the consumer to the local farmer. As a result, consumers are demanding more diversity in products, which differ from the products traditionally offered by corporate farms. Corporate farms have traditionally aimed to produce products that are uniform and efficient, often sacrificing flavor and variety in the process. When consumers buy straight from the farmer, the farmer gets to keep all of the dollars spent on food. None goes to the labor, packaging, and advertising involved in adding value.

See also: Additives and Preservatives; Advertising of Food; Children and Food; Diet Foods.

Stephanie Jane Carter

Farm to Table Mission Statement

Farm to Table is a nonprofit organization that encourages small farming and direct sales to the consumer through grass-roots activities and policy formation.

Farm to Table Mission Statement

Farm to Table is a nonprofit organization dedicated to promoting locally based agriculture through education, community outreach, and networking. Farm to Table enhances marketing opportunities for farmers; encourages family farming, farmers' markets, and the preservation of agricultural traditions; influences public policy; and, furthers understanding of the links between farming, food, health, and local economies.

Source: http://www.farmtotablenm.org/farm-to-table-faqs/.

FARMS, CORPORATE

The **U.S. Department of Agriculture** (USDA) defines a farm as "any operation that sells at least $1,000 of agricultural commodities or that would have sold that amount of produce under normal circumstances." In the 1950s, President Dwight D. Eisenhower's Secretary of Agriculture, Ezra Taft Benson, admonished farmers to "get big or get out." In the 1970s, President Richard M. Nixon's Agricultural Secretary, Earl Butz, told farmers to "get bigger, get better, or get out." Farmers complied and farms got much larger. Today, much of the farming land is owned by a few companies.

Critics of corporate-run farms cite drawbacks such as the possibility that corporations do not have a personal tie to the land and, therefore, are poor stewards of the land. Critics say that smaller, noncorporate farms often are owned by generations of the same family and are consequently managed in a more sustainable way. Another criticism is the tendency of corporate farms to become factory farms, raising livestock in confinement in large amount. Critics say that this causes pollution such as agricultural runoff, violation of worker rights, poor sustainability practices, and violation of animal ethics. They, in fact, operate like factories. The **Environmental Protection Agency** (EPA) defines certain farms as Concentrated Animal Feeding Facilities (CAFOs) in an effort to regulate the amount of pollution they cause because of the large amounts of animal waste. As fewer and fewer own more and more of U.S. farmlands, fewer varieties of animals and crops dominate more of the market. Monoculture is a word that is used to define the genetic similarity between crops and breeds. A farming culture that supports monoculture is usually concerned with large output, uniformity, and efficiency. These tend to be larger farms. The main criticism of monoculture is that it sacrifices flavor and variety to achieve these goals. According to critics, "monobreeds" of animals tend to be more susceptible to disease. Of course, it could be argued that it is the close quarters typically prescribed by factory farms that make animals, which may be mono-breeds, more susceptible to disease. However, it cannot go unnoticed that having too much of one thing can be the downfall of an otherwise prosperous society, as seen in Ireland's potato famine. Some theorists, such as ethicist Peter Singer, believe that monoculture will make the U.S. food supply highly susceptible to terrorists. Many believe that diversity is to be desired in all things. Moreover, 70 percent of the antibiotics in the United States are used not to treat human ailments, but to increase farm animal appetite and treat farm animal disease. By ingesting these antibiotics, the diseases they were formally used for evolve into more resilient strains.

Corporate farms that produce large amounts of animal waste claim that the waste is good fertilizer. This is true in small amounts. When this much waste is used as fertilizer, the ground cannot absorb all of it and it washes off into bodies of water, polluting them. Another argument by corporate farms is that their efficiency is necessary to feed a hungry world. However, the individuals often define a successful business as one that grows and becomes more financially sound. In some respect, corporate farms are the embodiment of this ideal in the farming industry. However, in cases where farms are used to grow animals for slaughter, the amount of protein needed to feed the animals exceeds the amount of protein that the animal provides a human, making a large animal production an inefficient use of land. Proponents of eating less meat argue that growing crops for food instead of animal feed would allow more people to be fed on less land.

Perhaps the argument can be summed up in terms of connection to the land. It is acceptable to own a lot of land. Many farmers make it a point to own land and farm it or treat it in a sustainable manner. Critics point out that the average number of acres in a farm has increased from 120 in the 1950s to over 500 acres now. It would be difficult to criticize a responsible landowner and farmer for owning and farming more land. The problem for some arises when the connection to land has been lost and the land is no longer farmed in a sustainable manner or treated in a respectful way.

See also: Clean Water Act; Farm Bill; Farm Labor Laws and Regulations; Farm-to-Table Pricing; Farms, Corporate; Growth Hormones; Humane Slaughtering Practices; Runoff, Agricultural.

Further Reading Foner, Eric. *Free Soil, Free Labor, Free Men.* New York: Oxford University Press, 1995; Headlee, Susan. *The Political Economy of the Family Farm.* Westport, CT: Praeger, 1991; McKibben, Bill. *Deep Economy.* New York: Times Books, 2007; Midkiff, Ken. *The Meat You Eat: How Corporate Farming Has Endangered America's Food Supply.* New York: St. Martin's Press, 2004; Singer, Peter, and Jim Mason. *The Way We Eat and Why Our Choices Matter.* Emmaus, PA: Rodale, 2006.

Stephanie Jane Carter

FARMS, FAMILY

The Economic Research Service defines a family farm as "any farm organized as a sole proprietorship, partnership, or family corporation." It excludes farms organized as nonfamily corporations or cooperatives, as well as farms with hired managers. Family farms are closely held (legally controlled) by their operator and the operator's household. A farm was defined in 1975 by the **U.S. Department of Agriculture** (USDA) as "any operation that sells at least $1,000 of agricultural commodities or that would have sold that amount of produce under normal circumstances."

The family farm system during the early 19th century has been defined as one "with enough land to support the family and no more land than could be farmed by the labor force of the family." A capitalist farm was a farm in which the family had more land than "they could operate and they did hire wage labor." Unlike in Europe, it was reasonable for the common person to desire to own land in the United States because land was so abundant and uncultivated. Another reason a common person could buy land was that the family farm community was able to win a struggle in Congress to continually liberalize land policy. The land was distributed in a relatively equal manner. The minimum parcel of land was reduced under Presidents Thomas Jefferson and Andrew Jackson so that a family could afford it. Today, the idea that a family can own a farm seems to be changing as an increasing amount of land is owned by large corporations. The defining factor of farm ownership in the United States was there were no heavy rents demanded by the aristocracy.

In the 1950s, President Dwight D. Eisenhower's Secretary of Agriculture, Ezra Taft Benson, told farmers to "get big or get out." In the 1970s, President Richard M. Nixon's Agricultural Secretary, Earl Butz, told farmers to "get bigger, get better, or get out." Farmers complied and farms got much larger. A lot of farming land is owned by a few companies, and there are significantly fewer farms. The 1980 Census Bureau did not even list farming as an occupation on its forms. In fact, many smaller farmers have contracted with large companies, which tell them how to raise their product. The farmers are not like the farmers of the past at all and maintain little of the control over the product and the land that once defined a farmer. In 1999, *The Baltimore Sun* described these farmers as "land-owning serfs in a feudal system." This is a major criticism of the "get big or get out" attitude and its effects on the family-run farm.

Corporate farms seem to have no personal connections to the land. Family-run farms are often passed down from generation to generation, giving the owners of the land a personal responsibility that is entangled in their past and their future. This responsibility is normally transferred to sustainable farming practices.

See also: Clean Water Act; Environmental Protection Agency; Farm Bill; Farm Labor Laws and Regulations; Farm-to-Table Pricing; Farms, Corporate; Growth Hormones; Humane Slaughtering Practices; Runoff, Agricultural.

Further Reading Foner, Eric. *Free Soil, Free Labor, Free Men*. New York: Oxford University Press, 1995; Headlee, Susan. *The Political Economy of the Family Farm*. Westport, CT: Praeger, 1991; McKibben, Bill. *Deep Economy*. New York: Times Books, 2007; Midkiff, Ken. *The Meat You Eat: How Corporate Farming Has Endangered America's Food Supply*. New York: St. Martin's Press, 2004; Singer, Peter, and Jim Mason. *The Way We Eat and Why Our Choices Matter*. Emmaus, PA: Rodale, 2006.

Stephanie Jane Carter

FEDERAL AND STATE LAW, CONFLICTS BETWEEN

Constitutional Powers Granted to the Federal Government

State law and federal law on a particular matter may be in conflict. This situation may arise in a number of ways. For example, there might be a change in federal law, resulting in a conflict between existing state law and federal law. If the matter falls under the constitutionally named powers given to the federal government, known as the enumerated powers, then a change in federal law that results in a conflict with state law triggers the need to resolve the conflict. Where the federal law differs from the state law, federal law will supersede or preempt state law.

Enumerated powers are those generally referenced in the U.S. Constitution in Article 1, Section 8. This clause is considered the basis of authority for the laws passed by Congress. In addition to this clause, the Constitution includes a clause known as the Supremacy Clause. This clause states that the "Constitution and the laws of the United States . . . shall be the supreme law of the land . . . anything in the constitutions or laws of any State notwithstanding." This clause gives these federal laws greater authority than laws passed by the states on these matters and allows the federal law to preempt the state law. This is referred to as the preemption doctrine.

Courts have recognized two forms of preemption: express and implied. When Congress passes a law that clearly is in contradiction to state law, the express preemption is not difficult to recognize. When the law is not directly contradictory, but merely has the effect of contradicting state law, courts may review the law and determine whether the federal law "occupies the field."

It is not enough that there is a contradiction; the powers must be part of the federally recognized powers, not a power reserved to the states.

An example of this rule is in the area of food labeling. Food labeling has been recognized as a federal function. If a labeling law, which may have a state law that mirrors it, is changed to require more stringent labeling or add new labeling requirements, the new federal law will preempt the state law. This rule of preemption also applies to local laws, such as those enacted by municipalities. The city of New York, for example, has enacted labeling laws for restaurants within its jurisdiction.

When a state or local government adopts legislation that is more onerous or stringent than the federal law, rule of preemption may permit the more stringent legislation to be enforceable. Thus, the city of New York can enforce its rules on restaurant labeling even when they conflict with federal restaurant labeling laws, by being more stringent than the federal laws.

The general rule is that when there is a conflict and the standard set by the federal law is a minimum standard, the competing law may avoid the doctrine of preemption if the competing law sets a higher minimum standard. Conversely, if the federal law sets a maximum standard, say in limiting **trans fat** in a product, a competing state law or local law can set a lower maximum standard within its jurisdiction.

In some situations, federal law specifically forbids state and local governments from deviating from the standard that it sets or in operating in the field.

Powers Reserved to the States

When the matter in question is one that has been traditionally reserved for the states to determine under the federal system of government, the matter is generally referred to as one of the reserved powers. The Tenth Amendment to the Constitution grants to the states the authority over those powers not specifically given to the federal government and not forbidden to the states. When the power over a matter is reserved to the states, the federal government does not preempt state or local law.

When Congress desires to impose a standard on the federal level in an area over which the states traditionally exercise their reserved powers, there must either be a constitutional amendment to change the law or the Congress must offer an incentive to change or a deterrent to not changing. An example of the need to adopt a constitutional amendment is Prohibition. The Eighteenth Amendment (1919) to the Constitution banned the sale of alcoholic beverages in the United States. Traditionally, control over the sale of alcoholic beverages was within the purview of each state. The Amendment was required to impose a single standard from the federal level on the entire country. And in recognition of the fact that this matter was still a state matter, the adoption of the Twenty-first Amendment (1933)—repealing the Eighteenth Amendment—specifically restates the power of the states to control the sale of alcoholic beverages. It allows the states to determine whether to allow the sale of alcohol, as well as determine other matters related to its sale. These include **alcoholic beverage control stores** and other forms of distribution.

The other method of imposing a federal standard on states that have competing or conflicting laws in areas that are traditionally reserved to the states is epitomized by the way the federal government handled the change in the **drinking age**. The federal government set a standard to raise the drinking age to 21 years. It enacted legislation that gave the states a deadline to amend the state law to adopt the drinking age of 21 years. If a state chose not to change the drinking age to comply with the new standard by the deadline, the federal government would withhold federal highway funds from the state. This is an example of using a disincentive to strongly encourage the state to comply with the desires of the federal government.

Conflicts of laws that are not conceded by the states must be resolved by courts, which apply the principles from the vast body of law known collectively as Conflicts of Laws.

See also: Appendix 1: *United States v. Fior D'Italia, Inc.*; Appendix 2: *Commack Self-Service Kosher Meats, Inc. v. Weiss*; Appendix 6: *United States v. Park*; Appendix 8: California Organic Products Act of 2003; Appendix 11: Bill AB 1437 Introduced into the California Legislature Dealing with Shelled Eggs.

Further Reading American Law Institute. *Restatement of the Law, Second: Conflict of Laws.* St. Paul, MN: American Law Institute, 1971.

Stephanie Jane Carter

FEDERAL ANTI-TAMPERING ACT

The Federal Anti-Tampering Act addresses the integrity of a product, with the safety of consumers in mind. Vandals or terrorists can tamper with products after the product has been safely packaged by the manufacturer without the manufacturer's knowledge or consent. Tampering is a crime, but the law also places a burden on manufacturers to package in a way that discourages tampering. It is thus a criminal act to threaten to tamper with a food product or to file a false report in which product tampering is alleged. The act mandates prison sentences as well as monetary fines for violations.

According to the act, a violation of the act occurs when the food product affects interstate commerce or foreign commerce. The interstate commerce provision of the law has been reviewed expansively by some courts and found to apply to sales losses or the need for an interstate investigation that results from the alleged tampering.

The act addresses food and drug safety and procedures that should be in place to thwart intentional acts of terrorism or vandalism. Other provisions regarding labeling and product packaging are monitored and reviewed by the **Food and Drug Administration** (FDA). For example, FDA anti-tampering regulations require that certain drugs and food supplements must be packed only in packages that are tamper-resistant. Product packages need to be "distinctive by design," and the label on the package should inform uses of the steps taken to make the package tamper-resistant. The purpose of the law is to help the user be more able to recognize a package that has been compromised, as well as to make the tampering more difficult to accomplish.

The law defines tamper-resistant packaging as packaging that has "an indicator or barrier to entry, which, if breached or missing, can reasonably be expected to provide visible evidence to consumers that tampering has occurred." The FDA gives examples of anti-tampering packaging. These examples include film wrapper seals often used when food is placed in a jar or bottle, tape seals used on soups and some drink boxes, break-away caps used on milk and orange juice containers, and foil or paper or plastic pouches, such as juice pouches.

The Federal Anti-Tampering Act was created in 1983 in

Tampering at Domino's Pizza

North Carolina has a tough anti-tampering law. Tampering is a Class I felony, which carries a maximum penalty of one year of incarceration, to knowingly make food available that may cause "mild physical discomfort without any lasting effect." In April 2009, two workers at Domino's Pizza in Conover, NC filmed themselves placing tampered food to be served to customers. One employee filmed himself placing a piece of cheese up his nose. The other waved a slice of sausage around his ear. They placed the film on YouTube. The video's "stars" were fired and arrested. The workers claimed that the video was a prank and that no contaminated food was served to customers. One worker pled guilty, while not admitting wrongdoing, and sentenced to probation. The other worker's case is still pending.

response to a 1982 incident in which seven people died of cyanide poisoning after taking Tylenol capsules that had been intentionally contaminated. Johnson & Johnson, the maker of Tylenol, was forced to recall $100 million worth of the product. Packaged food and food supplements were also included in the scope of the act. In more recent years the concern over food safety as an anti-terrorism measure has given even more meaning to this law.

The Product Packaging Protection Act of 2002 prohibits unauthorized materials from being affixed to the outside or inserted inside of packaged material in interstate commerce prior to sale to the consumer unless there is consent from the manufacturer, retailer, or distributor. The purpose of the law is to stop individuals or organizations with an agenda from damaging or altering food or drug packages or adding documents or other items to packaging to express a political opinion or otherwise comment on the product or a company's practices. This provision of the law was imperative because of situations where added items or altering of the package does not result in a foreign item actually touching the food. Before this provision, existing laws were not applicable to this situation.

The act was passed in response to several incidences in which people found offensive materials in packages of products that were purchased from the shelves of stores. This material was either pornography or stated political positions of those who tampered with the products. Because boxes can be easily tampered with, food in boxes, such as cereal, macaroni and cheese, and even frozen pizza, are often targets of tampering.

See also: Food and Drug Administration.

William C. Smith and Elizabeth M. Williams

FEDERAL CROP INSURANCE

Federal crop insurance is a form of insurance made available through the Federal Crop Insurance Program (FCIP). The FCIP is charged with providing tools to protect farmers against losses relating to agricultural commodities. Specifically, crop insurance protects against losses in crop yield because of disasters, such as drought, beyond the farmer's control; loss in value because of fluctuations in market price; and other adverse events, such as not being able to plant or a poor-quality harvest. Crop insurance is made available through the federal government under the Federal Crop Insurance Act, 7 U.S.C. 1501 et seq., Ch. 36. The purpose of crop insurance is to maintain economic stability in the agriculture industry and marketplace. The FCIP is administered by the Federal Crop Insurance Company (FCIC) within the **U.S. Department of Agriculture** (USDA), which in turn is managed by the Risk Management Agency (RMA) within the USDA. The FCIC is authorized to issue crop insurance contracts to producers on a subsidized basis to private-sector insurers to encourage private-sector participation in the crop insurance program.

Under a crop insurance policy, the farmer must be willing to insure the eligible acreage of a crop planted in a crop year. The reason that all the eligible acreage is required to be insured is to protect against adverse selection against the insurer. The insurer agrees to secure against loss the insured farmer during the crop year. Generally, the insurance pays out on a loss of yield higher than the deductible.

The FCIC was created on February 16, 1938, through legislation (7 U.S.C. 1501) passed by Congress to carry out the tasks of the FCIP, which was created to aid farmers in recovering from the economic loss resulting from the Great Depression and the Dust Bowl. Originally, it was created as an experiment and remained so until the Federal Crop Insurance Act of 1980. The Federal Crop Insurance Act of 1980 (P.L. 96–365) also expanded the program to include more crops and regions. However, the program was not as successful as the planners had wanted it to be due to competition from the free disaster coverage provided through the farm bills in the 1960s and 1970s. This act expanded the federal crop insurance to replace the free disaster coverage. Still, participation in the program was weaker than desired. Consequently, Congress passed four ad hoc disaster bills between 1988 and 1993. Desiring more participation in the FCIP, Congress passed the Federal Crop Insurance Reform Act of 1994, mandating the participation in the insurance coverage for farmers to be eligible for deficiency payments under certain FCIC programs. The Federal Crop Insurance Reform Act of 1994 also added catastrophic coverage. As an obvious result, participation in the FCIP increased with this act. In the mid-1990s, the FCIP became privatized so less government funding would be needed to administer the program and also to increase business in the private insurance sector. In 1996, Congress voted to repeal the mandatory participation requirement. The RMA was created to administer FCIC programs in 1996 as well. In 2000, the role of the private sector was expanded and the development of insurance products for livestock became unrestricted. Additionally, premium subsidies were increased to make the program more attractive and to encourage the purchases of higher insurance coverage. In 2010, a new draft of the

Standard Reinsurance Agreement, which is the financial agreement between the FCIC and approved crop insurance providers, began being drafted. The FCIC crop insurance contracts are found in the **Code of Federal Regulations**.

Some theorists believe that there is too little oversight of the FCIP. They point out that in 2005, only 100 people in the USDA RMA were charged with monitoring 2 million insurance policies. Others point out that the reason for expanding private-sector involvement in the program was so that the insurers would carry out some duties, such as overseeing the policies they manage. The issue in oversight is the possibility of fraudulent claims. The False Claims Act allows individuals to bring suit against anyone defrauding the U.S. government.

A new issue has arisen with the new draft of the Standard Reinsurance Agreement in 2010. The Government Accountability Office and the USDA have mentioned the discrepancy in the funds paid to insurance companies handling federal crop insurance compared with the number of policies. In 2000, there were 1.3 million insurance policies. By 2010, that number had dropped by 200,000. However, between 2008 and 2010, the amount paid to insurance companies handling federal crop insurance doubled. They also point out that banks often require crop insurance as a loan condition, making selling that insurance relatively easy. The insurance companies claim that the new draft proposals would cut the program by $6.9 million over the following decade, restrict the earning ability of insurance agents, and introduce "profit sharing" agreements. They claim that this weakens, rather than reforms, the program and limits marketplace competition. This, in turn, will make insurance agents less likely to write policies for high-risk areas, contradicting the intentions of Congress to make the program widely available.

Other issues include claims that the insurance policies may encourage growers to plant crops that require a lot of water in arid environments; that the program is too complicated and would benefit from fewer limitations on the products and the inclusion of insurance for farmers of high-risk specialty products; that it is possible to make a profit with the current program and the program should evolve into a cost-of-production program; and that unlike other insurance programs, the FCIP does not reimburse farmers for the costs associated with the loss.

See also: Agricultural Disaster Assistance Programs; Loans and Banking, Agricultural; Subsidies.

Further Reading Howard v. Federal Crop Ins. Corp. 540 F2d 695.

Stephanie Jane Carter

FEDERAL IMPORT MILK ACT

The Federal Import Milk Act (FIMA) was enacted in 1927 with two primary purposes. The U.S. dairy industry is protected and promoted by the FIMA. Importers of milk and cream are required to obtain a permit that authorizes the dairy products to enter the United States. The second purpose is to protect the milk-drinking public.

Before a permit is issued, several requirements must be met. Cows must be examined for disease and declared healthy before milk or cream from these cows can be imported into the United States. There is a specific requirement for a tuberculin test before importing raw milk or cream. Farms and processing plants must pass sanitary inspections, with specified minimum requirements. Milk must be inspected at importation and it may not exceed certain maximum bacterial counts. The importation and transportation requirement is that milk and cream cannot reach a temperature of more than 50°F.

If the cows that produce milk or cream for import have not been physically examined during the previous year, the milk and cream is deemed unfit under the law. Likewise, when there has not been a farm inspection during the previous year.

The act has come under attack from opponents because certain milk products are excluded from the application of the law. These exclusions are milk protein concentrate and casein. U.S. dairy producers say that because imports in general and specifically the importation and use by industry of those products that are excluded from the law the law should be amended to expand the umbrella of its protection. They claim that this protection is necessary because foreign governments are subsidizing dairy products that are imported, interfering with competition, and because some foreign dairy monopolies provide advantages in exporting. These excluded proteins and casein find their way into processed cheese and processed cheese food. Imported proteins offer producers these products at lower prices, thereby hurting the domestic market. Most of the domestic product has been used to make nonfat dry milk, which has lost favor with consumers. These imports are hurting the domestic dairy industry.

Critics charge that U.S. dairy farmers feel the loss of market with the importation of milk proteins. The requirements placed on the U.S. dairies make them uncompetitive. In addition domestic dairy product prices are dampened by the overproduction of replacement milk proteins and nonfat milk solids. Thus, there is a flood on the market and this further reduces market price for the product making the recovery from this situation very difficult.

On the other hand, other critics have charged that the FIMA is at odds with the free market, nonprotectionist practices espoused by the **World Trade Organization**. These critics claim that maintaining the current law risks reprisal by the WTO. Expansion of the law would ensure reprisals. In addition they claim that the enforcement of the FIMA is in direct contravention of the North American Free Trade Agreement. However, recent attempts to repeal the FIMA have been unsuccessful.

See also: Appellation d'origine contrôlée; Importation of Foods; World Trade Organization

William C. Smith and Elizabeth M. Williams

FEDERAL MEAT INSPECTION ACT OF 1906

The Federal Meat Inspection Act of 1906 (FMIA) requires inspection by the **U.S. Department of Agriculture** (USDA) when animals are killed and prepared for consumption by humans. All four-legged animals such as cattle, sheep, swine, goats, and horses are inspected. The law is designed to protect consumers from eating tainted or mislabeled food. The second purpose of the law is to protect consumer health by ensuring that livestock is processed under clean and sanitary conditions. This law is applicable to meat and meat products for import as well as domestic sales.

The act has a few general requirements. The first requirement is the health inspection of the standing livestock before the animals are killed. The animals must be individually re-inspected after they are slaughtered. Additionally the law sets minimum standards of sanitation at facilities that slaughter animals and/or process the carcasses. These facilities are subjected to USDA inspection to ensure that the standards are met.

The FMIA was enacted on the heels of the publication of a landmark muckraking work by **Upton Sinclair**, *The Jungle*, published in 1906. The work uncovered and publicized the unsanitary conditions in the slaughterhouses and meat-packing yards of Chicago. The book caused tremendous public outcry. President Theodore Roosevelt directed Commissioner of Labor Charles P. Neill and James Bronson Reynolds, a social worker, to make surprise visits to slaughterhouses. Roosevelt was incensed by the charges made in *The Jungle*, but he did not trust Sinclair, a socialist, and he wanted verification of unsanitary meat-packing conditions from trusted sources.

The meat-packing companies, tipped off before the pair could make their visits, engaged workers to clean around the clock for weeks before the surprise inspections could occur. However, when the pair made their visits to the meat-packing houses, they were appalled. The report they prepared, known as the Neill-Reynolds Report, confirmed the horrendous conditions at the meat-packing plants. Following the report, President Roosevelt began to support regulating the slaughterhouse and meat-packing industry.

The FMIA created the Meat Inspection Service of the USDA, which was later renamed the Food Safety and Inspection Service (FSIS). In 1910, the Meat Inspection Service created its first research center in Beltsville, Maryland, followed by seven other laboratories in various locations all over the United States. The labs were charged with inventing new tests and procedures that could detect the presence of disease.

Poultry Inspection

The FMIA did not apply to poultry. It was customary for people to purchase poultry either from a farm close to where they lived or from a store that had purchased the poultry from a local farm. This maintained poultry practices outside of the **interstate commerce** and thus subject only to state laws. This situation was found to be inadequate when in 1920 there was an outbreak of avian flu in New York City, which served as a major center for poultry distribution. After the outbreak, many municipalities implemented poultry inspection programs.

During World War II, demand for poultry increased sharply because of its availability and low cost. The U.S. Armed Services established their own minimum standards of sanitation inspection, because they wished to protect the health and safety of the troops as a part of readiness. Agents from the USDA regularly inspected poultry plants to determine whether operators were in compliance with its regulations.

In 1957, Congress passed the Poultry Products Inspection Act (PPIA). The PPIA paralleled meat regulations in that it called for the inspection of live poultry transported via interstate commerce, a second inspection of carcasses, and yet another inspection before any processing. Poultry from other countries was required to be inspected within the United States with inspection facilities established at points of importation. The PPIA also required that plant facilities be sanitary, that slaughtering and processing plants be inspected, and that product labels be accurate and truthful.

Other Important Inspection Legislation

As part of the Food, Drug, and Cosmetic Act of 1938, the practice of slaughtering animals and then transporting them to commercial plants for process was prohibited. Animals had to be brought alive to the slaughtering facility.

In 1946, the Agricultural Marketing Act (AMA) was enacted. It provided the USDA with the general authority to ensure that the food supply was safe and was what it claimed to be. Its powers included inspection and the ability to certify and identify agricultural products, especially those intended to be food. In 1981 the Agricultural Marketing Service was created and took over the responsibility of grading agricultural products, as well as identifying quality. The AMA also allowed the FSIS to perform laboratory and testing services on a voluntary basis for companies and organizations that requested them. The AMA also made it possible for the USDA to provide fee-for-service inspection of game animals and exotic food animals that must be inspected before human consumption.

Congress enacted the Humane Methods of Slaughter Act (HMSA) in 1958, amending the FMIA of 1906. The new law mandated that federally inspected slaughter plants adopt practices supporting the handling and slaughtering of livestock in a humane fashion. The law recognizes that animals are entitled to quick, painless deaths. They should be spared the anxiety of waiting for slaughter. This can be accomplished by stunning the animals to the point of unconsciousness before they are killed. The usual way of accomplishing the stunning is the use of electrocution and carbon dioxide for pigs and captive bolt stunning for other meat animals. Unconsciousness is achieved when the animal can no longer stand up and right itself, the "righting reflex." Once the animal is unconscious, slaughter can occur. The act provides exemptions for animals slaughtered in accordance with religious law.

The HMSA has been amended in response to the expansion of technology and the increase in production of meat. The enforcement powers have been increased to give inspectors the power to halt the slaughter line on the observation of cruelty in the treatment of the animals. The slaughter remains halted until abuse is corrected. The USDA has been consistently criticized for failure to enforce these rules.

Congress enacted the Wholesome Meat Act (WMA) in 1967, a piece of legislation promoted by consumer advocate Ralph Nader. The WMA is an amendment to the FMIA of 1906 that requires states to conduct more adequate inspections of meat not in interstate commerce, therefore raising quality standards. The WMA is referred to as an "equal to" law, meaning that states were given two years to develop meat inspection programs equal to those created at the federal level. If a state did not do so, the federal laws would be applied.

In 1968, the Wholesome Poultry Products Act (WPPA) was passed by Congress. Like the WMA, the WPPA mandated the coordination between federal and state agricultural agencies. It made the USDA the standard-setting agency, preempting the standards set by the states for both meat and poultry. The standards set by USDA regulation are applied by state agricultural agencies under the authority of the USDA. Should the USDA determine that a state is not properly carrying out the requirements of the law and regulation, or if the state does not develop and put in place a program of meat and poultry inspection and sanitation inspection, the USDA is empowered to step in and take over the state's duties. This is designed to maintain health and safety of all consumers and to protect the overall industry.

The 1970, the **Egg Products Inspection Act** was passed by Congress, which recognized the need to expand federal rules and standards to cover eggs and egg products. This is an extension of the control already established over the treatment, sanitation, and handling of poultry. It mandated that the USDA's Agricultural Marketing Service develop standards, conduct inspections, and continuously monitor facilities producing egg products in liquid, frozen, and dried form. In 1995, the FSIS became the USDA agency responsible for egg inspection. The **Food and Drug Administration** continued to have the responsibility for shell eggs.

Since the FMIA was enacted in 1906, inspection duties have been assigned to various agencies and have switched back and forth between agencies as needs and duties have evolved. When the FMIA was created, the federal government hired more than 2,200 inspectors for about 700 meat-packing plants. Currently, more than 7,600 inspectors are employed at 6,000 slaughter and food-processing plants.

See also: Appendix 5: *North American Cold Storage Co. v. City of Chicago.*

William C. Smith and Elizabeth M. Williams

FEDERAL TRADE COMMISSION

The Federal Trade Commission Act was passed in 1914 establishing the Federal Trade Commission (FTC). The Clayton Act, which dealt with antitrust laws, was also passed in 1914. Conceived by President Woodrow Wilson as an independent agency that could act against trusts and monopolies, the FTC, the trust buster, is an important consumer protection agency of the federal government. During its early history, the FTC was used to monitor trading with the enemy during World War I, and later was used by President Franklin D. Roosevelt to monitor certain New Deal activities. The Commission suffered from a great turnover of Commissioners in the early years, as the role of the FTC was constantly in flux. Finally after rule making through the **Administrative Procedures Act** (APA), the FTC was able to issue definitions and take public comment on its proposed rules and regulations. Its enforcement authority was finally settled also, paving the way for it to take action without a fundamental challenge to its authority.

In 1938 the Wheeler-Lea Act was passed, giving the FTC some enforcement authority. It allowed the FTC to describe unfair competition and "unfair and deceptive acts or practices" without having to show harm to competitors. This established the FTC as a consumer act, as well as an anticompetition monitor.

The Commission is made up of five commissioners who are appointed by the President and confirmed by the Senate. The President names the Chairman of the Commission who then acts as the chief executive and the chief administrative officer of the Commission. Commissioners serve for seven years, but their terms are staggered so that in any given year no more than one commissioner rotates off the commission. In some years there are no losses. In other years when a commissioner leaves the commission before the expiration of term, more than one commissioner may be appointed.to keep the number of commissioners at five.

The Bureau of Consumer Protection (BCP) is tasked with protecting consumers from fraudulent or improper business practices. The BCP does not monitor those consumer protections like food labeling under the jurisdiction of other agencies. However, any consumer fraud that might affect food, like sale of equipment, might be protected by the BCP.

The Bureau of Competition monitors business practices that are considered anticompetitive. This includes review of proposed mergers and acquisitions, and practices that may circumvent competition such as horizontal and vertical restraints. "Horizontal restraints" refer to competitors who agree to fix prices or engage in other activities that destroy competition. "Vertical restraints" refer to agreements entered into by people at different levels in the supply chain who arrange to limit competition.

In 1994 the FTC began investigating McCormick & Company, the largest supplier of spice to U.S. retailers, for possible anticompetition activities in selling its products for different amounts to different retailers. It was alleged that McCormick paid fees to certain retailers that were tantamount to a discount to these retailers. This would be a violation of the Robinson-Patman Act of 1936 over slotting fees in supermarket space. McCormick & Company is closely monitored by the FTC, because anything that McCormick does will affect the industry. The investigation revealed that 3 of 2,200 contracts over a three year period were flagged. Robinson-Patman allows suppliers to sell to retailers at different prices for various legal reasons, but when the supplier is doing so to kill a competitor in a price war and there is only one competitor, it is possible that a violation has occurred.

After four years of negotiations and investigation, the FTC and McCormick & Company reached a compromise settlement in 2000. There are several reasons why a company would seek a settlement instead of vindication in a lawsuit, if it thought that its actions were justifiable. One is simply the cost of **litigation**. A second reason is that litigation would expose business practices and other confidential and proprietary information. Finally a compromise settlement creates goodwill with the monitoring agency and usually results in a speedier resolution of the dispute. In the case of McCormick, the FTC determined that a workshop to explore the relationship between competition and slotting fees was in order.

The FTC reviewed the proposed acquisition by Whole Foods Market, Inc., of the Wild Oats Markets, Inc. Whole Foods, a retailer of organic and natural foods, purchased the chain of competing stores operating as Wild Oats Markets, Inc. The FTC brought suit against Whole Foods to undo the merger, claiming that it would hamper competition and create higher prices and less choice in organic foods. In 2009 Whole Foods reached a settlement with the FTC. It will sell 31 of the Wild Oats stores. These stores are located in 12 states. Whole Foods has also agreed to give up the Wild Oats brand. This settlement will leave 42 former Wild Oats stores with Whole Foods, stores that have already been absorbed into the Whole Foods brand.

In a similar move the FTC issued a complaint in 2008 against McCormick & Company for its attempt to purchase Lawry and Adolph's brands from Unilever N.V. If successful, the seasoned salt mixes sold under the brands Lawry and Adolph's would belong to McCormick. The FTC claimed that this move would be anticompetitive and would likely result in higher prices for consumers. McCormick and the FTC worked out a compromise settlement in which McCormick agreed to divest itself within 10 days of the acquisition of its Season-All line of seasoned salt to Morton International, Inc.

The FTC in both the Whole Foods Market, Inc., and the McCormick & Company cases was asserting its mandate to ensure that consumers have choices. It determines when and how to pursue its complaints by evaluating market share and projecting how market share will change because of the proposed merger or acquisition. The power of the FTC appears to fly in the face of the freedom to contract. In fact it does, but it has been determined that monopoly and anticompetition is a greater threat. Thus the FTC must walk the line between freedom and regulation and be able to justify that its actions are reasonable under its mandate and its authority.

One of the important functions of the FTC is to promulgate and enforce rules regarding the regulation of franchising and franchises. The law of franchises and their regulation is important in the field of food law because fast-food restaurants have proliferated throughout the country through franchising. Franchises like McDonald's, Taco Bell, Kentucky Fried Chicken, Arby's, and many other restaurants are regulated by the FTC. The FTC requires certain disclosure to prospective franchisees through the "Trade Regulation Rule: Disclosure Requirements and Prohibitions Concerning Franchising and Business Opportunity Ventures," or the FTC rule.

The FTC has the watchdog role of monitoring the limitations on advertising of alcoholic beverages. In particular the targeting of children has been a focus of their activities. The FTC has issued reports to Congress and has recommended industry self-regulation as a first method of enforcing the law. Only when self-regulation has proved to be unsuccessful has the FTC done more than issue basic rules. For example the FTC has focused on flavored malt beverages (malt beverages blended with spirits), which could be marketed to adolescents. But the FTC has found industry monitoring and self-regulation to be adequate at this time and has not recommended that Congress take any action on the matter.

On the other hand, the Center for Alcohol Marketing and Youth has criticized the FTC for praising the alcohol industry, claiming the advertising on television for alcoholic beverages has increased. Because the law prohibiting the advertising of spirits on television was passed before the rise of cable television, alcoholic beverage companies have used the opportunity to advertise spirits on cable television. The FTC did not recommend amendments to the law to close this loophole.

Another important regulatory function of the FTC is the oversight of advertising and marketing to children. The types of foods marketed to children and adolescents include soft drinks, breakfast cereal, and fast-food restaurants. Promotions include television, Internet, promotions related to movies, and promotional items, such as toys in children's meals. The FTC is currently urging more self-regulation in the area of advertising to children and it has not issued any of its own regulations with respect to children's advertising. There is concern that if the industry does not curb its direct appeals to children that the FTC will step in and create regulations and enforcement mechanisms that limit and regulate such advertising. The industry counters that it has First Amendment rights to advertise as it sees fit under the current law and that the FTC does not have statutory authority for actions against advertising to children. The FTC Commissioners have argued that Congress and the president could be supportive of new legislation that would limit advertising to children.

False Advertising

The FTC has the mandate to police truth in advertising. The enabling law is the basis for this authority. The FTC has promulgated the Deception Policy Statement, which covers omission of fact as well as an overt statement. The statement must not be misleading to a reasonable consumer. The law also details the evaluation of implied statements, which may not be overtly false but may leave the reasonable consumer with a false idea. Claims, direct or implied, must be based on solid evidence that is scientifically reviewable. The FTC has the authority to regulate truth in advertising, which may include labeling for some products, but not food. There is a line drawn regarding labeling of food which makes the FTC, the **Food and Drug Administration** (FDA), and the **U.S. Department of Agriculture** (USDA) loose partners in the monitoring, oversight, and enforcement of advertising, marketing, and packaging of food products.

Claims in advertising that are false are within the purview of existing regulations of the FTC. Recently the FTC took Kellogg's to task for its claims made in a national advertising campaign that included television, print, and Internet advertising that its breakfast cereal, Frosted Mini-Wheats, enhanced the attentiveness of children who ate it by 20 percent in clinical tests. The settlement would bar Kellogg's from continuing to make these false claims and contains record-keeping requirements that will allow the agency to continue its oversight of the situation.

A large area of activity for the FTC is the area of **dietary supplements**. Enforcing false safety and health claims in this area is a constant task of the agency. When an advertising claim is false, there is no need to establish that there was harm to anyone stemming from the false claim. There is no need to establish intent. If the claim is false, even when the advertiser has made a good faith error, there is a violation of law. The FTC has the power to use nonjudicial or regulatory means to bring the advertiser into compliance. In cases of good faith error, pointing out the error and requiring that the advertising stop, may be all that is done. The FTC can issue a cease-and-desist order and bring a civil court action. The FTC may obtain a court injunction to stop the advertising. The FTC also has the authority to order corrective advertising, with an admission of fraud or deception on the part of the advertiser.

Like other agencies, the FTC has a Web site that gives the consumer notices of its activities. Summaries of cases of false advertising are listed, as well as press releases that describe settlements and compromises with companies on the resolution of disputes. The FTC relies on its own investigations and observations, complaints and inquiries from consumers, and complaints from competitors to monitor false advertising. Although complaints from competitors may be inherently suspect, competitors have the most reason to monitor each other's activities.

See also: Advertising of Alcohol; Advertising of Food; Children and Food; Appendix 7: *In the Matter of McCormick & Company, Inc.*

William C. Smith and Elizabeth M. Williams

FEDERAL TRADEMARK ACT OF 1946

The Federal Trademark Act of 1946, also called the Lanham Trademark Act, creates the system for the registration of **trademarks**, trade names, and other identifying marks. The Federal Trade Mark Act is applicable to those trademarks, trade names, logos, and other symbols that are in use in **interstate commerce**. In addition to the registration process, the law creates a system of protection against infringement and interference for registered trademarks. The act provides for the enforcement of its terms against infringement, dilution, and false advertising either by the trademark holder or by the federal government. Before the Lanham Act, trademark was a common law protection. The law created a national system rather than the patchwork of state rules.

Trademarks are used to create an identity for a product. That identity or branding may take the form of a unique pictograph, symbol, or word or group of letters. This trademark makes it possible to recognize a product on seeing the symbol, word, or group of words. The protection of trademark can also apply to special packaging and labeling, distinctive colors or color combinations, unique designs of packaging or buildings, and what may be called the overall distinctive look of a product or its packaging. Only the trademark holder is allowed to use the trademark to identify its product.

There is a concept known as secondary meaning, which has developed in the law of trademark. Secondary meaning refers to something that is identified with a product, but that is not in and of itself unique. But with usage and the passage of time, the ordinary reference has taken on a secondary meaning that is an identification with a product. This concept is close in meaning to the concept of **geographic indicators**, which is a recognized and protected concept in the law of the European Union. Secondary meaning has also been recognized in packaging or trade dress. (Trade dress refers to the look of a product. It can refer to the product itself or to its packaging.) It is also possible to register and protect the identity or branding of services, as opposed to products. Such a protection is called a service-mark.

The act was sponsored by Fritz G. Lanham of Texas and thus bears his name. It was signed into law by President Harry S. Truman and it went into effect in 1947. It represents a modern view of the business utility of the trademark, and it reflects the importance of interstate commerce and the blossoming of the post

World War II economy. Prior to the enactment of the Lanham Act, there was a recognition of trademark; if a dispute arises that concerns pre-Lanham Act trademarks, it will be resolved in accordance with the prior laws. However, the Lanham Act brought together in one place all of the existing laws that referenced trademark and created a comprehensive law.

Despite the Lanham Act, common law trademark is still applicable when a mark is not registered. Additionally, most states have laws that protect trademarks in use within the state. These laws may also be common law and codified law. However, for a product that is sold in interstate commerce, state protection is not enough. Even when there is a long-established state usage and there is no Lanham Act registration, the registrant may be able to use the mark in all other states. Thus, national registration is very important in creating a product or service identity.

Registration under the Lanham Act and its amendments begins by an application for registration to the U.S. Patent and Trademark Office. It is not necessary under the act for the mark to already be in commercial use. In this way it is different from the common law. As are other rules and regulations of the federal government, the Patent and Trademark Office regulations can be found in the **Code of Federal Regulations,** Parts 1 through 7 in Title 37. Because a trademark must be unique, it is first reviewed by an examiner. If the examiner finds that it is unique and, therefore, unlike any mark already registered in its category, the mark is published in the Official Gazette of the Trademark Office. This publication will alert third parties of the application and the intent to approve the registration of the mark. This gives third parties the opportunity to oppose the registration if they find it to be confusing or too close to another already registered mark. If a decision by the Trademark Office is in dispute, there is an appeals process giving parties opportunity to provide addition materials in support of their position.

The genesis of common law trademark is to avoid and prevent unfair competition among businesses and to avoid confusing consumers. Instead of registration, common law trademark is established by usage. Besides the common law trademark most states have adopted some variation of either the Model Trademark Bill or the Uniform Deceptive Trade Practices Act.

The Lanham Act is divided into four subchapters: the Principal Register; the Supplemental Register; General Provisions; and the Madrid Protocol. Because of new developments in technology and mechanisms for identifying businesses, two new additions to the more traditional trademark law already have been created: one regarding intellectual property law and another that provides prohibitions against cyber-piracy.

Congress first passed federal trademark law in 1870 and amended that law in 1876. However the Supreme Court struck down the law in 1879, declaring it to be unconstitutional. There were two versions of trademark law that followed the decision of the high court, but they did not provide sufficient protection of trademarks and had little enforcement power. The Lanham Act recognized the types of trademarks actually in use in commerce. In addition it created an enforcement remedy that could be used by the holders of the trademark to protect themselves, allowing policing of trademarks to be the holder's responsibility and also in the holder's control. Finally the Lanham Act created rights in trademarks and for the trademark holders, which encouraged registration.

Although the law was enacted in 1946, it has been amended numerous times. Notably in 1988 the law was amended to allow for the registration of trademarks prior to their use. Such a change allowed for planning, but also made for protectionist registrations. This has been the most radical change from the common law concept of trademark since the enactment of the original act. See also Administrative Procedures Act, Food and Drug Administration, Interstate Commerce

---

Trademarked Characters Used in Food Advertising

- Jolly Green Giant, created for the Green Giant brand in 1928.
- Tony the Tiger, created for Kellogg's in 1953.
- Charlie the Tuna, created for the Starkist brand in 1961.
- Chiquita Banana, created in 1941 and first identified with Chiquita brand in 1963.
- Pillsbury Doughboy (originally known as Poppin' Fresh), created for Pillsbury in 1965.

Further Reading United States Patent and Trademark Office Web site: http://www.uspto.gov/

William C. Smith and Elizabeth M. Williams

FILLED MILK ACT

In 1923, Congress passed the Filled Milk Act, which banned the interstate sale of filled milk as a consumer product. Filled milk is reconstituted skim milk containing fats from sources other than dairy cows, like vegetable or coconut oils. Other filled milk products are used in such products as ice cream and whipping cream, but are filled with nondairy fats.

In the first half of the 20th century, milk as it is known today was not widely transported due to distribution and refrigeration issues. Filled milk was not considered to be popular as a beverage because of its unpleasant taste. But it is often used as a less-expensive substitute for evaporated milk in cooked or processed foods, like baked goods. Coconut oil frequently was used in filled milk and filled milk products, because it could be imported inexpensively, primarily from the Philippines. As a result, filled milk products containing coconut oil were able to undercut local products.

The act was passed partly as a protectionist law after pressure from the American dairy industry was brought to bear. The industry was facing fierce competition from foreign imports that were cheaper and plentiful. States became fearful of the loss of local industry and they joined in the protectionist legislation, banning and restricting sale of imported filled milk, as well as products containing filled milk.

The Filled Milk Act declares that filled milk "is an adulterated article of food, injurious to the public health, and its sale constitutes a fraud upon the public." The act goes on to prohibit the transport of filled milk in **interstate commerce** and contains penalty provisions if the law is broken.

In 1935, the Carolene Products Company was indicted in the United States District Court for the Southern District of Illinois for violating the Filled Milk Act, when it shipped "Milnut," a food made by combining condensed skim milk and coconut oil. It was designed to imitate condensed milk or cream. The indictment stated that Milnut "is an adulterated article of food, injurious to the public health." It stated further that Milnut was not a processed food, which would have been allowed under the exceptions provided for in the Filled Milk Act.

The Carolene Products Company filed a motion to dismiss, claiming that the charges were invalid because the law violated the U.S. Constitution. The defendant charged that there was no basis for the statement in the law that filled milk was unhealthy. In addition, the defendant claimed that because it was fortified with vitamins A and D, it was equivalent to regular evaporated milk. The Carolene Company argued that the Filled Milk Act was unconstitutional on two counts—it was passed in contravention of the Commerce Clause and substantive due process. The District Court for the Southern District of Illinois ruled for the defendant, and the Seventh Circuit Court of Appeals agreed with the ruling of the District Court.

In 1938, the Supreme Court ruled against the Carolene Products Company. Justice Harlan Stone, writing for the majority, stated that the health claims made by the Filled Milk Act were within the discretion of the Congress to determine, and it was not within the purview of the Court to second guess. The Court further held that there was sufficient evidence of the unhealthy nature of the product, and there was no basis to find the law unconstitutional.

Following the high court's ruling, several states struck down restrictions on filled milk. Despite the Supreme Court's ruling, the **U. S. Department of Agriculture** has failed to find filled milk products to be "in imitation of semblance of milk." Filled milk, including a popular brand known as Milnot, can be found in most supermarkets today.

United States v. Carolene Products Co. also is famous for a footnote penned by Justice Stone. Footnote Four, as it has become known, describes how the Supreme Court can interpret other kinds of regulation in light of the due process clauses of the Fifth and Fourteenth Amendments.

See also: Importing of Food, Interstate Commerce, U.S. Department of Agriculture.

William C. Smith and Elizabeth M. Williams

FIOR D'ITALIA V. UNITED STATES

Fior D'Italia claims to be the oldest Italian restaurant in America, founded in 1886 in San Francisco. The restaurant became the plaintiff in a lawsuit against the Internal Revenue Service (IRS) in a case that changed the way restaurants all over the United States reported tip wages, Federal Insurance Contributions Act (FICA) taxes, or Social Security taxes on tip wages.

Although a previous case established that restaurants and other employers of tipped employees had to pay FICA taxes on the tipped income, the restaurants paid the FICA taxes on what the IRS deemed to be under-reported tip income. The under-reporting was not being done by the restaurant, but by the tipped employees. Ultimately the Supreme Court of the United States posed the legal question whether the IRS could base the restaurant's assessment on the total amount of tips paid by the restaurant or the reevaluation of the tips paid by each individual employee.

In 1991 the Fior D'Italia's employees reported tip income of $247,181 and in 1992 they reported tip income of $220,845. In accordance with the law, the restaurant submitted FICA taxes based on the income reported by its employees. However, the IRS believed that, based on the income of the restaurant, the employees had under-reported their tips. According to credit card records kept by the restaurant, the patrons paid $364,786 and $338,161 in tips during the same years. Because of the difference in the restaurant's records and the reporting of the employees, the IRS determined that the restaurant had underpaid FICA taxes and assessed the restaurant the additional taxes.

To determine a reasonable estimate of the true total of tips left by patrons, the IRS calculated the average percentage of tips, based on the tips indicated on credit card receipts. Then it applied that same percentage to the total of the cash-paying patrons. The IRS then added the credit card tips and the percentage (approximately 14 percent) of cash totals to find the total amount of tip income paid to all of the tipped employees. This is called an "aggregate estimation." This aggregated figure is the amount that the government used to make its determination of the corrected FICA assessment.

The discrepancy was quite large. In 1991, $403,726 was the total of tipped income calculated by the IRS, that is, the total of tips reported on credit card receipts and the estimated tips that would have been paid by patrons who paid cash. This number is in contrast to the $247, 181 reported by tipped employees. A discrepancy also existed in the reported and aggregated tips for 1992. The IRS assessed Fior D'Italia $11,976 for unpaid taxes.

Although the restaurant paid the assessment, it claimed that the IRS owed it a refund and brought an action in court to collect the refund. The basis for the lawsuit was that the law does not support the use of aggregate estimation in determining taxes owed by the restaurant, since the aggregate estimation was on income earned and under-reported by the employees. Rather the IRS should make an assessment of the under-reporting by each employee individually and then determine the underpayment of the FICA tax. The District Court determined that there was no statutory basis for the use of this method of aggregate estimation, bypassing the individual determination of underpayment, finding for Fior D'Italia. The Court of Appeals affirmed the decision of the trial court. It found that the IRS would have to adopt rules that would allow it to apply the aggregate estimation method.

Because the various circuit courts had taken different positions on this point, the Supreme Court agreed to grant writs of certiorari to review the matter. On review, the high court reversed the two lower courts.

The Supreme Court found that the law, 26 U.S.C. section 6201(a), authorizes the IRS to make assessments of taxes owed but not paid. The method of determining the proper amount owed in this case was considered by the high court to be within the reasonable expectation of the law. The method selected was reasonable and defendable. The restaurant argued that the law specifically stated that FICA tax was to be paid on the amount earned by employees individually, thus the IRS must determine each person's true tipped wages, not make a mass estimate.

The Supreme Court found the restaurant's argument to be hair splitting, based not on the meaning of the law, but its grammar. In addition the "linguistic argument" was not even properly applied, according to the high court, because the language selected by the restaurant was found in the definition sections, not the actual substantive sections.

The Supreme Court also looked at the reasoning of the lower courts, which considered that if the IRS had used this method for determining income tax, it might be permissible. It found the use of this method for determining FICA tax to be improper. The high court rejected this distinction. In general, the high court found that the IRS acted reasonably and there was no reason to impose limitations on the reasonable actions of the IRS

Ultimately, this case stopped the tipped worker from being able to under-report income, by making the restaurants more carefully report tipped income themselves, to protect themselves from the underpayment of taxes of all sorts. The use of credit cards and the practice of leaving a tip on credit cards may mean that the patron may leave a larger tip, but it also means that there is a record of it. By correcting any underpayment, the IRS would not assess a penalty. If the restaurant cannot rely on the statements of its employees, then the restaurants must rely on their own records. Fewer and fewer restaurants are operating on a cash-only basis, making the under-reporting of tips more difficult.

There were a few other minor arguments made by the restaurant: that the IRS did not allow a discount for credit card commissions, they did not take into consideration that cash tips are usually less than credit card tips, and there was no general discount for those times when no tip had been paid. The high court simply rejected these arguments as minor and not making the entire process unreasonable.

See also: Court System; Appendix 1: *United States v. Fior D'Italia, Inc.*

Elizabeth M. Williams

FISH FARMING

Fish farming is a form of commercial aquaculture that raises fish in tanks or enclosures for food or other purposes. Intensive fish farming relies on an external food supply. Extensive fish farming uses local photosynthetical production for the food supply for the fish. Semi-intensive and super-intensive methods are also used. Within these types of fish farming are several more categories. Types of fish and seafood that are farmed include tilapia, shrimp, carp, salmon, catfish, sea bream, cobia, sturgeon, arctic char, perch, mussels, clams, trout, oysters, scallops, and conch. In 1970, fish farming accounted for 3.9 percent of the total amount of fish sold by weight. By 2000, fish farming accounted for 27.3 percent of those fish. Aquaculture is the fastest growing form of food production. According to one account, about 98 percent of all Atlantic salmon is farm-raised in countries including Chile, Canada, and Norway.

The aquaculture industry in the United States is regulated by many government sectors. The **Environmental Protection Agency** (EPA) established effluent limitations guidelines (ELGs) for aquaculture on June 30, 2004. The EPA has this power through the **Clean Water Act**. The EPA refers to aquaculture as concentrated aquatic animal production (CAAP). The guidelines aim to reduce pollution in U.S. waters and only apply to those CAAP facilities that create wastewater and deposit it into U.S. waters. Specifically, these facilities use systems that flow-through, re-circulate, or have net pens. They deposit unprocessed water and generate a minimum of 100,000 pounds of fish a year. Fish farms pollute waters with solid waste, nutrients, drugs which maintain the health of the fish, and cleaning products that maintain sanitary conditions in tanks and nets. The **U.S. Department of Agriculture** (USDA) has several units that focus on aquaculture. The Agricultural Research Service of the USDA conducts research to further the competitiveness and sustainability of U.S. aquaculture. The Animal and Plant Health Inspection Service provides programs on topics, such as global trade, aquatic diseases, pest prevention, and wildlife damage management, aimed at protecting the health of aquatic animals and plants. The USDA also provides an economic research service that reports on U.S. aquaculture production, its history, and its trade status. The National Agriculture Statistics Service publishes statistical reports and a census on aquaculture. The Center for Food Safety and Applied Nutrition focuses on drugs used in the aquaculture industry. It also provides information on Seafood **Hazard Analysis Critical Control Point** (HAACP). The HAACP plans are recommended or required for many industries, including individual restaurants. Seafood HAACP will help identify where a hazardous aquatic animal originated and where it was shipped, so as to mitigate the consequences of food-borne illnesses. The Center for Veterinary Medicine regulates drugs, devices, and food additives used in aquaculture. Other government agencies, such as the Joint Subcommittee on Aquaculture and the U.S. **Department of Health and Human Services**, are also involved in the aquaculture industry. Not all countries regulate aquaculture as much as the United States does. For this reason, consumers are encouraged to be wary of where seafood was farmed and what practices may, or may not, have been used. In several instances, it has been found that the Ramsar Convention, an international agreement signed by 141 countries to protect wetlands, has been violated.

There are several methods of fish farming, depending on the needs of the animals. Fish can be raised in open net pens or cages. They can be managed in ponds. Raceways and re-circulating systems are yet another method. Shellfish culture is another special method used for stationary mollusks. Open net pens and cages can be located near the coast in open water or in inland lakes. Most farm-raised salmon and tuna are farmed by this method. Many shrimp, catfish, and tilapia are raised in ponds. Ponds can be natural or human-made and hold fish in an inland body of fresh water or in open salt water near the coast. Rainbow trout are usually farmed in raceway habitats. Raceways are created by channeling water from an existing running source like a well or stream. The diverted water runs through the raceway where the fish are stocked, so that it looks like a water raceway. The government has established regulations to control the water quality of the near-by bodies of water. Re-circulating systems use enclosed fish tanks. Water is treated and re-circulated through the system. Shellfish culture is the method by which aquaculturalists raise shellfish on artificial reefs and suspend them in the water on various devices that allow water to flow around them. The animals raised with this method feed from the nutrients in the water that passes around and through them and they require no extra feeding.

Proponents of fish farming argue that it is a reasonable alternative to depleting the wild species. Although over-fishing has caused a large amount of alarm, farmed fish are not without issues. Each fish farming method raises concern among many critics. The most historically damaging and oldest form of commercial aquaculture, shellfish farming, has created an environment in which native species have been out-paced by foreign species with few native enemies. They use up natural resources and kill off native species. Re-circulating systems are lauded by many as the most sustainable method of fish farming. Fish cannot escape, so they will not interbreed with wild species or introduce disease and pests to the wild species. Also the wastewater is treated, preventing much of the pollution that critics of fish farming often cite. However, re-circulating systems may be prohibitively expensive for many to operate. Since so many fish are available for little cost, it is difficult to compete and recover the cost of the re-circulating system for some. Raceways create environmental concern because the fish can potentially escape, creating the possibility of interbreeding and thus compromising the wild species. Ponds also create alarm among environmentalists. Shrimp ponds constructed in mangrove forests have been responsible for the destruction of 3.7 million acres of coastal habitat formerly relied on by fish, birds, and human beings. The surrounding area can be polluted by untreated wastewater. Net pens and cages allow waste to pass freely from the fish into the surrounding environment. Because the fish are kept densely packed, a large amount of waste is created. It pollutes the surrounding water. This is similar to the issues of agricultural run-off in some forms of farming on land, such as in raising cattle in large quantities. Another issue with the open nets and cages is that the fish can escape. Because they are kept densely packed, they are more susceptible to diseases and parasites and can spread these among the wild species. Also, the farmed fish can interbreed with the wild fish, changing their genetic make-up.

In the aquaculture industry, shrimp farming is the fastest growing. Since the late 1990s, the amount of farm-raised shrimp has grown 400 percent. Thailand, Ecuador, Indonesia, the Philippines, and India produce most of the farm-raised shrimp. India led the shrimp farming industry in the 1990s. Because shrimp farming can harm the livelihoods and homes of humans living in coastal regions, Indian activists brought a class action lawsuit against the shrimp farming industry. Citing the pollution caused by fish farming, the Supreme Court of India ordered in 1996 that thousands of shrimp farms be destroyed. They also ruled that compensation be paid to workers who lost their livelihoods as a result of shrimp farming. In Bangladesh, there have been protests and violence over villagers displaced by the shrimp farming industry. The main markets for farm-raised shrimp are the United States, Japan, and Europe.

Salmon is another controversial farmed aquatic creature. According to data, for every 300 farmed salmon that are sold, only one is caught swimming freely in the wild. Moreover, as salmon are carnivorous, fish must be caught for them to eat. Some argue that this makes salmon farming inefficient. Some fish, such as tilapia, do not require meat or fish products in their diets.

Crawfish Farming

Until the late 1970s and early 1980s crawfish, or crayfish, were rarely eaten out of the spring-to-summer season. If one was not from the bayous around Lafayette, Louisiana, crawfish were exotic. After the advent of commercially viable crawfish farming, crawfish were available in a much wider area. At the World Exposition of 1984, travel and food writers ate crawfish in the Louisiana Pavilion; they then wrote about the availability of crawfish, manifested in many dishes, and helped Cajun cuisine explode on the American scene.

Proponents of fish farming note that they create a superior product because the fish can be quickly frozen, preserving freshness. However, farmed fish are kept in such tight conditions that they need numerous antibiotics and **pesticides**. In some instances, each fish has a space about the size of a bathtub in which to live. Fish, such as salmon, naturally spend their whole lives swimming freely over large distances. In fact, their entire lives are a trip from the place of their birth into the ocean and back to the place of their birth to spawn and die. Keeping them in dense conditions may cause a large amount of stress on the fish. The crowded conditions also mean that the fish have injures from rubbing against other fish. In the case of salmon farming, the fish must be fed artificial coloring so that their fish turns pink. Wild salmon have pink flesh because they eat krill. These factors must be considered when considering "superior products."

The fact is that people are eating more fish. This may be because it is considered healthy, because it is no longer so expensive, or simply because the world population is growing. While some fish farming can be a sustainable practice, it is far from being the norm. The sustainable practices cost more money, increasing the cost of the product. The low cost of the current product may encourage people to eat more than is sustainable.

See also: Runoff, Agricultural.

Stephanie Jane Carter

FOIE GRAS, BANS ON

In recent years, many municipalities in the United States as well as numerous countries have adopted or are considering adoption of laws that ban the delicacy known as foie gras, or goose liver pâté. Foie gras is the fattened liver of a duck or goose. It is produced by force-feeding ducks and geese during a two-week period before slaughter. The process takes advantage of the way in which ducks and geese store

Foie Gras in Ancient Egypt

The ancient Egyptians are said to have enjoyed foie gras. They took advantage of the natural tendency of ducks and geese to gorge themselves prior to migration. Dan Barber, chef of the restaurant at the Stone Barns Center for Food and Agriculture in Pocantico, New York, has spotlighted a farmer in Spain, Eduardo Sousa, who raises geese and produces so-called cruelty-free foie gras. Sousa won the International Food Salon prize in 2006 for his product Foie Gras—an ancient Egyptian delicacy—made from geese that feed on figs and olives.

fat in their livers prior to their winter migrations, in what is known as a pre-migratory gorge.

Foie gras is controversial because it involves a process known as gavage, which means "to gorge." During gavage, a tube is placed down the throat of the animals to receive a larger than normal mixture of corn boiled with fat to aid digestion. Birds do not reject the mixture because they have no gag reflex. The corn and fat mixture deposits a significant amount of fat to the liver, producing the buttery flavor sought by chefs and foodies. Foie gras is considered an expensive luxury dish.

Every major animal rights group, including People for the Ethical Treatment of Animals and the Humane Society of the United States, has condemned the manufacture of foie gras as cruel treatment of animals. The controversy has led to bans in some countries and municipalities.

The Chicago City Council voted in 2006 to ban the sale of foie gras and created fines of $250 to $500 for those who violated the ban. The council created the ban on the basis of animal cruelty perceptions. As a result of the action by the City Council several Chicago chefs filed suit to challenge the law and deliberately flaunted the law by selling foie gras. The city issued warning letters but no citations. One restaurant—a gourmet hot dog shop—was cited for violation of the law; the owner paid a $250 fine. Chicago Mayor Richard Daley called the ordinance "the silliest law" the council had ever passed. The city council repealed the ban in 2008.

In 2003, two California animal rights organizations brought an action against Sonoma Foie Gras in California alleging violation of the state's unfair business practices law, citing cruelty to animals. The California State Legislature intervened by passing a law that allows the business to practice gavage until the year 2012. After 2012, assuming that there is no additional change to the law, the sale and production of foie gras will become prohibited in the state of California.

The legislatures of other states—Oregon, Massachusetts, Washington, Connecticut, Hawaii, Maryland, New York, Illinois and Pennsylvania—have considered enacting bans on the production of foie gras or its sale. To date, none of these states has enacted such laws.

In the European Union, foie gras production is prohibited by treaty. There is an exception "where it is current practice." The applicable treaty is the Convention for the Protection of Animals kept for Farming Purposes. There are 35 signatory countries. The force-feeding of animals, including gavage, is prohibited in the Czech Republic, Denmark, Finland, Germany, Italy, Luxembourg, Norway, Poland, Ireland, Sweden, Switzerland, the Netherlands, the United Kingdom, and most of Austria. Though foie gras cannot be produced in these countries, it can be imported and purchased. Due to anticruelty laws that prohibit forced feeding of animals, foie gras cannot be produced in Turkey, Israel, or Argentina. In the past decade, the number of European countries that produce foie gras has been reduced by half. Five countries continue to produce foie gras. They are Belgium, Bulgaria, Spain, France, and Hungary.

See also: Appellation d'origine contrôlée, Legislation.

Further Reading "Welfare Aspects of the Production of Foie Gras in Ducks and Geese" Report of the EU Scientific Committee on Animal Health and Animal Welfare (1998) http://ec.europa.eu/food/fs/sc/scah/out17_en.pdf

William C. Smith and Elizabeth M. Williams

FOOD AID TO FOREIGN COUNTRIES

Food aid is internationally sourced food donations given to a country in need. The food aid program in the United States is extraordinarily complex, involving farmers, manufacturers, shippers, and numerous other entities on one side and nongovernmental and governmental organizations on the recipient side. It entails numerous national and international partnerships and a number of U.S. government entities, including the Secretary of the **U.S. Department of Agriculture** (USDA) and Foreign Agricultural Services Chair of the Interagency Food Assistance Policy Council (FAPC), which organizes food aid policies and programs. Representatives from the Office of Management and Budget, the U.S. Agency for International Development (USAID), the U.S. State Department, the National Security Council, and the USDA all make up FAPC. Additionally, the Department of Transportation is involved for the reimbursement of portions of shipping costs incurred through the transport of foodstuffs. U.S. food aid is authorized under three titles of P.L. 480, which is known as Food for Peace. Currently, Title II is the primary source of U.S. food aid shipments, whereas Title I had been the primary source for the first 30 years of the program. Title III funding was discontinued in 1999 but remains in existence if it becomes necessary. Congress funds the programs through annual and supplemental appropriations. Generally, there are three categories of food aid: program, project, and emergency or relief aid. "Program" aid is an intergovernmental form of aid, which is usually contingent on certain conditions being met by the recipient government. The recipient country may be required to sell the food for cash that will be used for development projects or agree to negotiate on certain matters. "Project" food aid is provided to the recipient government, its agent, or a multilateral development agency such as the World Food Program (WFP). "Emergency or relief" aid is used in times of crisis caused by such factors as war and famine. The United Nations WFP is the largest emergency response partner of the United States. The United States is also WFP's largest donor, with U.S. donations making up 60 percent of the WFP. In 2002 and 2003, 83 countries participated in the program and

U.S. contributions outweighed all other country's contributions combined. Most of the donations from the United States to WFP are in kind, whereas many other countries donate in the form of cash. The WFP is second in development funds only to the World Bank. The U.S. government claims that 300 billion people in 150 countries have benefited from US food aid since its inception.

U.S. food aid can be traced to 1812, when James Madison ordered emergency food aid be sent to victims of an earthquake in Venezuela. However, organized federal food aid stems from the Marshall Plan of 1947, which proposed aiding Western European countries devastated by World War II. The plan resulted in the passage of the Economic Cooperation Act of 1948 and was a temporary relief measure that ended on June 30, 1951. A more permanent food aid program was created in 1954, with the Agricultural Trade Development Assistance Act (P.L. 480) signed by President Dwight D. Eisenhower. The act was promulgated to export agricultural products overseas, prevent starvation abroad, and create jobs in the United States. The act provides for the direct donations of U.S. agricultural goods to countries worldwide, for both emergency and nonemergency purposes. In 1958, Eugene Burdick and William Lederer published *The Ugly American*, a political novel that addressed and criticized U.S. foreign operations. In 1960, U.S. aid to developing nations became an issue in the presidential election. John F. Kennedy and his administration became the architects of a new foreign assistance program. Congress passed the Foreign Assistance Act on September 4, 1961, and USAID was created under this act. The purpose of the act was to provide direct support to developing nations, without regard to a political or military imperative. In 1977, the Bellmon Amendment to P.L. 480 was passed to require that before food aid is sent, there must be assurance that there is suitable storage in the recipient country that will prevent waste and that food aid will not be a disincentive in recipient country. Wheat and other grains were produced in excess until the 1980s and constituted the bulk of U.S. food aid. After the farm reform programs of the 1980s, blended and fortified foods were also commonly seen in U.S. food aid shipments. Congress passed the International Food Relief Partnerships Act (IFRP) in November 2000, diversifying the sources of Title II food aid commodities. In 2001, President George W. Bush's management review listed U.S. food aid as one of 14 government agencies in need of reform. In 2008, the Agricultural Trade Development Act was renamed Food for Peace. The proportion of emergency, or relief, food aid is growing in relation to other food aid categories.

Food for Peace's stated mission is to reduce malnutrition and hunger by increasing food security. Food for Peace comprises three types of programs—one-year and multi-year assistance programs and international food relief partnerships. One-year assistance programs are usually performed through the direct distribution of aid in emergencies. Multi-year assistance programs are more developmental in scope and use a combination of direct assistance and monetization. International Food Relief Partnerships are authorized between Food for Peace, nonprofit organizations that prepare shelf-stable pre-packaged foods, and international organizations that establish and maintain the donated food in the recipient country. Food for Peace receives assistance from the Bellmon Estimation Studies for Title II

Project, the Famine Early Warning Systems Network, and the Food and Nutrition Technical Assistance Project. The Bellmon Estimation Studies for Title II Project were established in 2008 as a three-year pilot program. It performs studies to make sure that food aid programs comply with the 1977 Bellmon Amendment to the Food for Peace Program. The Famine Early Warning Systems Network uses U.S. satellite technology to detect early indications of a possible drought. The purpose of this network is to prevent the repetition of devastating famines on the Southern Fringe of the Sahara Desert and in Ethiopia. The Food and Nutrition Technical Assistance Project explores the role of food and nutrition in caring for people with HIV and AIDS. Additionally, Food for Peace coordinates with other U.S. government programs such as the Food for Work Program, Comprehensive Africa Agriculture Development Program, USAID Global Development Alliance, John Ogonowski and Doug Bereuter Farmer-to-Farmer Program, Presidential Initiative to End Hunger in Africa, USAID Center for Faith-Based and Community Initiatives, USAID Office of Economic Growth and Trade, and the U.S. President's Emergency Plan for AIDS Relief. The Food for Work Program gives food in exchange for work on agricultural, economic, community, and health development projects. Food for Peace reports that in 50 years, it sent 106 metric tons of food to other countries.

The definition of food aid can be oversimplified to mean the humanitarian donation of food. However, food aid is a complicated form of relief composed of a multitude of competitive goals by various groups involved in administering food aid. A major criticism is tied to U.S. farm policy, which is charged with getting rid of surpluses that often favor **corporate farms**. Some theorists argue that this goal often supersedes the supposed humanitarian goals of food aid. Although promoting U.S. agriculture is viewed as a worthy objective, there are many debates over whether U.S. farm policy does this in the best way. When those issues have not been settled, it seems to further the problem by using controversial farm policy to the detriment of humanitarian goals. Others point out that protecting farm incomes has always been a major objective of P.L. 480. In fact, Eisenhower signed the bill following major grain surpluses in the 1940s and 1950s. Another argument is that the Food for Peace program is a public relations venture more than anything, concerned primarily with marketing. In the 1990s, the United States made the controversial decision to provide food aid to Russia. Many theorists argue that the two main reasons for this decision were to garner Midwestern support in an election year following a surplus of U.S. wheat due to a recession in Asia and to appear more positive in the eyes of a former adversary. It is claimed that Russia's daily caloric intake at the time was actually in excess of the recommended caloric intake. Some Russians claimed that even though Russian farm production had declined, the ruble had collapsed, and their banking system was in shambles, the food aid actually hurt domestic producers and "distorted" the market. They claimed that the poor received little benefit from it. In fact, Russia exported half of the total amount that the United States was donating to them in 1999. The problem, according to them, was that the products would not sell in their domestic market and the donation of these products exacerbated this problem. The U.S. food aid program was the subject of criticism again in 2002, when it sent genetically modified corn to Southern Africa in response to a food crisis affecting Lesotho, Malawi, Mozambique, Swaziland, Zambia, and Zimbabwe. In October 2002, Malawi, Mozambique, Zambia, and Zimbabwe rejected the genetically modified corn. A debate regarding **genetic engineering** ensued during the crisis. Proponents of genetic engineering argued that there is no problem with genetic engineering and that it could be very useful in feeding the world. Opponents argued that the United States was simply using the crisis as a public relations tool for the biotechnology industry. There are numerous arguments against the implementation of U.S. food aid. A major argument is that food aid is only acceptable if the need is acute, local food is insufficient, and the markets in the recipient country do not function in a way that makes cash a more acceptable form of aid.

See also: Farms, Corporate; Seeds, Genetically Engineered; Appendix 17: World Medical Assembly Declaration on Hunger Strikers.

Further Reading Barrett, Christopher B., and Daniel G. Maxwell. *Food Aid After 50 Years: Recasting Its Role.* New York: Routledge, 2005.

Stephanie Jane Carter

FOOD ALLERGEN LABELING AND CONSUMER PROTECTION ACT OF 2004

Congress passed the Food Allergen Labeling and Consumer Protection Act (FALCPA) of 2004 in response to data that show that many adults and even more babies and children—2 percent and 5 percent—suffer from food allergies. This means that if a prepared or processed food contains an ingredient that is an allergen for that person, the person will react negatively. Ninety percent of food allergies are caused by one or more of the following: eggs, milk, crustacean shellfish, fin fish, wheat, peanuts, tree nuts, and soybeans. In addition to allergies, other food sensitivities, such as Celiac disease, are covered by the act.

The FALCPA is an amendment to section 403 of the Food, Drug, and Cosmetics Act (21 U.S.C. 343). Its provisions became effective in January 2006. It applies to processed or prepared foods. Agricultural products, fruits, and vegetables that are still in their natural state are not covered by the law. The law requires that the label state immediately after the nutritional content that the product "Contains . . ." followed by the name of the allergen. Contains must be printed with a capital C. With regard to the three major allergens, Crustacean shellfish, tree nuts, and fish, the label must actually name the type of nut, the type of fish, or the type of shellfish.

If the product does not contain the complete allergen, the label must notify the consumer that a certain ingredient is derived from the allergen. For example, if the product contains whey, and whey is listed in the ingredient list, the "Contains" portion of the label must reveal the word milk. This protects the consumer who does not understand that whey is made from milk. The law goes on to specifically require that colorants or other ingredients that were exempt from listing on the label are not exempt when they are derived from one of the listed **allergens**. Even if the allergen is listed in the list of ingredients, when a "Contains" label is required, the name of the allergen must be repeated after "Contains." The type size must be no smaller than the ingredient list type size. Failure to properly label in compliance with this law can result in civil sanctions, criminal prosecution, or both. The **Food and Drug Administration** (FDA) also has the power to have an improperly labeled product seized. It may also request a manufacturer to recall the product. The law applies to retail establishments, such as groceries, that process, manufacture, and package a product for retail sale. However, when a customer orders something and the clerk in the store packages it, FALCPA does not require labeling.

The use of the language "may contain" is called advisory language. It is often used when products that do not contain allergens are made in the same facility as other products that do contain allergens. The act does not require that advisory labels be used, only that it recommends that it be used. But when such labels are used by a manufacturer, they should be truthful. The FDA is required under the act to make a report to Congress. The FDA in 2006 reported that it was concerned that mandating the use of the advisory language could cause a manufacturer to be less careful about proper practices in keeping cross-contamination from occurring.

The FALCPA does not require minimum or maximum levels of allergens be set by the FDA. It is likely, however, that the FDA may have to consider these levels and their safety if a party applies for an exemption based on scientific evidence. Nor does FALCPA apply to accidental and nonintentional cross-contamination. Residue and other miniscule particles of an allergen will not result in a need for a "Contains" label. Not all cross-contamination takes place in the production facility. It also can occur during transport, harvesting, and storage. The FDA Food Code has been amended to reflect the definition of allergen used in the FALCPA.

Before this law, some ingredients were used in small quantities and were used as a seasoning, for example. Instead of being listed separately, the label might state "spices" or "seasonings." That might have been in conformity with the law, but it made it impossible for a consumer to know that an allergen that either affected the consumer or the consumer's family was contained in the product. The FALCPA only applies to those products that fall under the jurisdiction of the FDA. Meats, poultry, and egg products, regulated by the **U.S. Department of Agriculture**, are not covered.

When a manufacturer considers that a product should be exempt from this allergen labeling, even though it derives from one of the listed allergens, the manufacturer may apply for exemption. The burden to prove that the product does not cause an allergic or harmful reaction in humans is on the manufacturer/petitioner. The proof must be in the form of scientific study and not merely anecdotal evidence.

The act places the burden on the **Department of Health and Human Services** (HHS) to conduct inspections to make sure that products with no allergens made in the same facility that also produces products containing allergens do not cross-contaminate. The law also requires the development of a gluten-free labeling regulation. It even requires HHS through its offices to encourage restaurants to produce without allergens as an option for patrons, educating the chefs and wait staff regarding ingredients and eliminating cross-contamination.

The previous labeling law also stated that an ingredient must be listed by its common or its usual name. Sometimes a derivative of the allergen could have a name that was not obviously connected with the allergen. Once again this practice, while perfectly legal, made it impossible for a person reading the product label to know that it contained an allergen.

The law requires the HHS to ensure that trauma centers and emergency departments are prepared to deal with food allergies, both recognizing the symptoms of the allergies and knowing how to treat the condition.

See also: Labeling Definitions.

Further Reading "Food Allergen Labeling Initiatives of the United States Federal Drug Administration" (2008) http://www.allergenbureau.net/downloads/resources/international /AOAC_Labeling_FDA_Billingslea.pdf

Elizabeth M. Williams

FOOD AND AGRICULTURE ORGANIZATION OF THE UNITED NATIONS

The Food and Agriculture Organization of the United Nations (FAO), founded in 1945, has a mission to end hunger in the world. It is also often referenced by its French name, *Organisation des Nations Unies pour l'alimentation et l'agriculture* (ONUAA). One of the ways that it carries out this mission is to serve as an advisor to those nations that request assistance in making their agricultural and fisheries industries more efficient and modern. In November 2009, the FAO sponsored a World Summit on Food Security in Rome, the FAO world headquarters, at which the participating nations pledged to work to end world hunger.

One of the activities of the FAO involves projects that will improve the production of small farms in developing nations. Approximately 70 percent of hungry people live in developing nations. These projects can involve such things as helping to produce better and more viable seeds for agriculture or helping to improve distribution channels to more quickly and efficiently bring foods to market. Distribution requires an infrastructure, such as roads and communications, which are often either nonexistent or nonfunctioning in some countries. The FAO depends on the contribution of money and knowledge and people from its member nations to function. The 191 member nations of the FAO meet every other year to approve and assess the work of the organization.

The ability of a nation to produce enough food to feed its people is an important goal of nation building, as well as providing for the increase in nutrition-rich food. It means that food aid can be reduced and with it a reduction of dependence. It also means that the government can turn its attention to building the country without having to spend time feeding the people. It allows the country to begin focusing on education, infrastructure, and other matters that can bring a developing nation into the modern world. Such a country can, with improved efficiencies, begin to have excess food, and commerce can follow with the influx of money from food sales.

The motto of the FAO is *fiat panis*—let there be bread. With that goal in mind the FAO has created a project, The Special Programme for Food Security, through which it wishes to reduce hunger by half by the year 2015. Currently, it estimates that almost 1 billion people are hungry in the world. There are projects operating in 100 countries in support of this goal.

Another part of the FAO mission is to ensure food security. This part of the mission includes preparedness for emergencies and disaster response. The FAO both works with nations to create a plan for emergencies and disaster and helps with response after a disaster. In particular, the FAO serves as a world monitor highlighting warning signs of impending or potential food security problems such as food shortages due to drought or lack of reserves. The Global Information and Early Warning and Information System is the protocol in place to deal with the dissemination of information and predictions gathered from the regular monitoring.

The FAO works with developed and developing nations. The FAO is intended to provide a forum for all nations to discuss issues, resolve conflicts and differences, and create plans and projects. Sharing a border can make the problems of one country become the problem of another. Even without sharing a border, global travel makes the transport of animal and crop diseases and pests a constant issue for every country. This coordination and facilitation between and among nations is another responsibility of the organization.

The FAO works with local nongovernmental organizations (NGOs), governments, businesses, other UN organizations, universities, and other interested organizations in its attempt to eradicate hunger in the world. It is the scope of the problem and the difficulties of solving problems in various cultural environments that have caused many NGOs to complain that the FAO spends much money and lots of effort with no noticeable effect.

One serious concern under the jurisdiction of the FAO is the availability of clean potable water. Its program known as AQUASTAT is the ever-changing report of the water available around the world. Programs to assist and inform farmers of the problems with run-off into streams and the various methods of creating potable water are part of this program. This program is most important in developing nations.

CountrySTAT is another statistical analysis of the FAO that collects and merges data from multiple sources within various countries. It covers the acreage under cultivation and the production available from those acres as well as what is being grown. This information is useful, because it provides a synthesis of many sources of information and data bases. This information is useful for trade purposes, consumption, and production.

The FAO also maintains agricultural statistics, information about fisheries and production, the number of and production of livestock, and many other types of information that, because of its comprehensiveness, can be useful. It gives a very close approximation to the food, its movements, and the need and supply, around and across the world. These statistics make it possible to plan and map and predict changes in the world marketplace, as well as identify need.

The World Health Organization and the FAO have worked together to deal with certain basic health and nutritional issues. One in particular is the issue of infant formula. The problems that have been caused by unclean water mixed with infant formula include infant death, severe diarrhea, and low growth rate. In those countries with a high number of HIV- infected mothers, this problem is exacerbated. Infants of these mothers require infant formula but have less effective immune systems. Working with the standards given in the **Codex Alimentarius**, the FAO is attempting to solve the problems of developing nations, infant formula, and clean water.

See also: Codex Alimentarius, Importation of Foods, World Trade Organization.

Elizabeth M. Williams

FOOD AND DRUG ADMINISTRATION

The **Pure Food and Drug Act of 1906** marked the beginning of a series of reform legislation that laid the foundation for the consumer protection movement of the 20th century. The act protected consumers from false labeling of food and drugs and the sale of adulterated food. It was a great expansion of the powers created by the Commerce Clause of the U.S. Constitution. This law began to have teeth, allowed offending products to be confiscated and destroyed, and allowed individuals and companies to be fined and individuals to be sentenced to jail. This act contained the seeds of the current Food and Drug Administration (FDA), an agency that monitors, regulates, and oversees food, drugs, biologics, medical and radiologic devices, diagnostic agents, and cosmetics.

Currently the FDA exists under the umbrellas of the U.S. **Department of Health and Human Services** headquartered in Rockville, Maryland. The headquarters is supported by field offices and laboratories across the United States and its territories. Within the FDA there are offices that carry out the day-to-day activities of the various missions assigned to the FDA by law. The Office of the Commissioner supports the head of the agency. The offices that are most related to food are the Center for Food Safety and Applied Nutrition, the Office of Regulatory Affairs (ORA), and the Office of Criminal Investigations (OCI).

The ORA operates primarily through the field offices located around the country. It serves as an information-gathering arm of the agency. Inspections are conducted by investigators or Consumer Safety Officers, who are also spread through the country in the field. These offices are divided into regions, of which there are five basic geographic regions, subdivided into 13 districts. The support laboratories are also under the ORA.

In 2002 the OCI was established from the ORA to concentrate the enforcement powers and investigations of the FDA. The OCI agents are not involved with the day-to-day inspections, which make up the bulk of the ORA's work. The OCI agents uncover, investigate, and develop cases in criminal matters such as fraudulent labeling, intentional adulteration, intentional tampering, and other criminal acts. OCI agents are armed agents, not inspectors. Food Emergency Response Network, Strategic Partnership Program—Agroterrorism—and other programs are administered in cooperation with other federal agencies like the Federal Bureau of Investigation (FBI).

The FDA has jurisdiction over a large portion of the food in distribution and vitamin supplements in the United States. The Center for Food Safety and Applied Nutrition monitors ingredients, packaging, food safety, dietary supplements, and it coordinates packaging laws with the European Union and many other food-related activities. The FDA, the oldest consumer protection agency of the U.S. government, has become more important and more varied as the needs of the public have changed with increased technology. As more was learned about the toxicity of preservatives in food, for example, the FDA was tasked to protect the public. This required a marriage of science and administration that continues today to be the center of the agency's operation. The FDA maintains a recall Website for the benefit of consumers.

See also: Appendix 5: *North American Cold Storage Co. v. City of Chicago*; Appendix 6: *United States v. Park*; Appendix 10: Senate Bill Introduced into the 111th Congress, Amending the Food, Drug, and Cosmetic Act; Appendix 12: Excerpts from 21 United State Code Sections 341 and Others.

Further Reading Food and Drug Administration. www.fda.gov/.

William C. Smith and Elizabeth M. Williams

FOOD AND DRUG ADMINISTRATION MODERNIZATION ACT OF 1997

The Food and Drug Administration Modernization Act (FDAMA) of 1997 amends the Federal Food, Drug, and Cosmetic Act regarding the monitoring of food and drugs, devices, and biological products. By passing FDAMA, Congress expanded the power and purpose of the U. S. **Food and Drug Administration (FDA)** in ways that recognized new complexities created by new technological, trade, and public health issues. The highlights of the FDAMA are discussed in the following sections.

Prescription Drug User Fees

The law extends the authorization of the Prescription Drug User Fee Act of 1992 (PDUFA) for five additional years. The pharmaceutical industry gains from the extension of this program, because through the expansion of the number of people working in the drugs and biologics sections, approximately 700 additional people, the FDA has substantially decreased the time that it takes for a new drug to be reviewed

FDA Initiatives and Programs

This part of the new law affords patients with increased access to experimental and innovative medications and devices. This makes it possible for promising drugs and devices to reach more patients in a more timely manner. It also takes advantage of computer databases to track side effects and increases patient access to information about the new drugs and devices.

There is an additional portion of the law that allows patients using certain life-sustaining drugs or drugs that treat certain debilitating and serious diseases to be notified when a company intends to stop manufacturing that drug. The new law also applies the rules and regulations applicable to drugs to biological products, thus streamlining many processes.

Information on Off-label Use and Drug Economics

Sometimes a drug that has been approved for one purpose turns out to also have other applications. Sometimes the second inadvertent application is more significant than the original. Before this law, dissemination of information regarding unapproved applications of the drug and even medical devices was prohibited. The current law allows the dissemination of peer-reviewed articles in medical journals that discuss other implications of drugs and devices, if the company agrees to file another application for that use of the drug.

Another change is the ability of drug companies to disseminate information about the economics of drug decisions to organizations that purchase drugs and devices in quantity because they treat many people. The purpose of this portion of the law is to allow managed care organizations and formulary committees and the like to make informed decisions about the economic implications of their purchasing decisions. Currently such information may not be provided to individual health care providers.

Pharmacy Compounding

Certain drug therapies are not manufactured in commercial quantities. In such cases drugs must actually be compounded by hand by pharmacists. These drugs are excepted from the provisions of the law to ensure that pharmacists will continue to compound drugs needed by certain patients. To keep commercial manufacturers from avoiding the law by calling their activities compounding, the law states the definitions and quantities involved to minimize cheating.

Risk-Based Regulation of Medical Devices

The FDA, in an effort to place its resources where they are most needed, has created classes of medical devices. Those devices in Class I, that is, those that do not pose a large potential threat to public health if they fail or because they are not used in life-threatening cases, are exempted from pre-market notification. The law requires that the FDA focuses on monitoring those devices in the marketplace that present the highest risk to human health and safety. The FDA has put a reporting system in place and can give most of its attention to larger-scale facilities that use the devices regularly and in very diverse conditions.

The act also allows the FDA to contact with outside agencies, which it approves, to review risks and performance of Class I and some Class II devices. There are limitations to the work that may be done by third parties under contract with the FDA.

Food Safety and Labeling

The act does away with previous provisions that required that the FDA approve any substances that came into contact with food prior to its use. The current law allows the manufacturer to notify the FDA of the intent to use certain packaging materials. If the manufacturer does not hear that such an action is objectionable within 120 days of the notification, it may go forward with the use of the packaging. The new rules have not yet been implemented as the agency awaits new appropriations. There is also provision in the law allowing the FDA more flexibility in approving and reviewing health claims and nutrient contents claims.

Standards for Medical Products

The act provides for new efficiencies and allows for the setting of priorities in use of resources; however, the act does not lower previously determined minimum standards. This also applies to medical products and drugs. Certain regulations are codified into the law, including certain presumptions about safety.

The law allows intervention by Congress to prevent certain medical devices that have been approved by the FDA from entering the marketplace, when standards are grossly deficient and would thereby present a serious health hazard.

See also: Administrative Procedures Act, Fair Packaging and Labeling Act, Food Allergen Labeling and Consumer Protection Act of 2004, Labeling Definitions, Labeling International.

William C. Smith and Elizabeth M. Williams

FOOD AS A WEAPON

Food is used as a weapon when it is used as an instrument of force. The use of food as a weapon has been particularly apparent in times of war. In 1941, it was reported that Adolf Hitler used ration cards to manipulate German citizens. The ration cards that afforded the most food were given to the military, while the ration cards with the least amount of buying power were given to the Jews. People were encouraged to work toward positions that allowed them a greater ration. They established clear class distinctions based on Hitler's preferences. They also made clear what was considered by Hitler to be the best way to live. It was also reported that Germany would periodically cut supplies to make Germans think there was a serious situation and increase supplies to boost morale. All the time, the German government kept actual supply levels a secret.

During this time the U.S. government took the public position prohibiting the use of food as a weapon toward explicit military ends. However, it is not clear whether this public position was representative of the government's actual position. Theorists argue that all humanitarian deeds are done to accomplish something other than the goal of helping people. They claim that they are done to garner goodwill and support and as a strategic weapon. Others dispute this view, pointing to the work of the World Food Programme's work in Haiti following the 2010 earthquake. However, many theorists point out that it is possible that food should be used as a weapon. In certain areas, food that has been sent as humanitarian aid has ended up in the hands of militants. During the Clinton administration, Congress included in its final budget bill money for food aid that would be delivered to the People's Liberation Army in an effort to take a stand against the Sudanese government's treatment of the Sudanese. Previously, food aid had been provided to both sides of the conflict, but the food was distributed strategically by those creating the conflict. Some argued against this strategic use of food; others argued that it was previously being distributed in a way that aided the continuation of the war. Other reports demonstrate the U.S. food provided to Ethiopian refugees in Somalia was given to militants in the 1980s and that Saddam Hussein used food aid to trade for cash and weapons in 1989 in Iraq. In both of these cases, food was used as a weapon rather than aid.

Food has not only been used as a weapon by controlling who receives food, but also by denying food altogether or destroying food sources. In wars, crops and farmland have been destroyed, causing hunger and destroying economies.

A more recent development in the use of food as a weapon is the use of bioterrorism in food systems. Instead of destroying crops and farmland, an adulterant can be added to food to create illness and fear. Food-borne pathogens can be used as a form of natural weapons in food. Like the effects of the September 11, 2001, airplane hijackings on the psyche of the American public, an attack on the food supply could cause the same terror. However, use of food in war, whether cold war or active, is not only a practice by foreign forces, but by the United States in the case of boycott and blockade, as well as in supporting one side over another in foreign conflict.

See also: Boycotts; Food Aid to Foreign Countries; Appendix 17: World Medical Assembly Declaration on Hunger Strikers.

Stephanie Jane Carter

FOOD BANKS

A food bank is a nonprofit organization that obtains food donations from one source and distributes the food to another source. A food bank may distribute food directly or indirectly to low-income individuals. When it distributes food indirectly, it is normally done through charitable organizations such as soup kitchens, food pantries, and schools. The food obtained by the food bank is usually surplus or unsalable food. It may be unsalable due to a labeling mistake or other issue that does not affect whether the food is safe for consumption. Food can also come from donations from individuals or federal and state governments contracting with food banks to distribute **U.S. Department of Agriculture** (USDA) surplus commodities. It is not uncommon for food banks to also offer skills training and to distribute goods other than food, such as clothing and other grocery items. Additionally, they often partner with the government in disaster response endeavors. Food banks are created to make use of some of the food Americans throw away each year. A 1997 USDA study found that the United States discards a quarter of the food it produces each year. The discarded food weighs about 96 billion pounds.

St. Mary's Food Bank in Arizona, created in 1967, is considered to have been the first food bank in the world. The founder, John van Hengel, developed the idea from the deposit and withdrawal concept in banking. He had discovered that grocery stores often discard food that is in damaged packages or is near expiration. He started collecting that food for the dining room at St. Vincent de Paul. Since there was such a large amount of food, he developed the food bank concept. Individuals and companies could deposit food in a central location and the food bank would distribute the food to individuals and organizations such as St. Vincent de Paul. In 1976, van Hengel created a food bank development consulting organization, known now as Second Harvest. In 2008, Second Harvest changed its name to Feeding America. Feeding America is currently a network of more than 200 food banks, with locations in all 50 states. The 200 food banks are used by about 61,000 charities and 70,000 other programs. Feeding America reports that it provides food to more than 27 million low-income individuals in the United States every year. In 1986, van Hengel created a consulting organization for international food banks that is now known as Global Food Banking Network.

A major legal issue for U.S. food banks was the possibility that donors could be held liable for problems caused by the food they donated to the food banks and charitable organizations. Most state Good Samaritan statutes allowed **liability** if there was evidence of negligence. This issue was addressed with the passage of the Bill Emerson Good Samaritan Food Donation Act (Pub. L. No. 104–210, Stat. 3011 [1996]) signed into law by President Bill Clinton in 1996. The purpose of the law is to encourage the donation of food and grocery products to food banks and other charitable organizations by limiting liability in donating. According to the Bill Emerson Good Samaritan Food Donation Act, a donor will not be held liable for food and grocery products donated to nonprofits except in cases of gross negligence or intentional misconduct. This protects the donor from civil and criminal liability in case an item donated in good faith causes harm to its recipient. The act also made it much easier for companies to donate food by creating one standard. The donor no longer has to research liability issues in each state's statutes before donating food and grocery items. This act also limits the liability of the receiving nonprofit organization in the same way. By limited liability, the act is intended to encourage more food donations.

Tax incentives are another way individuals and corporations in the United States are encouraged to donate food. Those who donate to food banks are allowed a tax deduction based on their contributions. Originally, the deduction could only be the taxpayer's basis in the item donated, rather than its fair market value. However, the 1976 Tax Reform Act allows some corporations in some circumstances to take an increased deduction. The relevant regulation for these corporate tax deductions is IRC Section 170(e)(3). The amount of the deduction a corporation could take for a donation of ordinary property, property that is held by the donor to sell to clients or customers in the normal course of business, would be half of the unrealized appreciation plus the taxpayer's cost. However, the deduction cannot exceed two times the cost, not fair market value, of the item donated.

There are also several international food programs that operate as food banks. Two examples are the United Nations (UN) World Food Program and the World Bank's Global Food Crisis Response Program (GFRP). The UN World Food Program helps in and after emergency situations, such as natural disasters, civil conflict, and war. The GFRP aims to aid countries negatively affected by the high cost of food.

The world food banks have dealt with fraud and corruption when trying to distribute food. Following the earthquake in Haiti, they passed out **coupons** for food to alleviate the violence that occurred while people waited in line for food. However, coupons were counterfeited, preventing the fair allocation of food. In March 2010, the World Food Program encountered criticism when the UN Security Council's Monitoring Group on Somalia alleged that Somali businessmen holding more than $150 million in contracts were trading arms and not delivering the food to the hungry in Somalia. Many of the areas that need food the most are the most challenging places in which to deliver aid.

Some theorists argue that a world food bank funded by taxpayers, through actions such as buying surplus commodities from farmers, simply moves wealth from one entity to another, whether from individual to individual or from wealthy country to poorer country, unlike a real bank. They argue that the concept appeals to humanitarian impulses, while hurting taxpayers. Those theorists argue that all support of food banks should be through private donation. Other theorists argue that humans have an ethical responsibility to help and prevent further bad things from occurring through ethical means.

See also: Food Stamps, Liability, U.S. Department of Agriculture.

Stephanie Jane Carter

FOOD QUALITY PROTECTION ACT

Pesticides are used in the vast majority of U.S. agricultural production and much of agricultural production worldwide. According to the **U.S. Department of Agriculture**'s (USDA) Pesticide Data Program, 70 percent of U.S. produce samples contained detectable residues of one or more **pesticides** in 2008, most conforming to the limits set by U.S. law. In 1993, the National Research Council published a report that warned that the U.S. pesticide laws were failing to adequately protect children from harm to human health from pesticide chemical residues on food. In response to this report, other studies, and public attention to the issue, Congress approved the Food Quality Protection Act (FQPA) of 1996 that overhauled the federal pesticide regulatory framework.

FQPA was approved unanimously by Congress and broadly supported by both agricultural industry groups and public health and environmental advocates as a modernization of pesticide regulation. The FQPA amended the 1947 Federal Insecticide, Fungicide, and Rodenticide Act (FIFRA) and added more requirements to the federal registration process for pesticides to be legally sold, including labeling and other restrictions needed to protect human health and the environment. The FQPA also amended the Federal Food, Drug, and Cosmetic Act to regulate the maximum allowable levels of pesticides in food for human consumption, known as tolerances.

Both of these major regulatory standards—pesticide registration and control and setting tolerances for pesticides in food—are determined by the U.S. **Environmental Protection Agency** (EPA) as part of the pesticide registration process. The EPA manages the registration process, including the scientific regulatory process of setting the tolerance levels, also known as maximum residue limits. The **Food and Drug Administration** (FDA) (**Department of Health and Human Services**) enforces these pesticide tolerance limits for most foods, and the USDA enforces the tolerances for meat, poultry, and certain egg products through its Food Safety and Inspection Service and the Office of Pest Management Policy.

Titles I, II, III, and V of the FQPA amend the FIFRA pesticide registration and regulations for the use of pesticides in commerce. Title I deals primarily with pesticide registration. In general, FIFRA requires the registration of pesticides for sale. Each specified use for a pesticide generally requires a new EPA registration process under FIFRA. The EPA regulations specify the necessary data required based on the intended use of the pesticide and may waive some of these requirements for minor uses of certain pesticides. The FQPA requires the EPA to periodically review pesticide registrations with a goal of every 15 years to keep up with new scientific information about the potential health and environmental impacts of a pesticide.

The FIFRA also required re-registration for pesticides first registered before November 1984, and FQPA required the re-registration process to include a reevaluation of the tolerance levels of pesticide residues in food sold for human consumption. The act required the reevaluation of all tolerances within 10 years, which was generally completed by the end of 2008 and created a Scientific Review Board of 60 scientists to advise the EPA's existing Scientific Advisory Panel, which helps set pesticide tolerances.

Title II sets expedited procedures to review pesticides that reduce risk to human health and the environment. The act also creates a standard for minor crop protection pesticides, which have lower data burdens in the regulatory process. A minor pesticide means it is used on less than 300,000 acres or the economics do not otherwise support registration costs. Title II of FQPA also includes more detailed reform of the registration process for antimicrobial pesticides, including setting timelines for the registration of pesticides based on whether they are new, a new use for an existing pesticide, or similar to a registered pesticide. Antimicrobial pesticides are generally disinfectants or other sanitizers used to protect structures and products and generally do not require food tolerances as they are not usually directly applied to crops or food products.

Title III of FQPA improves data collection on food consumption and pesticide residue data in regard to effects on infants and children. It also improves overall data gathering on pesticide uses for major crops and crops of dietary significance and requires the EPA and USDA to coordinate to publicize the practice of

Integrated Pest Management (IPM). IPM refers to practices of managing crops and agricultural practices to naturally reduce pests and reduce the necessity of pesticide. It uses mechanical and biological controls, such as tillage practices or promoting pest predators, to combat pests before resorting to chemical pesticide controls.

Title IV of FQPA authorizes the EPA to collect fees to support the registration regulatory process. The FQPA's amendments in Title IV to the Federal Food, Drug, and Cosmetic Act represent a significant change in the regulation of pesticides in food for human consumption. The act creates a new health-based standard of reasonable certainty of no harm for pesticides tolerance levels. The standard requires the EPA to consider aggregate exposure to the pesticide residue, including both dietary and other nonoccupational exposure routes such as drinking water sources impacted by agricultural runoff. Before the FQPA, there were multiple standards that placed significant emphasis on the benefits of pesticides.

In setting the health-based standard, the EPA is required to consider the validity and reliability of the data on health effects, the nature of toxic effects, human risk information, dietary consumption information, including major consumer sub-groups, cumulative effects of pesticide residues, aggregate exposures, and endocrine or hormonal system disruption effects. To establish a tolerance, there must be a practical method of detection to ensure that enforcement is possible. In addition, the EPA may establish tolerances for unavoidable residues or lawfully applied pesticides that have since been suspended.

The act also changed the tolerance-setting process to require the EPA to assess risk based on consumption and special susceptibility for infants and children. Infants and children can face more risks from certain chemicals that impact neurological or endocrinal development. The EPA must also assess risk on the cumulative effects of multiple pesticide chemicals and other substances with common toxic effects, such as endocrine disruptors, on infants and children.

The EPA pesticide tolerance levels for agricultural and food products are listed in the **Code of Federal Regulations**. The USDA's Foreign Agricultural Service also operates a database that includes pesticide tolerance levels for crops and animal food products both for the United States and approximately 70 other countries. In conjunction with the University of Oregon, the EPA supports the National Pesticide Information Center, which provides a host of information about pesticides, including those found in food, online and through a toll-free number for the public. If a pesticide chemical residue exceeds the EPA's tolerance level for that pesticide, or no tolerance level exists, then the food product is deemed adulterated food under the Federal Food, Drug, and Cosmetic Act and cannot be sold or transferred in commerce in the United States, unless an exemption applies. If a pesticide metabolizes or degrades into another benign substance that does not have a tolerance level, then the food is not adulterated. Processed foods that include raw agricultural commodities with pesticide residues are permitted if the residue on the raw agricultural commodity confirmed to its tolerance or exemption. The EPA may establish, modify, or revoke tolerances either in response to petitions from the public or on its own decision.

The act also creates a category of "eligible pesticide chemical residues" that includes those for which the EPA cannot determine the level where exposure to a residue will not harm human health and the risk increases with quantitative exposure, such as for carcinogenic, or potential cancer-causing, chemicals. In this case, the EPA may set an aggregate exposure level tolerance for such a residue, meaning that the EPA may phase out the pesticide over time or allow a higher level than would otherwise meet the health-based standard if the pesticide protects from even higher risks to human health.

Pursuant to the act, the EPA collects fees from pesticide manufacturers to cover the agencies' costs in operating the tolerance regulatory system. The EPA is further authorized to require testing by pesticide manufacturers or importers and submit data to EPA for its use in the registration and tolerance setting process. The EPA also must publish an easily understandable document on pesticides in food for distribution to large retail grocers so as to inform consumers. The act also specifically allows states to require warnings on food treated with pesticides, such as Proposition 65 in California. To set different tolerance standards, however, a state government must petition the EPA for an exemption based on state-specific situations.

The FQPA allows any person to petition to set, modify, or revoke a tolerance or exemption for a pesticide residue. Petitions must be supported by data and information, including pattern of use data, safety and exposure tests, method of detection, proposed tolerance level, children- and infant-specific information, information about endocrine disruption effects, or residue removal methods. The EPA must publish a public notice for any petition that meets the requirements and act in response to the petition. The EPA may set, modify, or revoke the tolerance, in line with or differing from the petition, or it may deny the petition. If the petition would set a tolerance that is a lower risk than an existing tolerance for an "eligible pesticide chemical residue", then the EPA must act in response to the petition within one year.

In the approximately 15 years since its enactment, the act has led to the restriction and phasing out of a number of significant pesticides, such as some organophosphates, which have been used on fruits and vegetables and once accounted for a significant portion of pesticide sales. Rather than revoking registrations or tolerances, the EPA will more often restrict a pesticide's use or set a tolerance level and the industry will then sometimes cancel the pesticide's registration. Some agricultural industry and public advocacy groups are critical of the act and its implementation.

Environmental and public health advocacy groups are lobbying to restrict or ban the use of the popular weed killer atrazine, which is present in a large number of public and private drinking water sources. The Pesticide Action Network, another group, maintains the FQPA is flawed, arguing that the EPA rarely bans pesticides, relies too much on industry data and label restrictions, and does not place enough emphasis on cancer, endocrine risks, and differential sensitivity to pesticides among different people. The American Farm Bureau has been critical at times of the EPA's implementation of the FQPA when it phases out certain pesticides deemed important to fruit and vegetable production.

See also: Runoff, Agricultural.

Andrew G. Wallace

FOOD STAMPS

The Food Stamp Program (FSP), enacted in 1962, provides eligible households with special currency redeemable at authorized food stores for the purchase of most kinds of food. The purpose of the FSP is to aid low-income families in obtaining adequate and nutritious diets. Originally it provided food coupons, but it has recently begun distributing Electronic Benefit Transfer (EBT) Cards. The coupons and cards can only be used to purchase food. FSP is based on the belief that without food stamps, low-income households will not be able to purchase healthy foods and they will not be able to afford a nutritious diet. Of the federal food assistance programs, this is the largest.

Eligibility for benefits depends on on the size of the family or household, the value of household goods, and gross net income. A household must be at or below 130 percent of the poverty level in gross income. The level of food stamps one receives is based on the Thrifty Food Plan of the **U.S. Department of Agriculture** deemed low-cost and nutritionally adequate. The received benefit is the difference between 30 percent of the net income and the maximum allotment. It assumes that households spend 30 percent of their net income on food. Eligible households receive a monthly allotment of food stamps.

The FSP grew not only from a desire to support the nutritional adequacy of poor families, but also out of the government's need to dispose of surplus food commodities accumulated under legislation to stabilize farm prices in the wake of the Great Depression. The surplus was distributed to the poor instead of being destroyed. In this way it was similar in origin to school breakfast and lunch programs. The FSP has several uses. It has much support from agriculture, food processors, and food merchants, implying that it may support the market for agricultural goods. Having food stamps allows income to be spent on things other than food, so the FSP also serves as an income maintenance system.

Several issues concern the FSP. The first is the effect of food stamps on nutrition intake. With the increased availability of low-cost, high-calorie foods, there is a question of whether FSP is necessary. However, the goal

How Food Stamps Work

In 2004, the Food Stamp Program transitioned from a paper coupon program to a debit card-type program, with the intention of eliminating fraud and theft in the coupon system and to create a more efficient electronic system for record keeping. Paper food stamp coupons could be illegally sold and used by ineligible persons, and they could be stolen or even counterfeited. The goal of the new cards is to eliminate the possibilities for fraud and abuse and increase accountability. The card is swiped like a credit card, and the user puts in a personal identification number (PIN). This system also keeps change in the program on the card. Under the old system, change was given in cash or a combination of coupons and cash, because not all denominations of coupons were available. The card also eliminates the embarrassment of using the coupons, because they are used just like credit cards or debit cards.

of the FSP is to provide low-income families with nutritious diets, and these low-cost foods often do not support a nutritious diet. Some recommend that foods of minimum nutritional value should be eliminated from the program while others recommend incentives and nutrition education to promote the purchase of healthier foods. Also, in a discussion of public-sector assistance to the poor, a discussion of the cost of the aid follows. There is no constitutional guarantee to this sort of thing, although some argue that it falls under the obligation of the government to ensure individual life and liberty. Helping the poor is just one of many public policy goals, and they all compete for limited resources. Balancing benefit adequacy with budget constraints is an issue. Another issue is the effect on work incentives and welfare dependence. Since the benefits are determined by income, they decrease as income rises. Although this allows a higher proportion of benefits for the very poor, it also discourages beneficiaries from working for pay.

Further Reading King, Ronald F. *Budgeting Entitlements: The Politics of Food Stamps.* Washington, DC: Georgetown University Press, 2000; Ohls, James C., and Harold Beebout. *The Food Stamp Program: Design Tradeoffs, Policy and Impacts.* Washington, DC: The Urban Institute Press, 1993; Rossi, Peter H. *Feeding the Poor: Assessing Federal Food Aid.* Washington DC: The AEI Press, 1998.

Stephanie Jane Carter

FORAGED FOODS

With the new interest in eating local foods and in knowing what the origin of food is, there is also a renewed interest in foraging and eating foraged foods. Interest in foraging is even strong in urban areas. There are several legal issues related to foraging and eating foraged foods.

For the forager, a major issue is permission to be on the property where the foraging is taking place and permission to remove foods. When picking fruit on a farm where customers are encouraged to pick their own blueberries, apples, or other fruit, the customers/foragers are welcomed onto the property and obviously have permission to pick and remove fruits in exchange for a payment to the farm owner.

However, the more adventurous forager who picks wild berries and other fruit in fields, finds mushrooms in the forest, and finds greens by streams, will either be on privately owned land or on government-owned land. To avoid trespassing, the forager needs to obtain permission before entering privately owned land. In addition to obtaining permission to be on the property, permission to remove the foraged foods must also be obtained.

Foraging and removing vegetation are usually not allowed on government property, such as parks. On some federal facilities, such as parks, removing vegetation is a crime. Other government property may be foraged with permission. For example, it may be permissible to forage on an empty lot before it is prepared for development by a government entity. Picking dandelions from street medians or picking nuts that have fallen off trees onto a median or sidewalk will probably not result in prosecution, even if it technically requires permission. Taking fruit or nuts that have fallen from a tree is a different action from harvesting greens or cattails. If everyone were to forage, there would not be enough forageable food for everyone, and the foraged food supply could disappear. This creates an ethical issue, even if not a legal one.

In modern times, dumpster diving, that is searching garbage piles and dumpsters for discarded and edible food, especially dumpsters of restaurants and grocery stores, is considered foraging. The questions of legality are generally a matter of local law. In general, taking something from a garbage can, something that has been discarded, is not considered theft. Security guards may be expected to stop dumpster divers, but this may be because of concerns about liability for injuries while diving. When dumpsters are locked or held within a locked gate, breaking the lock is illegal damage to property. When a dumpster is on someone's property as opposed to being on the curb, going onto the property to enter the dumpster is trespassing. Thus, dumpster diving is not theft, but it could be trespassing.

Using foraged food in restaurants or selling foraged foods in markets is subject to local laws. Some health departments have raised health issues that may arise from eating foraged food, especially food found in urban areas. Certain bacteria that are found in animal urine, which may be present on medians and near sidewalks and parks in cities, can cause illness. Greens that are not properly washed or cooked or that are eaten raw may expose diners to illness. Mushrooms can be deadly poisonous. Some deadly mushrooms look similar to safe mushrooms. Buying mushrooms from unskilled or untrained foragers could be dangerous. These are issues that many health departments are beginning to address with the increase of foraging. Poison control offices receive calls about mushrooms each year during mushroom seasons, and people die from mushroom poisoning.

Buying foraged food, rather than foraging for it oneself, may mean that there may be no way to know where the food is from. For a forager to harvest enough food to sell, the food will probably come from several areas. In addition, if it is obtained illegally, the forager is unlikely to reveal its origin. If grocery labeling laws are applied to the foraged food, foragers may be unable to meet applicable rules.

Fishing and hunting may be considered forms of foraging. Fishing, frog gigging, collection of snails, shrimping, and crabbing can be undertaken by what may also be called sportspeople rather than foragers. Fishing done in public waters is usually regulated locally. A local fishing license is usually required. Local laws also generally limit the number and size of the catch. In some places, the type of equipment that may be used is regulated. Fishing is more regulated than foraging for vegetation. As more people forage, that situation may change. Sport fishing is only permitted for personal and family use. Fish that are caught by a person with a sports license cannot be sold legally.

Hunting for wild animals is yet another type of foraging. Hunting requires a license in most states and can only take place at regulated times. As with limited catches in fishing, there are limits to the number and maturity of animals that may be killed. These limits are imposed to ensure the sustainability of the animal and fish population. In some instances, redfish for example, have become so popular and so overfished commercially that sport fishing has been prohibited. In most states, the game that is killed through licensed hunting cannot be sold. A few states, however, allow special licensing to sell game to restaurants.

Food foraging is also becoming popular in England, Europe, and Australia. These areas are experiencing the same interest in foraged food, even in urban areas, that is found in the United States. Authorities there are also unprepared to answer all of the legal questions that are raised by the practice. As well, just like the foragers in the United States, European and Australian foragers must deal with vehicle exhaust settled on greens, herbicides sprayed on the sides of the highway, and other dangers that modern life imposes on foraging.

See also: Food and Drug Administration; Runoff, Agricultural; State Legal Systems.

Elizabeth M. Williams

FORBIDDEN FOODS

Food taboos can emerge for religious, cultural, or hygienic reasons. Religious prohibitions include permanent bans on certain foods, as well as rules tied to specific holidays or circumstances. Under Jewish law, many types of foods are forbidden or restricted, including pork, shellfish, and meat that has not been slaughtered according the kosher rules. Additional foods may be forbidden during holidays, such as the prohibition on leavened bread during Passover. Muslims are exhorted to eat only what is *halal*, or permitted. Some Hindus, especially high caste Brahmins, practice vegetarianism, and nearly all avoid eating beef. Nonviolent Jainists are vegetarians and tend to avoid onions, garlic, and other root vegetables. Many faiths prohibit the consumption of alcohol. The teachings of The Church of Jesus Christ of Latter-Day Saints are generally understood to prohibit the consumption of coffee, a rule shared by some Rastafarians and Seventh Day Adventists. In the Book of Isaiah, the terrible punishment that awaits eaters of forbidden food is described in graphic terms: "They that sanctify themselves, and purify themselves in the gardens behind one tree in the midst, eating swine's flesh, and the abomination, and the mouse, shall be consumed together, saith the Lord." (Isaiah 66:17) While the origins of religious prohibitions on certain foods are the subject of endless speculation, in practice food taboos serve to convey group identity and bind religious communities together.

Religious prohibitions often cross into secular law. The slaughter of cows is banned in most states in India, for instance, where Hinduism is the dominant religion, and there is perennial agitation to enact a national ban. Bans on alcohol are common in Muslim states or countries with large Muslim populations. Saudi Arabia bans the production, consumption, and importation of alcohol, under threat of lengthy prison terms and lashing. Other Middle Eastern states have bans with less severe punishments attached. Kuwait, Qatar, and the United Arab Emirates forbid most alcohol sales to citizens. Alcohol prohibition has a long history in the West, with some bans continuing into the 21st century. Absinthe production became illegal in the United States in 1912. The ban was lifted in 2007, and the first U.S absinthe brand, St. George Absinthe Verte, went into production at the end of that year. The sale of all alcoholic beverages to young people is forbidden in the United States under the National Minimum Drinking Age Act of 1984, which withheld federal highway funds from states lacking a ban on sales to anyone below the age of 21.

Other cultural prohibitions have evolved separately, sometimes due to concerns about animal cruelty and cleanliness. Sale and production of foie gras are slated to become illegal in 2012 in California, according to Sections 25980–25984 of the California Health and Safety Code, passed in 2004. Chicago banned the duck or goose liver delicacy in 2006 but legalized it again in 2008. Parts of the European Union not already producing foie gras were banned from doing so by virtue of their participation in the European Convention for the Protection of Animals Kept for Farming Purposes.

The consumption of animals traditionally kept as pets is a broad taboo, with the list of animals changing significantly from culture to culture. Although animal cruelty laws generally make an exception for the humane killing of animals for food, taboos on killing pets for food generally preclude even humane slaughter. Proscriptions on eating human flesh are generally not religious in origin and are extremely common, but not universal.

Preservation efforts have placed many foods off limits, including all animals on the endangered species list in the United States. In 2005, the U.S. Forest Service banned the picking of morel mushrooms in the wild, making foraging for the difficult-to-cultivate mushrooms illegal in parklands. In France, hunting the imperiled ortolon songbird brings a possible $12,500 fine and six months in prison. Ortolon is the centerpiece of a classic French dish, in which the bird is trapped, force fed, and then drowned in Armagnac before being roasted and eaten whole. A 1998 law outlawed the hunting of the bird, due to dwindling population figures. French president Francois Mitterrand famously requested ortolon as his last meal before he died in 1996. Whale preservation efforts led to the International Whaling Commission ban, which went into effect in 1982. In 1993, Norway resumed whale hunting, followed by Iceland in 2006. In the United States, the 1972 Marine Mammal Protection Act prohibits U.S. citizens from engaging in commercial whaling,

In addition to preservation concerns, other foods are forbidden for reasons having little to do with their place on the world's plates. Imports of Sichuan peppercorns, for instance, were banned in the United States in 1968 due to fears that they carried a canker disease that affected citrus plants. Would-be importers faced a $1,000 fine. The ban was lifted in 2005, on the condition that the seeds were heated before consumption.

Concerns about hygiene add another set of foods to the list of taboos. The sale of unpasteurized milk, or raw milk, is illegal in many states, due to concerns about food-borne pathogens like *Salmonella, E. coli,* and *Listeria.* The state of New York has forbidden *sous vide* cooking, where meat or other food is vacuum-sealed and cooked slowly at low temperatures, since a botulism scare in 2006. In Los Angeles, it is illegal to sell grilled hot dogs wrapped in bacon from a roadside stand, and street carts serving them are routinely busted by health inspectors. Importation of foods such as haggis, which contains sheep's lungs, and other kinds of offal were banned in the United States in 1989, in the wake of concerns about Bovine spongiform encephalopathy, the so-called mad cow disease. Living cheese, or *casu marzu*, which is made with larvae and eaten while the insects are still alive, is illegal for importation in the United States; however, it is protected under European Union law that allows traditional food practices to continue, even if they do not meet modern hygienic standards.

The notion of forbidden food has evolved at the end of the 20th century and now sometimes includes foods that an individual has chosen not to eat. In addition to the all-over ban on the consumption of endangered species, for instance, many people choose not to eat seafood that is over-fished or harvested in a way that damages marine ecosystems. The practice of nonreligious vegetarianism declared meat and fish to be forbidden. Veganism takes the same principle to greater extremes, with bans on dairy, eggs, honey, and other animal products. The Atkins diet, a popular weight-loss plan, largely forbids the consumption of refined sugars or carbohydrates. Extreme locavores eat only foods grown within a small geographical area, while freegans eat only food that they have not paid for. These schools of restricted eating often have ethical origins—concerns about environmental impact, income inequality, or animal cruelty—but can also simply be cases of personal taste, where the list of forbidden foods is flexible and idiosyncratic.

See also: Alcohol, In-State Distribution of; European Union Regulations; Foie Gras, Bans on; Kosher and Halal Labels; Appendix 2: *Commack Self-Service Kosher Meats, Inc. v. Weiss.*

Further Reading Simmons, Frederick J. *Eat Not This Flesh: Food Avoidances from Prehistory to the Present.* 2nd ed. Madison: University of Wisconsin Press, 1994.

Katherine Mangu-Ward

FRANCHISES AND RESTAURANTS

A franchise is a type of business organization that duplicates the successful and brandable elements of a mother organization through a special form of licensing. The organization that sells the franchise is known as the franchisor. The franchisee is the party that purchases the franchise. Many restaurants and fast-food facilities are independently owned franchises. Franchises are most successful when the business model is straightforward and can be re-created without significant differences in products in many locations. The franchise is most popular as a business model in the United States, which has laws protecting both the franchisee and the franchisor. Many countries do not have a legal infrastructure to support franchises, and in those countries the entire franchise agreement is spelled out by contract.

The Howard Johnson restaurant model was invented and executed by Howard D. Johnson in Massachusetts in 1932. He thought that his profitable restaurant could be replicated in exchange for the payment of a licensing fee. It allowed his business and identity to grow without additional personal investment. Once his idea was seen to be successful, others began to copy it.

The franchise has many advantages for the franchisee. The franchisee obtains a business model that has proven successful, the franchisee has the ability to benefit from total franchise marketing, and it usually means that the franchisee can obtain training and ongoing support from the franchisor. Although limited through the franchise agreement in some ways, the franchisee is still a business owner, whose hard work is directly rewarded. The business owner/franchisee also has an instant business without the need to build identity.

The advantages for the franchisor are also numerous. The franchisor grows its business through the entrepreneurship of others, meaning that others supply the capital and take the risk. The franchisor enjoys the benefit of licensing fees, but has the ongoing obligation to support the franchises. Both the franchisor and the franchisee have a financial incentive to want the other to succeed. Subway, Domino's Pizza, McDonald's, and Dunkin' Donuts are examples of restaurants that are franchised. Some companies, like McDonald's, have both company-owned outlets and franchised outlets.

In franchises, the franchisee pays a licensing fee or royalty to use the trademark and also pays for initial training. The royalty is an annual fee to the franchisor. But there can be other services offered to the franchisee, such as advertising. The franchise is a contract; therefore, it is for a stated time period. Franchises also usually describe a geographic area, known as the territory, in which no other competing franchise will be sold. Because the business is limited in time, although franchises are often renewed, franchises are considered a wasting asset for accounting purposes.

The franchisor not only has obligations to the franchisee, it has its own assets to protect. Once a franchisee begins to operate, it is in the best interest of the franchisor that it monitor the service provided by the franchisee to ensure that the trademark or brand is not diluted or sullied. Part of the standardization of the franchise operation and the protection of the trademark may extend to signage, uniforms, décor, and branding on packaging and wrappers. The franchisor may require the franchisee, through the franchise agreement, to use the recognizable signs, and so forth. When the franchisor owns the sign company, the napkin supplier, and other suppliers, there can be antitrust issues when the forced use of these suppliers eliminates competition. The risk of the franchise being a success for a particular franchisee falls entirely on the franchisee, and the franchise contract will almost always state that the franchisor makes no guarantees of success.

In the United States, franchising is regulated by the **Federal Trade Commission** (FTC). Franchises are governed by what is called the Franchise Rule found in the **Code of Federal Regulations**, Volume 16, Part 436. The basic document required by the Rule is the disclosure agreement. The Franchise Disclosure Document (FDD) includes audited financials of the franchisor so that the franchisee can judge the stability of the company that the franchisee will be buying into. Another important aspect of the FDD is that it includes the names and contact information of at least 100 other franchisees, in close geographic proximity if possible, so that the prospective franchisee can question others about their experiences with the franchisor and ask other pertinent questions. Fifteen states have additional requirements for information that must be contained in the FDD, which is called an offering circular. The FTC publishes a *Franchise Rule Compliance Guide* that is designed to make compliance with the FDD easier for the franchisor. The guide can also serve as a primer for the prospective franchisee who wants to understand the pitfalls and questions concerning the franchisor's role in the process.

The FTC regulations do not provide for a private action for violation of federal rules. There is a private action available for breach of contract, but failure to comply with the FDD can only be addressed by the FTC. Those states with disclosure requirements provide for a private right of action for violations of state disclosure rules that amount to fraud. There is no registry or filing of the FDD required by the FTC; therefore, the only reliable source of the FDD is from the franchisor itself. California, Hawaii, Illinois, Indiana, Maryland, Minnesota, New York, Virginia, and several other states require filing of the FDD.

The Franchise Rule is essentially a consumer protection measure to protect prospective franchisees from being fleeced by nonlegitimate temporary businesses. That is the reason that 100 purchasers of franchises are required in the FDD. It is difficult to organize that many "signers" to enable a fraud. Complaints against franchisors can be requested from the FTC through a Freedom of Information Act Request. Complaints against franchisors can be made to the FTC online or by mail.

See also: Contracts; Appendix 3A: *Pelman, et al. v. McDonald's Corporation*; Appendix 3B: *Pelman, et al. v. McDonald's Corporation*, Amended Complaint; Appendix 3C: *Pelman, et al. v. McDonald's Corporation.*

Further Reading Franchise Rule Compliance Guide. www.ftc.gov/bcp/edu/pubs/business/franchise/bus70.pdf.

Elizabeth M. Williams

FREE-RANGE FARMING

The current **U.S. Department of Agriculture** (USDA) requirement for the "free-range" label is that the producers must demonstrate that the poultry has access to the outside. It is not required that the animal actually go outside. The USDA has no specific definition for free-range eggs. Nor do they have a free-range definition for nonpoultry products. According to the USDA, in 2004, free-range chickens made up less than 1 percent of the billions of chickens produced annually in the United States. Organic growers are more likely to raise free-range chickens.

There are many criticisms to the USDA's definition of "free-range." Free-range does not tell the consumer about the bird's quality of life, whether the bird actually goes outdoors, how big the outdoor space is, how often the bird has access to the outdoor space, or what type of outdoor space it is. Moreover, the "free-range" label is often misleading to consumers who associate the label with rolling green, grassy hills. The "free-range" or "free-roaming" label can especially be abused in products that do not have legal definitions for the "free-range" label. For example, Rose Acre Farms of Indianapolis, Indiana, advertises their "free-roaming eggs which come from chickens that are kept in an open, cage-free hen house." According to meat industry critic Ken Midkiff, the chickens roam freely within the confines of a building crowded with thousands of chickens. This is not what most consumers think of when they purchase the eggs because of the advertising on the label. In fact, the Web site shows the "free-roaming" chickens inside on wire grates. Many companies raise their poultry and livestock in the way that many have traditionally defined as "free-range"—treating the animals humanely and providing a superior product that can be sold at higher prices to consumers who are willing to pay more for what they see as sustainable, humane farming.

The increased numbers of free-range chickens on the market are a direct response to consumer demand. For years, chickens were raised in the factory farm manner. It costs more to raise a chicken that roams freely, but many consumers were not only willing to pay a steeper price-they demanded it. Even large, corporate companies have realized that it is financially rewarding to qualify for the ability to use this label. This trend can be seen in the number of free-range meats and eggs sold at Wal-Mart. In fact, free-range foods are one of the fastest-growing agricultural sectors.

Chefs have helped in increasing the popularity of free-range animals. Menus often refer to and identify the specific farm that is the source of a menu item, such as a piece of meat or salad greens. Chefs do this particularly when that farm is known for its sustainable agricultural practices. Consumers may automatically believe in what the chef does and become interested in emulating it at home.

Although free-range animals are often considered more humanely raised and killed than conventionally processed animals, there is no real difference in rates of Salmonella between free-range chicken and conventionally produced birds, according to a study in 2004 by the Agricultural Research Service of the USDA.

See also: Foie Gras, Bans on; Growth Hormones; Humane Slaughtering Practices; "Natural" Labeling; Poultry Products Inspection Act; Pricing.

Further Reading Midkiff, Ken. *The Meat You Eat: How Corporate Farming Has Endangered America's Food Supply*. New York: St. Martin's Press, 2004; Singer, Peter, and Jim Mason. *The Way We Eat and Why Our Choices Matter*. Emmaus, PA: Rodale, 2006.

Stephanie Jane Carter

G

GENERIC FOODS

Generic foods have no brand name. When a food or food product has been patented, because it is a protected chemical, it is protected under federal patent law for the period prescribed by law. Currently that period is 17 years. For example the sweetener, Equal, was patented and could not be manufactured during the patent protection period by any other company other than Merisant. During the patent period Merisant garnered market share for Equal. Now that the protected period is over and the patent has expired, any company can produce and sell aspartame, which is the name for the chemical. Usually the generic is less expensive than the name brand product. In this case store-brand aspartame is usually cheaper than the brand name Equal.

The law protects the inventor—either an individual or a company—and allows the inventor an exclusive period in which to recoup the investment that has been made in developing the patented product and to reap the profits of the inventor's creativity and labor. However, after the patent period, public policy favors opening the door to the use of the invention to the general public. Not only does the company that produces the formerly patented item benefit, but also the general public benefits usually from the competition caused by additional companies entering the market. This often results in the cheaper prices.

In an analogous situation, store-brand products of all sorts are often less expensive than brand-name products. These no-name brands or store-identified brands are often packaged and named in a manner that is similar to the brand-name product. The brand-name product may have developed the product and established a demand for the product through advertising. The generic product usually sells for less than the brand-name product because the company does not advertise and does not have development expenses. An example is Cheerios. The manufacture of a breakfast cereal made of oats is not patented and is not protected in any other way. A generic brand of an oat cereal might call itself Oatios to let people know that the product is similar to Cheerios.

If the name of the name-brand product is trademarked, the name of the generic brand cannot be misleadingly close to that of the name brand. U.S. trademark law protects the company that has registered its trademark from "confusion" by competitors. And consumer protection law also protects consumers so that they buy the product that they think that they are buying.

Similar packaging or a similar name does not automatically mean that generic products are identical to the name-brand product. Equal is sold in a blue packet. Splenda is sold in a yellow packet. Sweet 'N Low is sold in a pink packet. All of these name-brand artificial sweeteners have generic competitors. These competitors sell under the chemical name of the sweetener in packages that are the same color as the name-brand products. However, in popular discussion consumers may ask for the blue stuff or the pink stuff, tacitly implying that they want a type of sweetener that is packaged in that color package. The brand of the product is irrelevant. When the product is a chemical, the truth in packaging requires that the products be the same.

The ingredients used in generic brands of processed foods are often identical to the name brand product. It is up to the consumer to determine whether the generic product tastes as good as or better than the name-brand product. An informal blind taste test may be the best way to make a quality determination.

In some instances there is a considerable difference in quality between name-brand and generic products. This distinction may be caused by freshness and handling, not just the ingredients. For example, cinnamon may be sold as a generic product. It may be wholesome for human consumption but have nevertheless lost its freshness, causing it to lose quality in level of flavor. In other instances, canned goods may be accurately labeled but still be of lesser quality. It is possible that some generic food may be packaged by the same contract packer or private label packers as the name-brand product. Milk is often bottled for a name-brand company and for a store brand, but the milk is the same. This is a matter for experimentation and personal taste.

In 1987 the U.S. Patent Office began to recognize and patent the invention of new life forms, including genetic seeds and special breeds of animals. The patent period of these inventions may begin to expire soon, and these life forms may pass into the public domain. When this happens the generic production of this food may begin.

Whether name brand or generic, the food must comply with all the same labeling laws, which should help make comparisons accurate. When comparing generic and brand-name foods, sometimes engineered food is matched with a processed food, the comparison is not one of equivalent products, even if the generic food is less expensive. Comparing a cheese food with natural cheese is not an equivalent comparison. However, for some purposes the cheese food may be sufficient. Because multicolored labels and having the evidence to support claims such as "no hormones" costs money, sometimes the consumer may not be aware that the generic brand is equivalent to the name brand, but no claim is made. Checking the label for the same packager may help the consumer figure out whether the generic brand has the desired qualities.

See also: Code of Federal Regulations, Labeling Definitions, Trademarks.

Elizabeth M. Williams

GENETIC ENGINEERING

Genetic engineering is a method of isolating DNA from different kinds of sources, combining DNA from these sources to make a "gene construct," and then introducing the gene construct into a living organism with the goal of transforming the organism in a specific way. The genes can be altered in such a way that a gene is removed or its operation is blocked. A gene from a different organism may be added to the food's DNA. Another form of manipulation is transgenic manipulation. In this case, genes are inserted from a different species. The technique is known as the recombinant DNA (rDNA) technique. Recombinant DNA is a form of DNA that does not exist naturally. The technique combines DNA sequences that would not normally exist together. This technique usually creates, or alters, traits in a species. The main types of genetically modified foods are currently corn, soy, cotton (used in cottonseed oil), and canola. However, one of the most famous genetically engineered foods is Golden Rice. This type of rice was genetically improved by adding beta-carotene, a substance which the human body converts to vitamin A. This particular crop has helped improve human nutritional deficiencies. Much of the world remains skeptical of genetically engineered foods, which are mostly being grown in the United States. Before a genetically engineered crop can be introduced commercially in the United States, the **U.S. Department of Agriculture** (USDA), the **Environmental Protection Agency**, and the U.S. **Food and Drug Administration** must be consulted. These agencies must ensure that the risks associated with genetically engineered crops are no greater than the risks associated with conventional breeding. They evaluate the genetically engineered crops with regard to effects on human and animal health, the potential for the crop to hybridize with a weed and become unmanageable, and the potential for the crop or its descendents to harm nontarget species. In 2003, 81 percent of soybeans, 73 percent of cotton, and 40 percent of the corn grown in the United States were genetically engineered. Two-thirds of all genetically engineered foods are grown in the United States. **European Union regulations** regarding genetically engineered foods are very strict.

There are many arguments for and against genetically engineered foods. The European Union spent the 1990s forming strict regulations regarding genetically engineered foods. By 1998, they stopped approving them at all. The European Union believes in taking a precautionary approach to genetically engineered foods. Its main argument is that even if genetically engineered foods appear safe, they must also be proven safe over the short-term and long-term. This approach is criticized by those who believe that it is not warranted in this case. They believe that this approach creates too much regulation, hindering good science and progress. Moreover, increased regulation drives up the cost of these crops that they believe are beneficial. They are quick to point out that crops have been modified over millennia. Since humans began growing their own food, they have chosen to grow things that suited them. They typically chose the biggest and the tastiest. For example, modern rice has little in common with the ancestral version. There are several ways that organisms have been modified over time. Hybridization is the technique of mating different plants of the same species. Wheat is commonly crossed with types of wild grass to improve traits. Tomato plants are often mated with wild species to improve their resistance to pathogens, fungi, and other potentially harmful things. Sometimes plants are sexually incompatible. In that case, "wide cross" breeding is employed. The embryos usually die when they are still immature, so the growing and harvesting are done in a controlled environment. Even then, they may produce sterile offspring. Chemicals are used to mutate, produce, and duplicate a set of chromosomes. Mutation breeding is a third type of alteration. It has been used since the 1950s. When a set of traits does not exist in a particular gene pool, breeders can mutate a plant with radiation or chemicals. Alternatively, they can also let the cells spontaneously mutate during cell division. The fourth method is modern bioengineering using rDNA. Proponents of genetically engineered foods argue that the rDNA method only alters a small part of the of a plant's genome, whereas these other methods alter a large part of a plant's genome. They argue that with the modern genetically engineered foods, it is possible to isolate the desirable trait without bringing over a number of other traits as well. Recombinant DNA was developed in the 1970s by Stanley Cohen and Herbert Boyer. Most scientists, including scientists from the National Academy of Sciences, American Medical Association, the United Nations Development Program, and 24 Nobel Laureates, have endorsed the technology and often say that genetically engineered foods are at least as safe as their counterparts. Still, it can be argued that genetically engineering an organism is not the same as grafting trees. If it were, there would be no need for genetic engineering. However, it is argued that genetic engineering has its own set of risks that must be considered.

A major argument in support of genetically engineered foods is that they will help to feed a hungry and growing world population by producing more food. Genetic engineering increases crop yields and allows more wilderness areas to be undisturbed. Proponents argue that they could be especially helpful in eradicating hunger in the developing world. Food can be engineered to be resistant to insect pests. Not having to use **pesticides** translates to less fuel needed to transport pesticides, less water needed, and no labor necessary to apply the pesticides. There would also be less of the environmental and health risks associated with pesticide use. Engineering crops to be herbicide-tolerant could allow for easier weed control. A farmer could spray large amounts of herbicide, killing everything except the desired crop. Since pests and diseases are much worse in tropical and subtropical regions, these crops could be helpful in these areas, especially in developing countries. Basically, genetically engineered crops promise to be more efficient. There are several arguments against this. The first is that pesticide resistance may not be a completely desirable trait. It remains a possibility that the genetically engineered foods may not only affect targeted pests. Monarch butterflies are shown to be at risk from a certain variety of genetically engineered corn known as Bt corn. However, it has also been proven that the risks to monarch butterflies are very small compared to the risks from conventional pesticides. Still, all the risks that genetically engineered foods pose to other organisms are not fully known. A second argument against these foods is that making herbicide-resistant crops may mean that farmers increase the use of herbicide because they can. In fact, as the use of genetically engineered foods has grown, so has the use of chemical pesticides. However, the use of herbicides as a moderate way is not a bad thing. The alternative to herbicide use is tilling the soil. Using herbicide instead of tilling the soil benefits soil conservation efforts; the soil is able to retain carbon. On the other hand, it is also arguable that genetically modified crops are bad for the soil. The Bt corn can release the Bt toxin into the soil through its roots, affecting the weight gain of earthworms, and finally affecting the soil negatively. Another argument is directly against the ability of genetically engineered foods to feed a hungry and growing world population. It is true that without any changes, the world's population will struggle to feed itself as its numbers swell over the coming years. However, it is questionable whether genetic engineering is the answer. Many critics believe that developing countries are not likely to benefit because the genetically engineered foods are controlled by large corporations that are profit-driven, rather than need-driven. They relate it to the likelihood of pharmaceutical companies working to create a cure for sexual dysfunction before finding a cure for malaria. The people who need the malaria cure are not the ones who can pay. On the other hand, Golden Rice has helped to reduce the vitamin A deficiency. The Rockefeller Foundation has promised to make it available at little or no cost. More convincing is the argument that the genetically engineered foods will not solve the hunger crisis because more food production is not the answer. In 2002, 16 million U.S. households reported food insecurity. In 2003, the United States exported 93 million tons of wheat, corn, and soybeans. Seventy percent of the grain harvested in the United States was used to feed chickens, pigs, and cattle. Since genetically engineered foods have not eliminated hunger in the United States, it points to the possibility that hunger has little to do with food production and more to do with money, social and economic policies, poverty, and food distribution. Moreover, the fact that most of the grain is fed to animals brings up another issue. Those animals produce much less protein than they consume, making them an inefficient food source. More food would be available if resources were not dedicated to this type of farming. If people consumed less farmed meat, there would be much more protein that could be devoted to human consumption.

Bioengineered foods are usually produced with the goal of having higher yields. Higher yields are usually the focus of corporate farms, at the expense of family-run farms. However, just because genetic engineered foods are produced on an industrial scale does not mean they have to be. A criticism of this high yield approach is that it normally results in monoculture and a lack of biodiversity. Critics of bioengineering call for more research because once these crops are released into the environment, it is impossible to reverse it. They are living organisms. Genetically modified fish, though not currently commercially available, could easily escape into the wild. According to a study published in 2004 by Purdue University, the genetically modified version could wipe out the native species in 40 generations, because even though they have a genetic mating advantage, the males are larger than nonmodified males, the offspring of modified fish are less viable; thus, in a few generations they may no longer exist. It is common for farmed fish to escape into the wild. Also, the fact that genetically engineered foods face a skeptical public means that they may be difficult to market. This not only affects farmers who are farming genetically engineered crops. These crops may breed with nongenetically engineered crops, causing those crops to become tainted and unmarketable as well. Millers who wanted a product free of genetically engineered foods would have to import the wheat from another country. Many brands will not use genetically modified ingredients in their products. These include Whole Foods, Wild Oats, Trader Joe's, and Gerber. In 2002, the "USDA Organic" labeling standards and certification program was implemented to ensure that consumers would trust that what they bought was held to legally enforceable standards. One standard is that plants and animals are not to be genetically engineered.

Genetic engineering has produced beneficial crops such as Golden Rice and crops that are salt-tolerant. Salt-tolerant crops mitigate the damage caused by irrigation, which leaves behind salt deposits that ultimately render land infertile. It has also produced some questionable products such as the FlavrSavr tomato, which caused stomach lesions in rats that would not eat it unless they were force-fed. Genetic engineering has been shown to have both positive and negative effects on the environment and human health, just as most things have. It may come down to deciding which way individuals would choose to help and harm different aspects of life. Perhaps the issues could be mitigated if genetically engineered foods were tested, labeled, and produced in a respectful way. During the last 50 years, global food output has doubled and the population has risen by at least 50 percent. Whether or not genetically engineered foods are positive or negative, the issue seems to be that something must change so as to feed the growing world population.

See also: Farm Bill; Farm Labor Laws and Regulations; Farms, Corporate; Farms, Family; Labeling, International; International Monitoring; International Trade Organization; National Organic Standards Board; Seeds, Genetically Engineered; Trade Secrets; Trademarks.

Further Reading Kleinman, Daniel Lee, Abby J. Kinchy, and Jo Handelsman, eds. *Controversies in Science and Technology*. Madison: University of Wisconsin Press, 2005; Singer, Peter, and Jim Mason. *The Way We Eat: Why Our Food Choices Matter*. New York: Rodale, 2006; Torr, James D., ed. *Genetic Engineering*. Farmington Hills, MI: Gale, 2006.

Stephanie Jane Carter

GEOGRAPHIC INDICATORS

Geographic indicators (GIs) refer to a developing group of laws that designate and describe certain products, including largely food and beverage products, that may label themselves has coming from a certain geographic area. These laws apply to agricultural products and prepared products. They may also refer to a method of making a product that is traditional and identified with that region. These GIs are identified with goods of a certain level of quality, as well as identification with a geographic area.

The GIs are distinct from **trademarks**. In fact trademarks based on geographic areas are considered "weak." Trademarks may be common law and based on usage, but the trademark law in the United States will not protect food that is known by a geographic indicator in its country of origin unless that name is registered as a trademark. Examples of such GIs are Vidalia onions or Idaho potatoes. These GIs are protected through state law, which licenses the use of the trademark.

Like GIs that are recognized by the **World Trade Organization** (WTO), these trademarked GIs in the United States protect the reputation of product and the producers who use the labels, as well as the consumers who can know that a particular product is what they expect. The physical location of the producer is an asset of the business.

The United States Patent and Trademark Office has an Office of International Relations to develop the policies that are consistent with U.S. law on how to deal with the reliance of other nations on GI law that is not protected by trademark. A number of issues in U.S. law have not been fully reconciled with GIs. For example, with agricultural products, it is possible to define a GI because the product has been grown within the geographic area that has been defined by law. But it is less obvious when the GI requires that something actually be manufactured within a certain area by certain methods.

California has laws that define the use of geographic names on wine bottles. The laws describe the geographic areas where the grapes must originate, where the fermentation and bottling must take place, but the method of fermentation, bottling, and aging is not a requirement.

A conflict exists between the law in the United States and champagne producers in France regarding the use of the word "champagne" in the United States as the generic word to describe sparkling wine. Wine makers in the United States use the name champagne regardless of whether the method of making the wine is the traditional method used in France, the introduction of carbon dioxide into the wine, or the method of secondary fermentation. In France the use of the word champagne is not only limited by geographic areas but also by the method of production. In France this regulation is the *Appelation d'origine contrôlée* (AOC). These "champagnes" produced in the United States cannot be imported into the European Union (EU), because the name violates the GI legislation of the EU.

As importation and exportation of food and drink become more and more prevalent, the resolution of the conflicts between countries over GI law becomes more important. But the United States, with no long tradition of regional artisanal products that not only are specialized because of region, but also reflect a certain way of life, is primarily driven by trademark law. Brand names and brand identity are not established by long years of tradition but by advertising.

The wine industry in California used place names in France, such as Chablis, to get instant identification with the quality associations of French wine. These names have been used for so long that they have become generic names for wine. Thus, a wine labeled Chablis may really just be a descriptor for white wine. It is questioned whether this use of Chablis or Burgundy is deceptive for consumers, as the French would argue, or whether it has become part of the usage of the industry that is easily understood by consumers.

The Bureau of Alcohol, Tobacco, Firearms, and Explosives (ATF) is the agency that regulates wine production in the United States. In 1978, the ATF began the appellation regulation system. The system divides the GIs into three categories. The "generic" category refers to a wine descriptor that has become a general referent to wine even when the word also has a secondary specific geographic meaning. "Semi-generic" is a word that refers to a type of wine and a place. The semi-generic geographic meaning is foremost. An example of this is the word champagne. When a name is semi-generic the label must include the actual place of origin so that it is clear what geographic area the wine is from, for example, California champagne. "Nongeneric" names, such as Champagne, are only associated with the geographic area.

The International Agreement of Trade-Related Aspects of Intellectual Property Rights (TRIPS) was negotiated in 1993 and became effective in 1996. The United States is a signatory to this agreement. It has an important component that deals directly with alcohol-related GIs. All signatory nations agree to conform their own laws to protect wine and spirits GIs. However, the agreement allowed those existing trademarks to continue even if they were in conflict with GI laws.

In 2006 the Agreement on Trade in Wine was negotiated. This agreement was considered necessary, because the EU was not satisfied that the United States was properly protecting its GIs, believing the exceptions to the TRIPS to be too liberal. But the new agreement allows the importation into the EU of wine made by methods not allowed in the EU and also provides for the EU recognition of certain geographic regions in the United States, such as Napa. Although the new agreement does begin the process of forbidding the use of semi-generic names in labeling in the United States, it still provides for exceptions for those labels that had certain approvals prior to the signing of the agreement. The wine makers in the EU have not been satisfied with this agreement, not only because of the exceptions to the GI rules, but also because of the exceptions based on wine methods that are not allowed for wine manufactured in the EU. Even the 2006 agreement is still subject to interpretation. In addition, not all U.S. vintners agree that GIs add value to their products.

GIs apply to the traditional methods of production of certain goods, like cheese, wine, and charcuterie, which form a part of the requirement for the labeling of various GIs in the EU. The GI adds value not only from the location, but from the method of production. Most of the agreements regarding GIs have addressed the simple and straightforward issue—location. The more complex issues of methodology, protection of the way of life, and tradition are only now being approached. Even in the EU questions of what types of modern technology may be used and still retain a GI are being debated.

That the GI flies in the face of trademark law is being slowly addressed as the United States and other strong property rights nations like Australia develop traditions. These traditions make it more possible to appreciate the traditions of the EU. But protecting a way of life and the traditional methodology may not be so easy to accommodate. There is a cultural resistance in the United States to keeping something the same for the sake of tradition alone.

Ultimately, the legal difference between the GI and the non-GI label is that the GI label describes a geographic area, not the specific brand. Thus, the use of Florida in Florida oranges is not owned by any particular Florida grower. It is a designation that can be used by any qualified Florida grower. That may be a tool for joint marketing of individual growers. It also may make it easier for a large producer to take advantage of the market created when it buys from a number of different farms. But when the product is identified by its own brand and not by its place of origin, GIs may not actually add any benefit. It has been argued in France, for example, that wines produced on the border of an AOC region are just as good, but much less expensive, because they have not received the protection of the AOC. Vintners often petition to expand the territory of the AOC so that they benefit from the marketing and the reputation of the GI.

See also: *Appellation d'origine contrôlée,* World Trade Organization.

Elizabeth M. Williams

GOVERNMENT, CITY AND LOCAL

Local systems of government are based on an authorization that is usually created in a state constitution. The different states have different types of local governments often depending on their size. Some states have several types of local governments, one adapted for rural areas and another for urban areas. Very often the geographic and political boundaries defined by local government were established when travel by horseback was a standard means of transportation. Often districts are too small for efficiency and they have overlapping jurisdiction. Instead of expanding the power of an existing district, new boards were often created when each new and developing need was established. Thus, a local board of health might have the authority to inspect a restaurant that stands alone but not have the authority to inspect a food vending facility located within a gas station. That power might fall within the authority of a transportation board.

Local systems of government mirror the three branches of federal and state government: legislative, executive, and judicial. They must conform to requirements of due process and other constitutional rights granted to citizens. But the scale of city and local government reflects their smaller nature as compared to state and federal government. Sometimes the legal systems cross from local to state, because there is no applicable parallel local system in place. For example, a small-town restaurant cited for improper sanitary facilities might have to appeal the citation to a state court, even though the citation was issued by a local authority, when there is no local infrastructure for appeal.

Legislative Branch

Cities like Chicago and New York have city councils that pass laws, known as ordinances. The jurisdiction of city councils is limited to the geographic area of the city. The city council in Chicago, in its concern for the reputation of the city, passed a ban on serving **foie gras** in restaurants. The Illinois Restaurant Association challenged the ordinance in court. This court challenge took place in state court, because that was the court with the appropriate jurisdiction. The trial court ruled that the city council did have the authority to pass the ordinance. Before an appeal on the matter could be heard, the city council repealed the ordinance.

Other types of local legislative bodies are based not on city limits but on the county (parish in Louisiana) limits. A County Board of Supervisors, for example, may be made up of representatives elected from the entire county. Many times some members of local legislative bodies are elected from defined areas within the local area, and others are elected at-large. This ensures that the usually one chambered body represents both the individual districts within the locale, but also the local as a whole. Zoning, determining which type of business can be located where, is an example of a local legislative prerogative. A restaurant or bar may be located in only certain parts of the community, often not near a school or church.

As in the relationship between federal legislation and state legislation, state legislation generally preempts local legislation. The exception to this is something called home rule. When a state constitution grants home rule to a municipality, the city has the authority to pass certain laws even when in conflict with state law.

Sometimes state constitutions reserve certain authority to each county and counties vote on these matters. An important example of this county-by-county authority deals with the sale of alcohol. Many states still reserve this power to each county, and in these states there are dry (alcohol-free) counties where alcohol cannot be purchased and wet counties where alcohol is available.

Executive Branch

The **executive branch** in local government may be a mayor or a county president. The various agencies in the executive branch of local government run things on a day-to-day basis. The mayor may be the only official in a city or town who is elected by all of the people, so he or she may have much personal power. Also in an attempt to keep government small, some government entities outsource local responsibility such as garbage collection, parking ticket administration, and restaurant health and sanitary inspection, giving the mayor additional power in the ability to grant contracts. Very often the detail that might be found in the regulations at the federal or state level is not to be found in local regulations. This can make it difficult to comply and often leaves much to the discretionary decisions of inspectors and licensing officials. The quality of the training that inspectors receive is also inconsistent from city to city.

Special Boards

Local government has a system that mirrors not only the federal three-branch system, it also has additional boards, many of which are elected, which are independent of the mayor and city council. For example, school boards, which may administer school breakfast and lunch programs, are usually elected from defined school districts. The school board members have authority over the limited matters related to schools and education. Most school boards are independent and not subordinate to the city or the mayor.

Other special boards may be taxing boards, dock boards, library boards, and other boards whose members are appointed by various elected officials, but who have authority to issue contracts and perform oversight of those contracts. This autonomy is not paralleled in other levels of government. These types of special boards are known as special districts.

Inspection boards can be created by appointment or be made up of employees. There is no model that is mandated universally. This means that boards that are creating restaurant health and sanitary standards may be politically appointed in some cases, but be made up of specialists in others.

Streets, utilities, law enforcement, fire protection and hazard protection, emergency medical services, local zoning, health inspection, libraries, and traffic management are all the responsibilities of city and local government. Many of these governments were established in the 19th century and they have not been updated in decades. Competing taxing districts and special districts that may have begun as independent bodies have come to have conflicting missions. The complexity of running cities, complying with federal and state requirements and finding the funds to make the city run, is growing all of the time.

With limitations on their ability to tax, cities sometimes levy fees for services, such as regular inspections or application fees, that more than pay the cost of the services. This practice can make the cost of applying to open a restaurant or a grocery very expensive.

Judicial Branch

The local judicial branch of government is probably the least developed. Small claims courts, justices of the peace, or special tenant courts are the usual gamut of local courts. When an ordinance or regulation is challenged, it is often necessary to bring the action in a state court.

See also: Children and Food; Executive Branch and Executive Orders; Foie Gras, Bans on; Appendix 2: *Commack Self-Service Kosher Meats, Inc. v. Weiss;* Appendix 5: *North American Cold Storage Co. v. City of Chicago;* Appendix 6: *United States v. Park;* Appendix 8: California Organic Products Act of 2003; Appendix 14: Enabling Act of the Zoning Laws of the City of Boston, as Amended.

Elizabeth M. Williams

GRAS

GRAS is an acronym used by the U.S. **Food and Drug Administration** (FDA) for foods that are "generally recognized as safe." The Federal Food, Drug, and Cosmetic Act was amended in 1958 to require substances intentionally added to foods, also known as food additives, to be reviewed and approved by the FDA before those substances could go to market. This regulation appears in section 201(s) and 409 of the act. The GRAS designation means that the substance does not have to go through the same approval process. The GRAS designation only refers to food additives.

There are generally two ways a substance can achieve the GRAS designation. The first is through "scientific procedures" and falls under 21 CFR 170.3(b). The FDA claims that this method of achieving GRAS designation requires the same type of scientific evidence that is required of substances used as food additives. It further states that this is "usually" based on published studies, but proof can also come from unpublished studies, data, and information. If there is widely available information on its safety and that information is held reliable by qualified experts, then it could be considered GRAS. Another route to GRAS status, found under 21 CFR 170.30(c) and 170.3(f), is through "common use in food." This applies to substances that were used in food prior to 1958. Moreover, the substance must have been consumed as food by a significant number of people. The FDA states that the substance must be demonstrated or widely accepted to be safe in its intended use.

Interestingly, the FDA does not approve GRAS substances. In fact, the FDA does not have to be notified if someone has determined a substance to be GRAS. The GRAS substances can be marketed without the notification or approval of the FDA. Notification is strictly voluntary. A substance has a GRAS designation if a community of qualified experts has "widespread" knowledge of this. The FDA publishes some lists of GRAS items, but as it has little to do with the designation, it is impossible for them to know of all GRAS substances. If the FDA is notified that a substance will be called GRAS, it can respond in writing. There are three typical responses to a GRAS notification. One is that the FDA does not question the basis for the GRAS designation. Another is that more evidence is needed to show that the substance is GRAS.

There are three types of GRAS status. The first is "self-affirmed" GRAS status. This is the quickest way to claim GRAS status because it requires nothing from the FDA. The substance is supposed to have to the same level of evidence proving that it is safe in the intended use for human consumption as a substance that is approved as a food additive. Another status of GRAS is "FDA-pending." This status is used for substances that have submitted the information to the FDA for a response. The last designation is "no-comment," reserved for substances that have been submitted to the FDA and to which the FDA has responded with no challenges or comments. As GRAS substances require no pre-market approval, claiming or obtaining GRAS status is the quickest way to get a substance to market.

The way a substance becomes GRAS has changed in recent years. Originally, a petition with scientific evidence demonstrating a consensus of acceptance among qualified experts would be submitted to the FDA. The FDA would then publish an affirmation of its agreement that the substance was, indeed, GRAS. In 1997, the FDA expressed concern that an excessive amount of funding and resources were being used in this process. Rather than an approval process, it is a voluntary notification process. Although the new procedure was proposed in 1997, it has not been finalized. The FDA has adopted the procedure as an interim policy and used it since 1997. Critics of the new procedure claim that this allows companies to escape pre-market approval altogether for substances that most people would not consider GRAS. This is an issue, but the FDA has argued that it is an organization with limited funding. With growing concern over the food system, the FDA becomes increasingly strained in finances, personnel, knowledge, and other resources.

However, the Government Accountability Office (GAO) published a report in February 2010 that encouraged the FDA to improve the way it treats GRAS substances. The report found that the GRAS status was less credible since the new notification process had not been approved. The GAO also expressed concern of the lack of monitoring of GRAS substances since the FDA does not even have to be notified when a substance has been designated as such by a community of qualified experts. Further, they expressed concern that there was no formal oversight confirming that the requirements for GRAS had actually been met. The FDA states that GRAS status can be revoked if new scientific evidences emerges demonstrating that the substance is not GRAS. The GAO criticized the FDA for failing to review GRAS substances in light of new evidence. The GAO said that the FDA had not responded to requests for reviews of certain GRAS substances, including **trans fat**. Another issue raised by the GAO regarded nanomaterials. Canada and the European Union require all engineered nanomaterials to be submitted to them before they enter the market, yet the U.S. system does not even follow which nanomaterials have entered the food supply. Ultimately, the GAO found that the FDA's approach to GRAS is a detriment to the safety of the food supply.

The FDA does periodically challenge GRAS foods. In 1972, it removed saccharin from the GRAS list until it could be proven safe for its intended use. In 2001, it sent letters to several companies warning that herbal additives may not be GRAS. They did this in response to the popularity of adding herbal substances to food and beverages. The industry had grown from $20 million to $700 million in annual sales between 1997 and 2001. However, with the number of new substances entering the market, from herbal additives to fat and sugar substitutes, it is difficult for the FDA to monitor all of them in a reasonable amount of time.

See also: Additives and Preservatives; Pure Food and Drug Act of 1906.

Further Reading Gaynor, Paulette, and Sebastian Cianci. "Regulatory Report: FDA's GRAS Notification Program Works." *Food Safety Magazine* (December 2005 and January 2006).

Stephanie Jane Carter

GREEN MARKETS AND TAXATION

A "green market," also commonly known as a farmers' market, is commonly defined as a public market where farmers and other producers can gather to sell local produce, crafts, and/or prepared foods directly to the consumer. Green markets are often held outdoors. The definition varies widely with many different types of operations calling themselves green markets.

Green markets are beneficial in several ways. They allow small farmers to sell directly to the public. This interaction with the public raises public awareness of where and how food is produced and introduces the concept of farming to an urban environment and landscape. They often incubate new businesses. It is not uncommon for a business to start as a producer at a stand at a farmers' market. As the product and brand becomes recognized, these businesses grow. However, it is very difficult to achieve that without the existence of green markets.

Green markets, or farmers' markets, have grown considerably in the United States between 1994 and 2009. The **U.S. Department of Agriculture** (USDA) publishes a National Directory of Farmers' Markets and tracks the number of these markets operating each year. Between 1994 and 2004, that number more than doubled with an increase of 1,568. Between 2004 and 2009, the number of green markets operating in the United States increased by 1,949. In 2009, the USDA reported 5,274 of this type of market operating in the United States. Interestingly, as of 2009, Maine was the only state with a legal definition of a farmers' market or green market.

Although an outdoor public market where farmers sell fresh, local produce is the common conception of a green market, it is not uncommon to see places as varied as roadside stands, **community-supported agriculture** programs, green markets that are publicly owned and operated, and green markets that are privately owned and operated all considered green markets. In fact, the term has become so popular that one may even see a section of a large supermarket called a green market or farmers' market for marketing purposes, although that is not what most would consider a green market. Many people include in their definition of a green market the distinction of nonprofit status. As demonstrated by the various entities that refer to themselves as green markets, not all are necessarily fulfilling requirements to achieve nonprofit status.

A green market is not always as easy to define as it may seem, and the definition, purpose, and activities of any particular green market is imperative to how that organization will be taxed by state and federal governments. A nonprofit organization can be defined as a legally existing entity that is incorporated under state law as charitable or not-for-profit. It is designed to serve a public purpose rather than to make money and has achieved tax-exempt status according to the Internal Revenue Service (IRS). Any particular green market must not have in its governance structures purposes that demonstrate self-interest or private financial gain. The organization must demonstrate this to the state and federal governments to achieve tax-exempt status. If a market is operating as a nonprofit, it may be more than a place that just sells food and crafts. It may have goals that support the public good such as education or promoting sustainability. Nonprofit status is legally associated with state law and organizations apply for it through their individual states. Although benefits for nonprofits at the state level vary from state to state, they may include exemption from paying state sales tax, property tax, and income tax. To qualify for federal income tax exemptions, an organization must apply through the federal government. Requirements for federal income tax-exempt status are found in the Internal Revenue Code. With the many different green markets that exist, not all exist in forms that qualify for tax-exempt status.

Private Letter Rulings, written decisions by the IRS in response to a taxpayer request for guidance, are only binding between the IRS and the taxpayer who has requested it, but they can offer insight into the different incarnations of a green market. On February 8, 2008, a green market was held not to be a tax-exempt organization by the IRS (Priv. Ltr. Rule. 200818028) because the organization was deemed to exist for the purpose of financially benefiting those selling products there. The IRS determined that it was indistinguishable from a commercial entity. The amount the operator of the market made from renting the booths to vendors was more than 90 percent of the operator's revenue. Seventy percent of the operator's expenses were for advertising with the rest for operating expenses. From this, the IRS determined that the market was mainly a location to sell goods and to promote sales activity of those goods. The market had no evidence of engaging in any activities expressly for the public good, such as education or economic development activities. The IRS determined that this organization did exist for a private interest, making it ineligible for 501(c)(3) status.

Whether or not a green market is considered a nonprofit does not only affect how that organization pays taxes, but whether donors can deduct from their own taxes their gifts beyond the cost of goods and services to the organization. If a green market is a 501(c)(3) organization, a taxpayer can donate time, gifts-in-kind, or financial gifts to the organization and deduct those from their taxes.

Taxes are relevant not only to the type of organization a green market is, but also to the types of goods it is selling. States differ in the way they tax goods sold, but tax requirements may be based on what a particular vendor is selling. For example, Virginia taxes "every eligible food item." For that state, food from grocery stores, food from farmers' markets, prepared food, and produce are all taxed. Other states do not tax produce but do tax prepared or value-added foods. This means that a whole watermelon is not taxed but a sliced one is taxed. Once a vendor washes and chops lettuce, it is consider value-added and is taxed. The peaches at a farmers' market may not be taxed, but the artisanal bread sold there is. Many green markets sell cut flowers and crafts. Those are taxed differently from food. With so many different types of products being sold at farmers' markets by so many vendors, a main issue is how the markets or market managers will collect the taxes at the end of each day. This is difficult because each vendor or stand is essentially its own business and consumers pay the person operating the stand directly. It would be difficult for the market to know how much is being sold because there is no main check-out area, as is found in a grocery store, to track goods sold. For this reason, many green markets have written rules that require individual vendors to be responsible for reporting and paying taxes on their own.

Additionally, a green market may have to pay business and occupation taxes, depending on state requirements. Purveyors at green markets may have to pay income, employment, sales, and use taxes depending on the federal and state laws that apply to them. Other than state and federal taxes, farmers' markets or green markets may be required to pay local business taxes. For example, Philadelphia taxes gross receipts and net income of farmers' market sales.

See also: Groceries, Taxes on.

Further Reading Hamilton. Neil D. "Farmers' Markets: Rules, Regulations and Opportunities." National Agricultural Law Center. 2002. www.nationalaglawcenter.org/assets/articles/hamilton_farmersmarkets.pdf; Spier, Jess Anna, and Jill E. Krueger. "Understanding Farmers' Market Rules." 2006. Farmers' Legal Action Group Web Site. www.flaginc.org/topics/pubs/arts/FarmersMarket.pdf; Wolf, Thomas. *Managing a Nonprofit Organization in the Twenty-First Century*. New York: Simon and Schuster, 1999.

Stephanie Jane Carter

GROCERIES, TAXES ON

Taxes on groceries are a kind of sales tax imposed by state or municipal governments on food products meant for home consumption. Since taxes on groceries are a tax on an item rather than an individual, they are considered indirect taxes.

Groceries are typically defined and taxed differently from prepared foods. Although definitions of grocery and prepared food vary from state to state, there are some common, general definitions. Groceries are generally foods meant to be consumed in a location other than the location of purchase. A prepared food, in contrast, is typically defined as a food prepared for immediate consumption at the place of purchase. A prepared food can be considered a grocery item if it is a cold, prepared food meant to be reheated at home for home consumption. For states that tax these items differently, a grocery store with a dining area may have to charge sales tax on the items meant to be consumed there and no sales tax on the typical grocery items. Grocery tax varies by state and local government.

West Virginia became the first state to impose a sales tax in 1921. By 1940, 30 states had a sales tax. By 2009, 45 states and the District of Columbia imposed a sales tax. Many of these states exempt prescription medications, over-the-counter medications, and/or groceries from the sales tax requirement. Thirty-one states and the District of Columbia exempt grocery items from the sales tax. Arkansas, Mississippi, Tennessee, Utah, Virginia, and West Virginia tax other products higher than they do groceries. Hawaii, Idaho, Kansas, Oklahoma, and South Dakota all tax groceries at the full state sales tax rate but offer rebates and credits for people who qualify. Alabama and Mississippi charge groceries at the full state tax rate and offer no relief. Some states tax groceries at their regular tax rate, but other states eliminate, reduce, or offset grocery taxes. Methods of offsetting grocery taxes are credits or rebates. The five states with no sales tax, and therefore no food tax, are Alaska, Delaware, Montana, New Hampshire, and Oregon.

Whether states have a sales tax is a separate issue from whether local governments have a sales tax. Most local governments have no sales tax on food if the state has no sales tax on food. Arizona, Louisiana, Georgia, North Carolina, and South Carolina fully or partially exempt groceries from sales tax but have local governments that charge a sales tax on grocery items. Even if a state does not tax groceries, a local government may.

Prepared foods, and sometimes foods termed junk foods, are considered a separate category of food by many states. For example, North Carolina taxes groceries at a reduced rate while taxing prepared food, candy, and soft drinks fully. States do not share definitions of terms like grocery, prepared food, or candy. Wisconsin includes granola bars in its definition of candy. Wisconsin also fully taxes beverages that are not 100 percent juice. Pennsylvania imposes the full sales tax on drinks that are less than 24 percent juice, while Texas imposes the full sales tax on drinks with less than 99 percent juice. In most states, ice cream is a dairy product that qualifies as a grocery item. In Wisconsin, ice cream is a candy subject to full sales tax. Texas requires that sales tax must be paid on individually packaged foods that are sold at the same register as prepared foods meant to be eaten on the premises if the store has a dining area. The idea is that the consumer also intends to eat these on the premises. In Texas and many states, a bakery item is not taxable until it is sold with a plate or eating utensils. Texas requires that sales tax be charged on all food kept hot and food sold with plates or eating utensils. Texas charges sales tax on food mixed from at least two ingredients and sold by weight or volume. Salad bar items are such items. Frozen sandwiches are exempt from sales tax in Texas, while other sandwiches are not. If food is expected to be reheated at home before consumption, Texas does not charge sales tax. Items that would qualify are the prepared food dinner items stored in a cold case. Those items are meant to be reheated and consumed at home. If food has simply been cut, pasteurized, or repackaged, it is not subject to sales tax. Local governments may also have varying views regarding what food items should be taxed. The Chicago Department of Revenue puts extra taxes on bottled water and fountain drinks.

Grocery taxation is a contentious issue. Some theorists argue for or against it based on its designation as an indirect tax. Some believe that indirect taxes are fairer than direct taxes because consumers are taxed based on how much they use. Direct taxes such as income tax are imposed on income before it is used. Some view the food tax as a way to evenly spread the tax burden. An argument against the grocery tax is that it hurts the poor because they spend more of their income on groceries. Others argue that this is more of an argument against sales tax in general, because the poor spend more of their income on any purchase. Others point out that spending a greater proportion on something does not mean spending more on something. The wealthier buy more and spend more doing it. They pay more sales taxes. Another argument is that it is unfair to tax a necessary item, such as food. People have to buy certain things no matter what the cost and this tax burden hurts the poor. They cannot choose not to buy food. Others respond with what has become known as the "food stamp" argument. They claim that the poorest are able to buy groceries that are not only tax-free, but free, through the food stamp program. However, there are many financially needy people who do not qualify for **food stamps**. The burden is still great to them. Critics of the grocery tax say that it takes away money that could be otherwise used to stimulate the economy. However, that could be an argument against most taxes. Oklahoma recently considered exempting food from sales tax. The cities responded by claiming that the sales tax, much of which comes from groceries, accounts for 37 percent of the city tax base. It was claimed that getting rid of the grocery tax could cost the state treasury over four million dollars each year.

See also: Sweetened Drinks, Taxes on.

Stephanie Jane Carter

GROWTH HORMONES

A growth hormone is made of protein and contains 190 amino acids. In the body the hormone is synthesized and secreted by cells called somatotrophs in the pituitary, a pea-sized structure at the base of the brain. It stimulates the synthesis of protein and the growth of the long bones of the limbs. It fuels growth and helps maintain tissues and organs throughout life.

Recombinant bovine growth hormone, or rBGH, is a synthetic hormone, manufactured by Monsanto, that is injected into cattle to stimulate the production of milk. It is marketed under the brand name POSILAC. Use of this hormone stimulates cows to increase by 15 to 25 percent, their production of milk. Monsanto and the

Food and Drug Administration (FDA) have stated that milk that has been treated with rBGH is identical to untreated natural milk. They claim that it is safe for both dairy cattle and drinkers of milk.

For more than a dozen years, dairy products drunk and eaten by Americans have contained rBGH. The FDA does not require labeling of foods containing rBGH. Many consumers have not been informed that a growth hormone is present in their milk, cheese, and yogurt.

Animal rights activists and health care advocates contend that significant health problems develop in cows treated with rBGH, including increased risk of lameness (leg and hoof problems). In addition, there are a greater number of udder infections (mastitis), and there is an appearance of serious reproductive issues such as infertility, cystic ovaries, fetal loss, and birth defects. Cows subjected to injections of rBGH often suffer from malnourishment, because the nutrients are lost from the cow into the cow's milk and are not adequately replaced through feed. This weakens their ability to resist diseases.

Activists also assert that since cattle treated with rBGH have more disease, they are more often treated with antibiotics, which in turn also can be found in milk and other dairy products. Some people are allergic to these substances. It is also said that widespread administration of antibiotics through dairy products is partly responsible for the development of strains of antibiotic-resistant bacteria. This is a human public health issue.

The European Union, Japan, Australia, and Canada prohibit the use of rBGH because of concerns for animal health as well as concerns regarding the implications for human health. The FDA promulgated regulations in 1994 that prohibited dairies from making claims that hormone free (free from rBGH) milk was different from milk from rBGH-injected cows. This decision has caused considerable controversy that continues today.

The Pennsylvania Department of Agriculture in October 2007 outlawed the practice of hormone-free labeling, claiming that labels on dairy products were "false" and "misleading" to consumers. By executive order in January 2008, Governor Ed Rendell allowed "hormone-free labeling" to be used again as a result of public outcry.

Ohio Agriculture Director Robert Boggs, in February 2008, approved the use of labels that assert that milk is rBGH-free in those instances where the FDA's disclaimer, "no significant difference has been shown between milk derived from rbST-supplemented and non-rbST-supplemented cows," also appears on the label. (Recombinant bovine somatotropin, also abbreviated rbST, is a synthetic BGH.) This position was revised in March 2008. The Ohio Department of Agriculture interpreted the law to prohibit labels that claim that a product is free of something ("compositional absence claims"), rather one may only make affirmative claims ("production claims"). If rBGH appears on a label, it must also include the FDA's statement about hormones.

House Bill 1300 passed in the Indiana House of Representatives, effective July 2008. The bill prohibits synthetic hormone-free labeling. It defines a product as "misbranded" if "compositional claims cannot be confirmed through laboratory analysis."

Other states currently are engaged in battles over labeling practices, especially since many large grocery store chains are now deciding to cease sales of dairy products containing rBGH.

See also: Food and Drug Administration; Labeling Definitions; Milk, Organic.

William C. Smith and Elizabeth M. Williams

H

HAZARD ANALYSIS CRITICAL CONTROL POINT

Hazard Analysis Critical Control Point (HACCP) refers to a seven-principle system of maintaining food safety and identifying points at which biological, physical, and chemical factors can be controlled. With these points identified, biological, physical, and chemical hazards can be prevented, eliminated, or reduced to safe levels. When a problem occurs, a HACCP plan makes it easier to identify and manage the hazard at the appropriate point. The **Food and Drug Administration** (FDA) oversees mandatory HACCP plans for the seafood and juice industries, and the **U.S. Department of Agriculture** (USDA) oversees mandatory HACCP plans for the meat and poultry industries. In general, HACCP plans are voluntary but recommended for all other food industries. The National Restaurant Association and the FDA encourage all restaurants to have HACCP plans. However, HACCP plans are required in establishments that smoke or cure food as a method of food preservation, use additives to preserve food, package food with a reduced-oxygen packaging method, offer live shellfish from a display tank, custom-process animals for personal use, or package unpasteurized juice for sale to the consumer without a warning label. When a HACCP plan is required, the USDA and FDA can shut down an establishment that fails to have a HACCP plan in place. To do this, they file a decree with the appropriate court. If the company does not abide by the terms of the decree, the company can incur civil or criminal penalties. Controlling hazards throughout the flow of food is necessary in ensuring food safety. The longer the chain is from farm to table, the more critical HACCP plans are.

The HACCP plans for food were conceived in the 1960s as a group of scientists and Pillsbury worked with NASA to produce food that would not crumble under zero gravity and also be safe to eat for the first manned missions. The HACCP plan was based on NASA's critical control points (CCPs) for engineering management. Pillsbury adopted a HACCP plan for its commercial production of food after developing the plan for NASA. In the 1990s, the outbreak of *E. Coli* O157:H7, a food-borne illness that sickened or killed hundreds of people, caused the USDA's Food Safety and Inspection Service to propose the Pathogen Reduction/Hazard Analysis and Critical Control Point (HACCP) Rule. The final rule, published in 1996, aims to reduce the risk of food-borne illness associated with the meat and poultry industries by the implementation of HACCP plans. The HACCP programs in the seafood industry became mandatory in 1997. The FDA published the Federal Juice HACCP rule in 2001. The **Codex Alimentarius** Commission, held in Switzerland in 1993, adopted guidelines for the application of HACCP, demonstrating that HACCP is now an international system of food safety management.

HACCP plan operates on seven principles. The first principle is to conduct a hazard analysis. This principle requires an examination of the flow of food and how it is processed. It requires an examination of the biological, physical, and chemical hazards and an identification of ways to prevent these hazards. For example, *salmonella* may be identified in this step as a biological hazard for cut melons in a grocery store. The second principle is to determine CCPs. The CCPs are the points in the flow of food where hazards can be controlled by prevention, elimination, or reduction. In the case of the cut melons, this means keeping them on ice or refrigerated at proper temperatures. The third principle is to establish critical limits that will prevent, eliminate, or reduce the hazard to a safe level. The proper temperature to hold the cut melons is 41 degrees Fahrenheit or lower. Holding the cut melon at the maximum temperature for long periods would be identified as a critical limit. The fourth principle is to establish monitoring procedures. Once the CCPs have been identified and the critical limits have been set, a monitoring process must be established to ensure that the critical limits are consistently met. To monitor the temperature of the cut melons, the grocery store may routinely check the temperatures of its refrigerators to ensure that they are no warmer than 41°F. They may also keep a log of the temperature at each investigation. The fifth principle is to identify corrective actions. If a critical limit is not met, there must be a predetermined plan to correct the failure. If the refrigerator were discovered to be warmer than 41 degrees, the log would reveal the last time that the product was held at the correct temperature. If the melon has been in the temperature danger zone (41°F to 135°F) for longer than four hours, a time-temperature abuse has occurred. The corrective action would be to discard the melon and correct the refrigeration issue. The sixth principle is to verify that the systems in place actually work. On reviewing the storage temperature logs, the grocery store may notice that the temperature of the refrigerator is routinely recorded during one shift as warmer than the temperature desired. On investigation, the manager may find that employees during that shift are leaving the door of the refrigerator open so that they can quickly move in and out of it. The management would then know that their team does not understand the importance of maintaining proper temperature of food. By educating the staff, management may prevent more egregious transgressions and prevent the loss of more product and money. The final principle is to establish procedures for record keeping and documentation. The store would decide how long it needs to keep the

---

Regulating Molecular Gastronomy

A developing area of health regulations that has not yet reached every restaurant or local authority concerns the techniques of molecular gastronomy. This technique is still developing and is known for its creativity; thus it is hard for regulations to keep ahead of the new ideas. Special freezing with liquid nitrogen, vaporization, and crystallization, use of lasers, and unusual chemicals are all examples of techniques that are used in molecular gastronomy. It is unknown whether the trend is going to expand to a point that makes the development of model rules necessary. It is such a creative process and so cutting edge that its techniques become obsolete as soon as they are perfected, making codifying applicable safety rules difficult.

logs. The existence of a functional HACCP plan can help mitigate damages when food safety standards are breached.

Many food establishments voluntarily use HACCP plans, regardless of whether they are required to implement a plan. Among many industry professionals, HACCP is a sound system to reduce the risk of food-borne illness. The benefits of instilling a HACCP plan are typically seen to outweigh the costs. For a restaurant, a food-borne illness incident can result in diminished reputation, loss of customers and sales, lawsuits, increased insurance premiums, and embarrassment in the press.

HACCP is typically considered a sound plan to mitigate the hazards associated with food production, but there is a growing drive to reduce the number of steps from the origin of food to the table, thereby eliminating the number of hazards to which food can be subjected. The growing number of farmers' markets and the amount of literature written on simplifying the food chain reflect this trend.

See also: Liability; Litigation.

Stephanie Jane Carter

HEALTH AND SAFETY REQUIREMENTS FOR GROCERY STORES AND FARMERS' MARKETS

Grocery stores have particular health and safety requirements. Grocery stores handle, process, sell, and have to ensure that food is properly stored. Specialized stores such as butcher shops and bakeries are not generally considered grocery stores. All of these stores must comply with health and safety requirements that protect employees and customers.

Farmers' markets may have relaxed rules regarding certain matters, but as public health and safety in food handling are still the primary concern in the sales of food, basic requirements are still necessary. These matters usually involve holding temperature, wearing of gloves, and inspection of food preparation sites.

Employee training in safety requirements is essential in limiting employee injuries in a grocery store. Employees in a grocery store may be required to unload trucks and load shelves. This requires training in lifting and carrying and grabbing. When some of this work is done with forklifts and pallets, special training in the use of the forklift is necessary. Training includes use of proper equipment such as thermal gloves when loading freezers or moving frozen food. In addition, the workplace should allow workers to naturally stand and work in the proper positions. This may include installing foot rests, having adequate toe room at counters, and the placement of cushioned mats. Counters of the right height, stools, and other equipment that makes work smarter can help keep injury to a minimum.

Many people working in grocery stores can suffer from repetitive trauma injuries, because they repeat many activities. Cashiers and those working in deli cases, butcher shops, and seafood counters are all areas where proper safety and ergonomic devices can reduce these repetitive trauma injuries. Because so many young people work in groceries, some injuries are caused by lack of judgment and experience. This makes training and established procedures even more important.

To ensure that the safety and health permits necessary to operate can be obtained, all local requirements must be met. These include zoning, parking, and space requirements and can include plumbing, fire, and building requirements, and a health inspection and permit. The food safety inspection involves compliance with regulations that control how fresh food is held and the conditions under which it can be displayed for sale.

If food is prepared on site for sale for immediate consumption or to be taken home for consumption, the food code also applies to the food preparation areas, the food holding areas, and dispensing areas. If food can be consumed on site, those areas will also have to conform to laws and regulations concerning food safety. This includes a deli section of a grocery where salads, cooked chickens, and prepared sandwiches may be held for self-service, including **Hazard Analysis Critical Control Point** (HACCP) and other rules and regulations. In most cases the licensing authority will require both a retail food license and permit and the license and permit for prepared foods. Retail food stores that do not prepare food on site and sell prepared food that is wrapped and prepared by a licensed food preparation facility may not have to have a special license. When food is consumed on site, there may be additional restroom requirements for patrons that are not typically required for groceries.

Grocery stores must also comply with food labeling laws in their areas. These requirements could mean labeling fish as wild or farmed, giving the source country for fresh produce, or listing the ingredients and nutritional information on foods that are prepared in-store.

Although each state has its own variation of the law, most states have certain basic requirements that reflect federal government suggestions. Ready-to-eat foods that are consumed raw, such as salad and certain fruit, should not be handled by bare hands. This is applicable in a grocery store and in farmers' markets. The foods may not require additional refrigeration. Those raw foods that are better hosts to pathogens, such as certain cut fruits, sprouted seeds, seafood, and egg, require a maximum temperature for holding.

Some foods pose a high risk for pathogens, like botulism, that grow in an anaerobic environment. Such foods are often bottled or jarred. These foods must be prepared at a licensed facility and must be inspected by the local board of health. Soup sold at a farmers' market, for example, should be prepared in a commercial kitchen off site.

Food that is provided for sampling within a grocery store or at a market will also have to be handled properly. This means no direct hand contact with food, maintaining hot food hot and cold food cold, and clean and sanitized utensils.

Some of these rules will also apply to food **cooperatives.** Some of them are open to the public and must comply with regular health and safety requirements of grocery stores and food handling. There may be relaxed standards applied to buying clubs.

Safety and permits will also require the compliance with **Americans with Disabilities Act** (ADA) requirements, whether for patron access—motorized carts, ramps, special grabbing devices—or for employees. For those employees with illnesses transmitted by handling food, the ADA and **Food and Drug Administration** and **U.S. Department of Agriculture** regulations apply, as they do in restaurants.

Safety for patrons also includes the maintenance of hazard-free floors and proper stacking and accessibility of items. The grocery store should have a procedure for hazard monitoring that is independent from an alert. Store personnel should have a procedure for responding to either type of hazard. Stacking of items should be undertaken only by those who have been trained. Patrons who remove cans or other heavy items from a stack should not face the hazard of a collapsing stack or falling items. In addition, if items are place too high on a shelf or on a high shelf that is also deep, patrons may climb the shelving to obtain the item, and this can cause either the collapse of shelves or the overturning of shelves.

See also: GRAS.

Elizabeth M. Williams

HEALTH REGULATIONS, LOCAL RESTAURANT

Local health regulations are usually based on the Food Code of the **Food and Drug Administration** (FDA). The Food Code is developed to help health departments develop regulations for food service inspection programs. It is written by the FDA with help from the Conference for Food Protection and is updated every four years, with the most current revision in 2009. By modeling their food safety rules on the FDA's Food Code, local, state, tribal, and federal regulators are able to be consistent with the national food regulatory policy. However, although the FDA recommends adopting the food code, it cannot legally require it. Forty-eight states and U.S. territories have put food codes in place, modeled on one of the versions of the FDA Food Code. Those that had adopted these food codes represented 79 percent of the population.

Although the federal government writes the Food Code and inspects food service operations that cross state borders and inspects food-processing plants, most of the regulations that affect restaurant and food service operations are written at the state level. The state regulations are enforced by local (city or county) or state health departments. Usually, health inspectors conduct food service inspections.

Most food codes cover handling and food preparation. Those terms refer to a myriad of activities such as purchasing and receiving, proper storage of both raw and cooked food, proper display of food where applicable, transportation, and issues affecting personnel like employee hygiene, uniforms or clothing, and proper health of employees. Additional matters cover equipment and utensils, installation of appliances, storage of tools, types of materials used, and restaurant and kitchen design. Cleaning and sanitizing of the facility and the equipment are covered. Types of utilities, such as required sewage, plumbing, and waste disposal services are also part of these codes. The number and condition of restrooms is usually covered. Safe methods of pest management are stated. Proper lighting and ventilation are prescribed. Procedures for review, inspection, and closure are given. The Food Code includes recommendations on how restaurants should be built, maintained, and inspected, including the number of times and regularity. Usually stated is the minimum training required to be given to inspectors. There are standards for kitchen equipment like refrigerators and dishwashers. There are minimum cooking temperatures for meat, poultry, eggs, and fish. There are prescribed temperatures for holding hot, cooked foods and prescription of rules to caution consumers of raw or undercooked foods.

When health inspectors inspect restaurants, they normally look at several different parts of the facility. For example, food must come from approved sources and it must be fit for consumption and stored in accordance with regulations. Many local health regulations require that food be stored six incheds from the floor. All areas of food, whether cooled or stored, must be properly organized and maintained. Refrigeration is typically required to hold food at 41°F or lower. Some jurisdictions allow refrigeration to be set at 45°F or lower. Most regulations require food to be stored on particular shelves in the refrigerator. Raw poultry should be stored on the lowest shelf in the refrigerator. Raw, ground meat should be stored above the poultry. Whole, raw meat should be stored above the ground meat. Whole, raw fish should be stored above the whole, raw meat. Cooked and ready-to-eat food should be stored above all of these things. The purpose of this is to prevent food-borne illnesses caused by food dripping onto a lower shelf. Since cooked and ready-to-eat foods will receive no further cooking, they cannot be dripped on by a more hazardous item, like raw poultry. Usually, a local health inspector checks to make sure thermometers are present in refrigerators and freezers and that the temperature on them is consistent with the temperatures required by local health regulations. Foods must also be wrapped properly. The inspector may also check that foods are thawed in accordance with local health regulations. Produce must be washed before it is prepared. The health inspector may also check to see if hand-washing sinks are available, easily accessible, and stocked with soap and clean towels. The health inspector will also check to make sure handling of ready-to-eat foods is in accordance with local health regulations. This varies according to the jurisdiction. A food that will not be cooked any further is considered ready-to-eat. New York State is very stringent, requiring all ready-to-eat food to be handled with utensils or with gloved hands. One of the reasons for this is that some believe that food service professionals do not reliably wash their hands. Critics of this believe that cooks do reliably wash their hands and that the requirement to wear gloves is wasteful. The health inspectors may check that food is being cooked and reheated properly and that equipment, floors, walls, and ceilings are clean. They will also check for rodent infestation. Another aspect of an evaluation is the evaluation of the staff. The inspector will make sure that employees are in compliance with regard to eating, drinking, and smoking practices in the kitchen. They will also make sure they follow health, hygiene, and dress code.

The Food Code is widely accepted by food service professionals. The National Restaurant Association (NRA) believes that local and state regulators should adopt the FDA Food Code. According to the NRA, "a nationally recognized, widely accepted, reasonable and science-based food safety code that states can adopt or local health authorities can use as a template can have a substantial and positive effect on public health in the United States." Although the NRA does not believe the FDA Food Code is perfect, it supports having a uniform food code.

Indeed, most agree that uniform food safety standards can increase the efficiency and effectiveness of the food safety system in this country.

One of the more controversial issues in local health regulations is smoking. Many local health boards are empowered to enforce smoking bans. Some have decided to enforce smoking bans in all public places. Others have restricted smoking in restaurant dining areas. Some have restricted smoking in bars as well. Proponents of these regulations note that restricted smoking may lower health care costs, reduce the risk of fires in areas with explosives, increase the cleanliness of restaurants, reduce ventilation needs and the costs and energy associated with them, and provide smokers with an incentive to quit smoking. Some critics say that a ban on smoking in restaurants prevents establishments from meeting the desires of their customers. Bars, particularly, have claimed reduced profits following smoking bans.

See also: Government, City and Local; Smoking and Restaurants and Bars.

Further Reading Curran, William J. "The Preparation of State and Local Health Regulations." *American Journal of Public Health Nations Health* 49, no. 3 (March 1959): 314–21; Lambert, Thomas A. "The Case Against Smoking Bans." *Regulation* 29, no. 4 (Winter 2006–2007): 34–40.

Stephanie Jane Carter

HOSPITAL FOOD, REGULATION OF

Hospital food regulation differs from regulation of food in the general marketplace because of the presence of individuals with weakened immune systems and increased risk of infections. Hospital food service facilities must be extraordinarily sanitary and strictly follow food safety guidelines. Food-borne illness can be detrimental in the hospital environment.

Hospitals generally follow several guidelines to ensure that the food served in their facilities causes no harm. When composing menus, hospital food service providers must closely monitor foods that commonly carry food-borne pathogens. A common pathogen is *Listeria monocytogenes*. The **U.S. Department of Agriculture** (USDA), the **Department of Health and Human Services**, and several medical associations recommend that pregnant women not eat smoked fish, uncooked lunch meats, or soft cheeses, among other things. This recommendation also applies to transplant recipients and other immune-compromised individuals. Often, increased presence of pathogens are periodically found on common foods. *E. coli* 0157:H7 is most commonly associated with undercooked beef but is also found on foods such as lettuce, spinach, and sprouts. Although this may not cause a problem for an individual with a healthy immune system, the effects of this pathogen can be catastrophic for individuals with compromised immune systems. Norovirus has been regularly found in hospitals in the United Kingdom. It can be transmitted in several ways, including through contact with an inanimate object. Additionally, hospital food service providers must closely monitor the **Food and Drug Administration** (FDA) recalls to ensure that food thought to cause harm is kept out of the facility. A **Hazard Analysis Critical Control Point** plan is imperative in hospital food service, allowing issues to be controlled, monitored, and reduced to safe levels before they cause deleterious effects. It is recommended that hospital food service facilities be inspected monthly. In addition to monitoring the quality and sanitation of the food that the food service facility serves hospital patients, careful cleanup and disposal of food items waste are required. Patients eat in their rooms and the soiled eating utensils, plates, cups, bowls, and waste must be transported through the hospital in such a way that does not spread infection. Infection-control is not only an ethical concern but a financial concern as well.

Normally, physicians regulate the specific diet of patients while in the hospital. If this diet is not administered correctly, lawsuits that are quite similar to malpractice lawsuits can arise. In one instance, a patient sued a hospital for providing solid food for three consecutive meals when his physician had ordered that he take no solid food. The night nurse had made a mistake and the meals were delivered. When he complained to the nurse on duty, she assured him that no mistake had been made. He ate two of the meals and became severely ill. Eventually, he needed a double-barreled colostomy and could not return to work for five months after the surgery. The court said that the hospital was negligent, but the need for the surgery could have been caused by at least two other factors. The lawsuit (*Lenger v. Physician's General Hospital, Inc.*, 455 SW 2d 703-Tex. Supreme Court 1970) demonstrates the importance of close monitoring and hospital food regulation. In the hospital setting, food takes the role of therapy in some instances.

In addition to providing food for patients, hospitals also provide food for staff and visitors. The prevalence of unhealthy food, including fast-food burger franchises, has been a source of criticism of hospitals. The American Medical Association recommends "health-promoting" foods in hospitals. New physicians have also called for healthier food to be served in hospitals. In 2006, the American Medical Student Association campaigned to remove the non-nutritious foods from hospitals. However, hospitals want the eating establishments to produce revenue. Some hospital administrators claim that the unhealthy food is more popular and more profitable. Others, such as the Institute for Agriculture and Trade Policy, claim that a well-publicized switch to healthy, sustainable foods can create positive publicity for the hospital and differentiate the hospital from its competitors. Moreover, many point out that a hospital, ethically, should be a health-promoting venture in all areas. Studies also show increased obesity and chronic disease rates among hospital workers, which could result in a less productive, less profitable workforce. Still others say that changing what they serve will not necessarily change what workers eat. In 2006, Kaiser Permanente, the largest nonprofit health system in the Unites States, organized farmers' markets in some of its locations. In all of its locations, it stopped serving milk that had synthetic hormones. Healthcare Without Harm, a health care organization, asked that hospitals sign a pledge to serve healthier, more sustainable food. By May 2008, 122 hospitals in the United States had signed the pledge.

Where eating takes place is also a major concern of hospitals. The Occupational Safety and Health Administration prohibits food and drink in areas where contamination is likely in its Bloodborne Pathogen Standard. Under LD.1.30, no food can be consumed in clinical areas.

Further Reading Kolasa, Kathryn M , Jeff Dial, Scottie Gaskins, and Russ Currie. "Moving toward Healthier-Eating Environments in Hospitals." *Nutrition Today* 45, no. 2 (March/April 2010): 54–63; Silverman, M.R., M. B. Gregoire, L. J. Lafferty, and R. A. Dowling. "Current and Future Practices in Hospital Foodservice." *Journal of the American Dietetic Association* 100, no. 1 (January 2000):76–80.

Stephanie Jane Carter

HUMANE SLAUGHTERING PRACTICES

Almost all animals killed for food in the United States are slaughtered in federally inspected slaughterhouses. The primary federal law regarding slaughter is the Humane Methods of Slaughter Act (HMSA) of 1958, which would therefore be applicable to most animals killed for food in the United States.

The HMSA requires that all techniques of killing animals for food must be humane. Nonhumane slaughtering techniques are not in compliance with public policy and are not *pro bono publicum* (in the public good). If a nonhumane method of slaughtering is used, the facility cannot be certified under the HMSA.

The HMSA provides for two approved humane techniques:

(a) in the case of cattle, calves, horses, mules, sheep, swine, and other livestock, all animals are rendered insensible to pain by a single blow or gunshot or an electrical, chemical, or other means that is rapid and effective, before being shackled, hoisted, thrown, cast, or cut; or

(b) by slaughtering in accordance with the ritual requirements of the Jewish faith or any other religious faith that prescribes a method of slaughter whereby the animal suffers loss of consciousness by anemia of the brain caused by the simultaneous and instantaneous severance of the carotid arteries with a sharp instrument and handling in connection with such slaughtering. (7 U.S.C.A. § 1902)

HMSA is considered limited by animal rights activists because it covers only livestock killed for food. Animals used in scientific experiments and killed for their fur are not covered by the HMSA. No law protects them from inhumane slaughtering methods.

The regulations deriving from the law mandate that animals be held and moved with minimal "discomfort." This means that places of gathering and holding, such as pens, and pathways and ramps that are used to channel and move the livestock be well maintained. They cannot be dangerous or unsafe for the animals in a ways that would threaten them.

There are four methods that the HMSA authorizes to kill animals: the use of carbon dioxide for smaller livestock like pigs, calves, and sheep; the captive bolt method for all types of animals; the use of a gunshot for all animals; and electrical stunning for all animals. The regulations mandate that if violations are found and observed by inspectors, these violations must be made known to the administration of the slaughterhouse. Should the administration fail to correct the violations within a reasonable time, the agency has the power to stop the operation of the facility until appropriate corrections have been made.

The HMSA outlines two methods of enforcement: stopping the line and/or imposition of criminal penalty. Inspectors have the option of stopping their inspections of a facility. This is a serious step, but an easy one to take. Meat must be inspected in order to be sold. By suspending inspection, the inspectors in effect stop the line, because the management of the slaughterhouses does not wish to continue to produce meat when it cannot be sold. Criminal penalties can be imposed through the normal criminal process. Fines may be $1,000. Imprisonment for up to one year, as well as fines, are authorized by the Federal Meat Inspection Act.

The HMSA was amended in 1978. The killing and stunning techniques that had been approved in the original act were made mandatory in those facilities that were federally inspected. This means all facilities involved in interstate commerce. The 1978 amendment gave enforcement powers of the HMSA to the **U.S. Department of Agriculture**. Although the 1978 did not specifically state that it was applicable to states, it has been interpreted by extension that it is also applicable to the states.

Animal rights activists have consistently charged that the USDA has been lax in enforcing provisions in HMSA.

See also: Appendix 2: *Commack Self-Service Kosher Meats, Inc. v. Weiss*; Appendix 9: Twenty-Eight Hour Law of 1873 as Amended in 1994.

Further Reading The Humane Methods of Slaughter Act, 7 U.S.C.A. § 1901 et seq.

William C. Smith and Elizabeth M. Williams

IMITATION FOODS

A food that is a substitute for, and resembles, a food, but is nutritionally inferior to that food, is considered an imitation food. Imitation foods must be labeled as "imitation" followed by the name of the food that it is imitating. Labeling for foods changed as regulatory approaches and societal norms have changed over time. The **Pure Food and Drug Act of 1906** sought to use labeling to protect consumers from economic harm. The 1938 Food, Drug, and Cosmetic Act replaced the 1906 act and sought to use labeling to prevent misleading information from being conveyed to the consumer. It created standards of identities for food, which were to resemble recipes. Imitation foods originally were defined as a deviation from the standard of identity for the food items they imitated. If a food deviated from that standard recipe prescribed by the **Food and Drug Administration** (FDA), that food had to be labeled as an "imitation." The first food standards to be issued under the 1938 act were for canned tomato products. Over time, food science allowed fortification and enrichment of foods, as well as substitutes for regular ingredients in those foods. This challenged the definition of "imitation." The definition of "imitation" was debated over a couple of decades. Over time, companies were encouraged to develop imitation foods, or substitutes, to create healthier alternatives to certain foods. For example, a sugar substitute would not cause the weight gain and problems associated with regular sugar. Those foods, even if they were considered healthier alternatives, would have to bear the "imitation" label. "Imitation" was not a highly marketable term. In the early 1970s, the American Heart Association began to argue that "any existing and regulatory barriers to the marketing of such foods be removed." In 1973, the FDA repealed the 1938 regulation for imitation foods. The new ruling was that as long as the imitation product was not "nutritionally inferior" to the product it claimed to imitate, it did not have to be labeled with the word "imitation." Foods that had originally been labeled "imitation" could now be marketed without that term and their popularity increased. Instead of calling a product, "imitation sour cream," companies could promote it in positive terms such as "low-fat sour cream."

Foods that imitate other foods, without regard to their nutritional inferiority, include fat substitutes such as Olestra; meat substitutes such as Boca Burgers; sugar substitutes such as Splenda; milk substitutes such as soy milk, rice milk, and almond milk; imitation cheese such as Velveeta; Surimi imitation crab meat; Cool Whip; margarine; and imitation juices such as Kool-Aid, Tang, and Crystal Light. The intended, as well as unintended, uses of these foods varies. Imitation foods have historically been created to offer cheaper alternatives, "healthier" alternatives, substitutes for a food forbidden in an individual's diet (such as meat or dairy), or more convenient alternatives. In the case of Velveeta's role in Tex-Mex cuisine, an imitation food became a small, but integral, part of a cuisine. Although science and industry have largely driven the U.S. food industry and the United States consumes a large amount of imitation foods, the United States does not alone rely on imitation foods. In fact, where Americans have imitation meat products, so do other countries. For example, Austrian supermarkets are well stocked with imitation meat (imitation wiener schnitzel and knockwurst), but they are not stocked with imitation chicken nuggets and burgers.

According to the FDA rule, as long as a product is not nutritionally inferior to the one it simulates, it does not have to carry the imitation label. However, most people consider these foods imitations. Over the last several decades, imitation meat products have grown in popularity. Companies like Morningstar and Boca make products like "Chik'n," Italian sausage, and ground burger. However, not one of these products contains meat. Instead, soy protein imitates meat. Since soy is widely considered to be a healthy product and vegetarianism is widely thought to be a healthy lifestyle, these products are thought by many to be part of a nutritious lifestyle. In fact, Boca's Web site asks, "On the menu tonight? A healthier household." While these imitation meat products are healthier than their counterparts, it is important to ask what their counterparts are. Conventional frozen chicken nuggets are not very healthy at all, making the vegetarian version the lesser of two evils, as the vegetarian version is a highly processed food. Because of the wide availability and clever marketing of these products, they are gaining in popularity. Since consumers spend less time in the kitchen and less time reading product labels, consumption of this healthier "junk" food has increased. The irony is that the vegetarian lifestyle is thought to be more natural, but it is becoming a lifestyle of processed foods. These products, like **diet foods**, may encourage consumers to eat things they would not have eaten before simply because they carry the concept of health. Most vegetarians would never eat a burger or chicken nuggets. Many now eat the imitation meat products daily. Even most meat eaters do not eat processed chicken and burgers on a daily basis. These companies have come up with products that imitate processed foods but can claim all the glory and health associated with vegetarianism. In the defense of these products, they offer a healthier alternative to their counterparts and it may behoove some people to choose this version when they are craving the original.

One of the most controversial imitation products has been Olestra. Olestra was approved by the FDA for use as a food additive in 1996. It was originally used in potato chips under the WOW brand by Frito Lay. In 1998, WOW chips were marketed nationally and sales were over $400 million. By 2000, sales were half that due to an FDA-mandated health warning label. The label said, "This Product Contains Olestra. Olestra may cause abdominal cramping and loose stools. Olestra inhibits the absorption of some vitamins and other nutrients. Vitamins A, D, E, and K have been added." In 2003, the FDA decided that this warning label was not warranted, but the public perception of Olestra had already been damaged. The loose stool side effect caused much of the public disapproval, and many people also thought Olestra was simply too fake, too manufactured. However, many critics note that consumers have already accepted as common, and even natural, items that their great-grandparents would not have recognized as food.

Although thinkers in the 1970s encouraged the development and marketing of imitation foods as healthier alternatives, modern thinkers support the 1938 legislation with its stricter regulations on "imitation" food labeling. In fact, identities of products have been so drastically changed by these products that would have been labeled "imitation" by the 1938 rules, they are no longer even recognized as imitations. Food theorist Michael Pollan is quick to point out that low-fat sour cream really has nothing to do with sour cream. Instead of being labeled "low-fat," it should also be labeled "imitation." Moreover, Pollan notes that the 1938 ruling was repealed by the FDA, rather than by Congress. He believes that the FDA's actions were extralegal in this case. Imitation fats and sugars are often criticized because they often carry side effects. Olestra products carry a warning that they may cause loose stools. Moreover, these foods encourage consumers to eat more of something that is not particularly nutritious. Instead of eating Olestra potato chips, nutritionists argue that the consumer should eat fewer potato chips and find a vitamin-rich, nutritious alternative. Another criticism of imitation foods is that they increase the distance from the food source. Imitation foods normally have so many ingredients that they do not really resemble the original food. Commercial mayonnaise is highly popular in the United States. Most consumers have never made mayonnaise from scratch. Many people are surprised to discover that mayonnaise is simply eggs, oil, salt, pepper, and vinegar. These are all products that consumers regularly have in their homes. However, some commercial mayonnaises contain so many ingredients that it is reasonable to think that it could only be created in a laboratory. It seems that the repeal of the imitation food law in the 1970s has created some confusion among the public about what real food is.

See also: Appendix 4: *Arnett, et al. v. Snyder*; Appendix 13: Excerpts from the Code of Federal Regulations Regarding Cheese and Cheese Food.

Further Reading Berdanier, Carolyn D., Johanna T. Dwyer, and Elaine B. Feldman. *Handbook of Nutrition and Food.* Boca Raton, FL: CRC Press, 2008.; Curtis, Patricia A. *Guide to Food Laws and Regulations.* Oxford: Wiley-Blackwell, 2005.; Pollan, Michael. *In Defense of Food: An Eater's Manifesto.* New York: Penguin Press, 2008.

Stephanie Jane Carter

IMPORTATION OF FOOD

Importation of food stuffs into the United States is governed by the U.S. Federal Food, Drug, and Cosmetics Act. The act places the burden on the importer to comply with all laws imposed on the sale of food, including food safety, sanitation, and other requirements, and food package labeling. Federal law is applicable to all imports as imported food is all considered to be in **interstate commerce** even if it is imported into and remains in the same state. The law places the imports under the jurisdiction of the **Food and Drug Administration** (FDA), which does not license importers or certify that food is safe or sanitary or

Tare Rates Allowed by the Customs and Border Protection Tare

In determining the quantity of goods dutiable on net weight, a deduction is made from the gross weight for just and reasonable tare. "Tare" is the allowance for a deficiency in the weight or quantity of the merchandise caused by the weight of the box, cask, bag, or other receptacle that contains the merchandise and that is weighed with it. The following schedule tares are provided for in the U.S. Customs and Border Patrol (CBP) Regulations:

Apple boxes. 3.6 kilograms (8 lb.) per box. This schedule tare includes the paper wrappers, if any, on the apples.

China clay in so-called half-ton casks. 32.6 kilograms (72 lb.) per cask.

Figs in skeleton cases. Actual tare for outer containers plus 13 percent of the gross weight of the inside wooden boxes and figs.

Fresh tomatoes. 113 grams (4 oz.) per 100 paper wrappings.

Lemons and oranges. 283 grams (10 oz.) per box and 142 grams (5 oz.) per half-box for paper wrappings, and actual tare for outer containers.

Ocher, dry, in casks. Eight percent of the gross weight; in oil in casks, 12 percent of the gross weight.

Pimentos in tins, imported from Spain. Depends on size of tins—drained weights:
[#,32]?>3<?show kilos, 13.6 kilograms (30 lb.)—case of 6 tins
794 grams (28 oz.), 16.7 kilograms (36.7 lb.)—case of 24 tins
425 grams (15 oz.), 8.0 kilograms (17.72 lb.)—case of 24 tins
198 grams (7 oz.), 3.9 kilograms (8.62 lb.)—case of 24 tins
113 grams (4 oz.), 2.4 kilograms (5.33 lb.)—case of 24 tins

Tobacco, leaf not stemmed. 59 kilograms (13 lb.) per bale;
Sumatra: actual tare for outside coverings, plus 1.9 kilograms (4 lb.) for the inside matting and, if a certificate is attached to the invoice certifying that the bales contain paper wrappings and specifying whether light or heavy paper has been used, either 113 grams (4 oz.) or 227 grams (8 oz.) for the paper wrapping according to the thickness of paper used.

For other goods dutiable on the net weight, an actual tare will be determined. An accurate tare stated on the invoice is acceptable for CBP purposes in certain circumstances. If the importer of record files a timely application with the port director of CBP, an allowance may be made in any case for excessive moisture and impurities not usually found in or upon the particular kind of goods.

otherwise in compliance with the law. However, importers must register production facilities as well as storage and handling operations with the FDA under the Bio-Terrorism Preparedness and Response Act of 2002. The FDA has the power to detain any food shipments that it determines are not being imported in compliance with U.S. law, that is, the same laws that are applicable to food produced in the United States.

The FDA does not inspect most meat, poultry, and egg items. These items are inspected and monitored by the **U.S. Department of Agriculture** (USDA). Dairy products are inspected by the USDA and the FDA. Raw agricultural foods, such as fruits and vegetables, are also subject to the USDA Food Safety and Inspection Service for inspection and certification.

U.S. Customs and Border Patrol (CBP), a division of the Department of Homeland Security, has the responsibility of dealing with the customs aspect of imports. The authority derives from the Customs Modernization Act (Title VI of the North American Free Trade Agreement Implementation Act [P.L. 103–182, 107 Stat. 2057]), which came into effect in 1993, and from the Trade Act of 2002. The Customs Modernization Act is often called the Mod Act. The Trade Act shifted the burden from the government to the importer to declare the traditional customs information, that is, value, rate of duty, and the classification of the items. These laws apply to all imported goods, not just foods. The CBP operates within a system of "informed compliance," which means that the CBP has the responsibility of keeping the importer informed of changes in the law and regulations and the importers have a responsibility of altering their actions to comply with changes in the law.

Importers must declare the point of origin of the materials imported, the value of products, the purpose of the importation, as well as other information. When the materials are perishable and cannot safely wait in the custody of the CBP, such as raw food, the law provides for a special permitting system that essentially allows the imported goods to bypass the standard waiting and inspection, although all documentation must be filed and applicable duty paid.

Importation of alcoholic beverages is governed by the Alcohol and Tobacco Tax and Trade Bureau (TTB) of the U.S. Treasury Department, which issues alcohol import permits. The alcohol must comply with all U.S. regulations regarding labeling and proofs.

There are hundreds of U.S. trade agreements and amendments with various countries that create special exceptions to the general rules or confer "most favored nation" status. Most favored nation status means that no other nation has a more favorable relationship on a particular matter regarding trade with the United States. These agreements are in constant flux regarding individual commodities, so they must be monitored to ensure up-to-date information. Many of these agreements also give the USDA the ability to investigate, in cooperation with the parallel organization in other nations, when there has been a suspected breach in food safety, such as an *E. coli* outbreak due to imported vegetables or fruit.

See also: Bioterrorism Act of 2002; Fair Packaging and Labeling Act.

Further Reading U.S. Customs and Border Patrol. *Report of Customs and Border Protection, Importing into the United States.* http://www.cbp.gov/linkhandler/cgov/newsroom/publications/trade/iius.ctt/iius.pdf.

Elizabeth M. Williams

INTERNATIONAL PLANT PROTECTION CONVENTION

The International Plant Protection Convention (IPPC) is an international agreement designed to protect the world from the spread of plant diseases and also to prevent the spread of agricultural pests. This Convention was first promulgated in 1952 by the **Food and Agriculture Organization of the United Nations** for consideration by the nations of the world. The Convention coordinates the collection of information regarding the spread of pests and disease and helps to track the methods of prevention and other forms of aid between the member nations regarding agricultural pests and disease. Over 170 nations currently are participants in the work of the IPPC.

The IPPC is governed by the Commission of Phytosanitary Measures. The Commission recognizes that in a world where imports and exports of agricultural products cross hemispheres, continents, and oceans, agricultural pests and plant diseases are constant threats to world agriculture. Within the IPPC there are regions that coordinate and gather information about the issues that are of interest to and threaten each region.

Another important task of the IPPC is to settle disputes between and among member nations. Although the decisions of the dispute resolution of the IPPC are not binding on the parties, the parties may resort to taking their dispute to the **World Trade Organization** (WTO), whose decisions are binding. It is likely that the WTO will give weight and consideration to the recommendations of the IPPC. The IPPC also issues standards regarding plant safety and the prevention of the spread of pests. Especially when a dispute is related to the question of standards, the IPPC's recommendation will carry weight.

In 2005 under the IPPC the Subsidiary Body on Dispute Resolution was created. Each of the seven regions of the Commission is represented. The group approves and recommends technical experts, works with the WTO, and also reports on decisions of the resolution of disputes.

The IPPC is committed to lending technical assistance to member nations so as to help developing nations become a part of the international marketplace. This includes help with capacity building and also with advance identification of areas of possible dispute and planning for the avoidance of disputes. Developed nations are also expected to lend aid in emergency situations to protect the health of agriculture.

The IPPC has found that even the best intentioned programs, one in particular called "Plants for Planting," have the potential for spreading pests. The spread of aquatic species of plants that have few natural predators to new areas can cause loss of other plant and animal life in their new locations. In developed nations, invasive plant species and pests have been released through aquariums, for example. When those pests have nothing to keep them in check, they can choke streams and kill wildlife. The failure to stop certain transfers for pests has been the cause of criticism of the IPPC.

See also: Pesticides;   Appendix 16: World Trade Organization Ministerial Conference Decision.

Further Reading International Plant Protection Convention. https://www.ippc.int/file_uploaded//publications/13742.New_Revised_Text_of_the_International_Plant_Protectio.pdf.

Elizabeth M. Williams

INTERNET SALES

Internet sales continue to grow year by year. In 2002 U.S. online retail sales were $48 billion. In 2006 online retail sales were more than $130 billion. In 2001 each buyer was spending $457 each year online. In 2006 that figure had grown to $784. Food products are part of the growth of Internet sales. The growth in sales is accompanied by growth in online fraud and other illegal activity.

The Fair Credit Billing Act (FCBA) was enacted by Congress in 1986 as an updating of the Truth in Lending Act. It is designed to protect consumers from unfair and disadvantageous billing practices. In addition, it contains a provision to deal with legitimate billing errors. The FCBA applies only to accounts considered to be "open-ended" such as a credit card account or charge accounts issued by department stores. It applies to purchases made through PayPal and other online payment systems. The act does not apply to installment loans. The **Federal Trade Commission** (FTC) is the general enforcement authority for the FCBA. Bank billing errors are covered under banking regulations.

The FCBA outlines many different types of billing errors that might result in a dispute. One such consumer protection deals with unauthorized charges. Consumers are protected in that they do not have to pay for unauthorized charges beyond $50. This places the burden on the company to protect itself against these charges. There are procedures to resolve issues of charges that list the wrong date or the wrong amount. There are procedures to resolve disputes over charges for goods and services that were not received as promised. Those accounting issues like addition errors, not posting payments and credits, such as returns, are also covered by the FCBA. There is a procedure for bills sent to an old address. There is also a procedure that allows the consumer to inquire about questionable charges, ask for a written proof of purchase, claim an error, or ask for an explanation of a charge.

Consumer invoices must list an address identified for "billing inquires." To take advantage of the law's protections, the person claiming a dispute must write to this address. Using the address to which payments are made may mean that the dispute has not taken place within the time frame stated in the law. The claim must state the name and address of the claimant, as well as the account number. There must be a written description of the error or dispute. The consumer has 60 days from the date of the error billing to have the written claim received by the creditor. Proof of mailing by using a certified letter with a return receipt is recommended.

The law provides that creditors must send a written acknowledgment of a complaint no later than 30 days after receipt or resolve the issue. The creditor has two billing cycles in which to resolve the matter, but in no case can the matter take more than 90 days to resolve.

Consumers are not required to pay the amount that forms the basis of the claim or dispute during the period of investigation. But all amounts not in dispute must be paid including any finance charges or interest. The consumer cannot refuse to pay the entire bill, just because a portion of it is in dispute.

Mirroring the consumer portion of the regulations, creditors may not impose finance charges on the challenged amount or try to collect it while the matter is under investigation. To protect the creditor from consumer misconduct or fraud, the credit line may be limited by the disputed amount.

No action may be taken against the consumer during the investigation, including affecting the credit report of the consumer or claiming that the consumer is late in paying bills. The creditor may state that the bill is in dispute. The Equal Credit Opportunity Act provides that consumers may not be punished for taking advantage of the rights established in the FCBA.

After investigation, if the creditor does confirm an error, a written report of the manner in which the error will be corrected and the account rectified must be provided. The creditor may not charge finance charges or interest when there is an error and the creditor must remove the incorrect charge. If it is determined that some of the bill is owed by the consumer, this determination must be explained in writing.

It is inevitable that sometimes there will be no error found. The creditor must so inform the consumer in writing of this finding with an explanation of the findings. If the consumer continues to believe there is an error, the consumer may request documentation of the error. Such a finding allows the creditor to impose all finance charges and interest, including those that were not charged during the investigation period. A minimum payment will be due by the consumer.

When there is continued disagreement about the dispute and the investigation by the creditor indicates that the money is owed, the consumer may inform the creditor within 10 days, reasserting the claim. If the consumer refuses to pay the disputed amount under these circumstances, the creditor may begin collection procedures and take other reporting action. If the creditor does make a report to a credit bureau about the consumer, the creditor must inform the bureau that the consumer still disputes the invoice and that this is the reason the consumer has not paid. The creditor must also inform the consumer of those to whom these reports are sent.

Creditors failing to act in accordance with these rules are prohibited from collecting the disputed charges (except for the basic $50) including finance charges and interest. This is the case even when it is determined that there is no error and the invoice is accurate. This is an incentive in the law to make the creditor comply with the law and regulations.

The FCBA provides a consumer remedy, allowing those creditors who violate the law to be sued by affected consumers. If consumers prevail, remedies include a damage award as well as a penalty of two times the finance charge amount, limited to between $100 and $1,000. The creditor may also have to pay attorney's fees and costs.

More and more food is being sold over the Internet, often escaping sales tax and other regulation. The need to collect sales tax on sales by mail or other method of shipping outside of a particular state was addressed by the U.S.

Supreme Court in the case, *Quill v North Dakota* in 1992. The high court ruled that sellers who have no nexus (physical presence in a state) with a state need not collect sales tax from that state. Requiring retailers to collect sales tax from each state would represent such a burden that it would interfere with **interstate commerce**. Although this case dealt with mail order catalog sales and fax orders, its decision impacts internet sales. Companies selling grass-fed meat, organic fruits and vegetables, specialty ethnic foods, and other products over the internet are selling to consumers who often do not pay sales tax. Congress has not required Internet sellers to collect sales tax where there is no nexus with the state. This advantage over local sales may actually make some unusual food economically available to consumers over the Internet.

Yet another issue with Internet sales that directly affects food is that, especially from small operations or when sold in foreign countries, food may be sold that does not comply with health and safety requirements of the **Food and Drug Administration** or the **U.S. Department of Agriculture**. Because companies selling food and beverages can number into the millions all over the world, these companies can accept funds through credit card sales and mail or otherwise send food anywhere. It may not be possible for improperly labeled packages to all be checked by customs officers. Internet sales may make it possible for consumers to order and obtain alcoholic beverages and fresh foods and processed foods that escape regulation. For example, there are special regulations about the sale of cheese made from unpasteurized milk. Many people like these cheeses and will order the cheese directly from France or another country, hoping that it will slip into the country and be delivered.

See also: Food and Drug Administration, Interstate Commerce, U.S. Department of Agriculture.

William C. Smith and Elizabeth M. Williams

INTERSTATE COMMERCE

In today's world, despite the locavore movement, which advocates consumers buying food grown locally, most food and food producers are not involved in interstate commerce. Interstate commerce refers to goods that are transported from the state in which they are grown or produced to another state, another country, or another place within the same state when it passes through another state during transport.

Interstate commerce was originally the basis for the U.S. Constitution's jurisdiction over activities that would normally have been controlled by the states. The Constitution specifically grants power to the Congress in matters that involve interstate commerce in Article 1, Section 8, Clause 3. (This clause grants additional commercial powers to Congress.) It is a fundamental enumerated power and forms the basis for legislation and regulation regarding food, beverages, organics, transportation, labeling, and almost everything that Congress regulates. Without this clause, each state would be passing and enforcing different laws. This means that for goods to pass from one state to another, the goods could only go where they conformed to another state's laws. This would severely inhibit the movement of foods and beverage, and, thus, severely inhibit commercial activity in general.

Another clause in the Constitution, the Necessary and Proper Clause, is also a clause used in conjunction with the Commerce Clause, which expands the power of the Commerce Clause alone. This means that Congress has the power to do what is necessary to accomplish what the constitution gives it the authority to do. Thus, if the Commerce Clause gives it the authority, the Necessary and Proper Clause allows Congress to pass laws to accomplish its goals.

Use of the Commerce Clause blossomed in the 20th century. Its use has grown as interstate commerce has itself grown. Today large food producers ship their products all over the country. These products are made of raw materials and agricultural products that also come from all over the country. These companies and their products are regulated under the interstate commerce powers of Congress.

With the regulation of commerce on a national basis, a company can conform to one standard and know that such conformity will allow it to transport and sell its products around the country. This allows small companies to know what must be done everywhere in order for them to expand. Federal law also preempts state law in many matters, thus often conflicting state laws will not inhibit interstate commerce.

Now it is established that in addition to the actual transportation of goods over state lines, the commerce clause also includes advertising that crosses state lines. This is the basis for national regulation of children's cereal, banning the advertising of certain alcoholic beverages on television, and other types of advertising. Labeling laws apply to foods in interstate commerce. In addition, interstate commerce refers to transportation and packaging. All of these matters affect food safety and the cost of food. Interstate commerce also regulates food and beverages that are imported from foreign countries. Import laws, labeling laws, and safety laws also apply to what is brought legally into the United States. These laws affect local products and what may be available to consumers. Labeling will identify country of origin and allow consumers to be informed.

Internet commerce has caused changes in attitudes toward interstate commerce. This is particularly true as it applies to states sales tax. In the early days of the nation, states actually imposed import taxes on goods that came into one state from another. The states treated each other like foreign countries. This practice was outlawed by the U.S. Supreme Court. However, within a given state, tax on the sale of goods was permitted. Many states rely heavily on the revenue generated by sales tax. A use tax, which is a tax levied by a state when goods are registered in a state, is another type of tax that affects interstate commerce. An example of this tax is the cost of registration of a vehicle in a new state, when the vehicle was previously registered in another state. When trucks are reregistered from one state to another, the additional costs may be seen in increased costs. Small farmers moving from state to state are most likely to be affected by this. These taxes are based on point of sale and point of registration.

States have been affected by **Internet sales** of all goods. These sales are virtually impossible to regulate and monitor, and when the seller does not sell in the state to which the goods are shipped, no taxes need be collected. With the increased sale of foods over the Internet, those states that collect sales tax on foods have complained that taxes have been negatively affected. Congress has resisted allowing the imposition of sales tax on internet sales for several reasons. The primary reason is that it will create a chilling effect on the development of Internet commerce. But in addition Congress is motivated by the difficulty of monitoring these sales, the increased burden that might be imposed on sellers and thus the increased cost of goods that would be passed on to the consumer.

> ### The Commerce Clause
>
> Article 1, Section 8, Clause 3 of the Constitution of the United States declares that the Congress shall have the power "to regulate commerce with foreign nations, and among the several states, and with the Indian tribes. . .." This power was written into the Constitution but was not found in the Articles of Confederation. The Founding Fathers considered this a shortcoming of the original document and added this clause, which has become one of the foundations of power for the economic regulation of the nation, enabling the United States to act as a nation. It has affected the development of the relationship between the federal government and the states, as well as the relationships between the three branches of government.

All of these issues are based on interstate commerce and the interstate commerce clause, the primary clause used to regulate the economy of the United States. Food and beverages are one of the most highly regulated areas of commerce. As the law of food changes, as policies and attitudes toward eating evolve, interstate commerce and the commerce clause must be flexible enough to reflect these changes.

See also: Advertising of Alcohol; Appendix 7: *In the Matter of McCormick & Company, Inc.*; Appendix 9: Twenty-Eight Hour Law of 1873 as Amended in 1994.

Elizabeth M. Williams

INVENTIONS AND PATENTS

There is an interesting history of food products that have been patented. A patent is a special status of protection that is extended to an inventor. The government extends this exclusive right to produce the patented invention in exchange for the public declaration of the invention. The patent grants the patent holder the time to exclusively benefit from the use or sale of the invention for a limited period of time. When the patent expires, then anyone can benefit from the invention. To be patentable an invention must be new, not obvious, and either useful or have some industrial application. There are four types of patents recognized by the law in the United States: software patents, biological patents, chemical patents, and business methods patents. The basis for U.S. patent law is found in Article I, Section 8 of the Constitution.

The patent allows the patent holder to exclusively benefit from the patent; however, the patent holder can also keep others from benefiting during the patent period, even when the patent holder does not benefit. The usual patent period is between 17 and 20 years, with a renewal fee. The patent is a form of property right. Thus, as a property right, it can be sold, licensed, or mortgaged. A patent can be owned by a real person or a corporation.

The government grants a patent and its special protections to encourage innovation. The patent also encourages the innovation to become part of public knowledge. Without the special protections and exclusivity, an inventor would tend to keep the innovation secret. That would mean that the public would not benefit from the invention. The period of exclusivity allows the inventor the opportunity to recover the costs of development of the invention. Those who copy the invention only invest in the cost of production, not the cost of development.

Patent law has been criticized on several fronts. One criticism is based on the biological products and knowledge that exists in some traditional cultures. Many plants and practices are generally known within some cultures to affect cures for certain conditions and diseases. Developed nations have been criticized for learning about these practices, not unknown or unfamiliar in the traditional society, and taking the plant, often an herb made into a tea or other infusion, and the knowledge to the developed nation. The researcher develops an invention from the plant, armed with the knowledge from the traditional culture. The researcher patents the invention and benefits from it, but the entire traditional culture that has known about the beneficial plants receives no benefit. This situation is one that favors the property rights of the developed world over the sharing of traditional knowledge in cultures without the same type of property rights.

Another area of criticism is the biological patenting of seeds that have been genetically engineered. In such cases, seeds that are saved from a crop grown from patented seeds cannot be used by the farmer without paying a fee to the patent holder. The patent holder owns the right to control the use of the seeds. The patents of developed nations have been protected against challenge by the **World Trade Organization.**

The food industry has been inventing and patenting products for years. Some companies, like Coca-Cola, have avoided the public disclosure required by patents by maintaining their secrets as just that, trade secrets. The formula for Coca-Cola is not patented. As long as the secrets remain secret, they do not expire. George Washington Carver (1864 to 1943) is credited with inventing crop rotation, hundreds of uses for peanuts such as peanut butter and peanut oil, as well as uses for sweet potatoes (flour and sugar), soybeans (paint), and pecans. Despite the number of his inventions, he only held three patents.

A grinder to make peanut butter was patented by John Harvey Kellogg of Battle Creek, Michigan, in 1895. Kellogg was the brother of the cereal manufacturer W.K. Kellogg. In 1922, Joseph L. Rosefield patented a method for churning—rather than grinding peanuts—to create a smoother peanut butter that remained stable on the shelf. The Rosefield method allowed a container of peanut butter to remain good for up to a year. In 2004 inventors assigned their patent for cereal bars to General Mills. It is a layered cereal bar, application number D/183322.

Splenda, the commercial name of sucralose, is patented by Tate & Lyle, which holds 32 patents related to the product. Some of the manufacturing patents have expired, threatening the company's ability to continue to manufacture the product. Wal-Mart has begun manufacturing a product that it markets as Altern. Altern is chemically identical to sucralose. Altern is sold for less than Splenda. The laddered expiration of the sucralose series of patents illustrates how important patents can be in preserving the exclusivity of benefit for the patent holder. When even one patent expires, the net of protection may be lost.

There are patents for various types of high fiber pasta, methods for cutting the time needed to cook pasta, making pizza crust crispy, and thawing frozen foods. Clarence Birdseye received 168 patents in the late 1920s for this quick-freezing method, which revolutionized freezing food for storage and transportation. This series of patents revolutionized the quality of frozen food, and made the food retain its flavor, texture, and color. Yet today, after the expiration of the patents, quick-frozen foods have been improved and have created an entire frozen food industry.

Patent violations are not pursued by the government under criminal statutes. In the United States patent violations are private actions, handled in civil court. In some countries, blatant patent infringement may be prosecuted as a crime. In the United States, it is thought that the patent holder is the most interested party to protect and monitor patent infringement.

See also: Seeds, Genetically Engineered.

Elizabeth M. Williams

IRRADIATION

Irradiation is a procedure that is applied to food to extend its life and retard decomposition or retard ripening. The procedure uses ionizing radiation to bombard the food. The irradiation of other things, such as medical equipment and tires, to sterilize the object or impair the ability of microorganisms to grow, is commonplace. It is food irradiation, however, that engenders health concerns and controversy. Food was irradiated by X-rays as an experimental method of preservation in the early part of the 20th century. It has progressed to the stage of implementation and adoption today.

Living organisms contained in food, which have been irradiated, have their DNA altered by the process. This change in the DNA negatively affects the organism's ability to reproduce. This could mean insects, as well as viruses or bacteria. Without reproducing, the organisms cannot consume or deteriorate the food. The DNA of the food is also altered, which affects ripening and sprouting. The radiation levels used in the process are high. The effects thus produced cannot be duplicated by other means. Heat or pasteurization, for example, is a method of achieving this effect in liquids. Heat cannot achieve this effect in solid foods without totally changing the texture or cooking the food.

The **U.S. Department of Agriculture** (USDA) has issued regulations approving the use of irradiation in low doses as a pesticidal treatment for fruits and vegetables. The primary insects affected are fruit flies and certain weevils. As a part of its work with the **Food and Agriculture Organization of the United Nations**, the USDA works with developing countries that have adopted policies approving the irradiation of fruits and vegetables. The USDA has promulgated simplified importation regulations that allow this irradiated product to enter the United States. The waiting period to eliminate incoming insects is thus shortened by the assurance that irradiation will not allow the proliferation of foreign or dangerous insects. Another example of approval of irradiation is the treatment of meat patties to reduce the growth of *E. coli*. This approval is found in the regulations of the **Food and Drug Administration** (FDA).

The European Union (EU) only permits irradiation for dried herbs and spices, as well as dried vegetables intended as seasoning. In the United States, the highest levels of irradiation are also approved for dried herbs and spices. Basically this level of irradiation makes the herbs and spices free of pests of all types and changes the DNA of the herbs and spices to the extent that they do not deteriorate. The EU regulations allow the member nations to promulgate their own regulations and laws regarding irradiation in accordance with the scientific positions adopted by the EU. Several nations, notably France and Italy, allow some irradiated food into their food supplies. In Europe, one of the concerns has centered on setting an upper limit on the amount of irradiation that can be allowed. The **Codex Alimentarius** has proposed the elimination of the upper limit of irradiation, but that position has not been adopted.

Markets in the United States carry irradiated food. Tropical fruits and herbs and spices are likely to have been irradiated. Many ground beef products are irradiated to eliminate the threat of *E. coli*. The U.S. labeling requirement is the use of the Radura at the point of sale. The Radura is the internationally recognized symbol—a green dot and leaves within a partially broken circle. The United States has not adopted regulations that consistently allow labeling that informs the consumer of the level of radiation used. All that is required is the phrase "Treated by radiation" or "Treated with irradiation." One reason for the lack of standards in the field is its rapidly changing technology, as well as the difficulty of creating one standard. Different foods react differently to different levels of irradiation. New technologies are also complicating the attempts at standardization. There are also, of course, political differences regarding setting standards of irradiation.

The FDA has been considering allowing some foods to be sold without the radiation label when the food is not materially changed by the application of the process. The agency is also considering allowing alternative phrases that make less explicit reference to radiation to be used, such as cold pasteurization or electronic pasteurization. The Nuclear Regulatory Commission is the organization that regulates the safety of irradiation facilities. Applying **Hazard Analysis Critical Control Point** (HACCP) principles allows irradiation of food before it reaches the consumer to be a control point.

Some people welcome irradiation as a way to ensure food safety when foods come from countries where growing and handling practices can allow for importation of products with food-borne contaminants. Yet others see the use of irradiation as a way to not enhance the practices of other countries, ignoring the food safety issues that affect developing nations. Other concerns are more practical, such as the fear that food that is spoiled will be irradiated. The process may halt further deterioration, but it may not be fit for consumption with toxins that exist in the food not destroyed by the irradiation. The usual signs of spoiled food, such as an offensive odor or obvious signs of insects, would be masked. Others are concerned that irradiation will affect taste and texture.

Scientific studies of irradiation have been ongoing since the 1950s; however, changes in technology continue to make the studies and the long-term effects of irradiation elusive. Possible areas for study include the concern over vitamins being less easy to absorb or the feeding of irradiated foods to animals that are consumed by humans. Animal food may be irradiated at levels not currently allowed for human consumption. If the animal is negatively affected by eating irradiated feed, consuming the animal may pose a health danger to humans.

Alternatives to food irradiation exist. The use of various gases, use of ultraviolet rays, and heat pasteurization are all proposed by opponents of irradiation as safer and reasonable alternatives to irradiation.

See also: European Union Regulations; Pesticides.

Elizabeth M. Williams

JACOBSON, MICHAEL (1943–)

Michael Jacobson is one of the founders and now secretary of the watch group **Center for Science in the Public Interest** (CSPI). Started in 1971, the organization has advocated for healthier foods throughout the United States, raising awareness through nutrition labels, warnings, and independent scientific studies. Jacobson grew up in Chicago's North Side neighborhood, attended Von Steuben High School, and went on to earn his Ph.D. in microbiology from the Massachusetts Institute of Technology. He then went to work for Ralph Nader's Center for the Study of Responsive Law. He and co-workers Albert J. Fritsch, a chemist, and James B. Sullivan, a meteorologist, wanted to team up to create a public-interest advocacy group that would address concerns through scientific research. Since their areas of expertise were quite varied, the organization initially focused on everything from toxic chemicals and nuclear power, to food additives and nutrition, as well as highways and air pollution.

The scope of CSPI's projects narrowed considerably when Fritsch and Sullivan left to pursue other projects in 1977. Jacobson became the executive director, and food and nutrition became the main focus. The organization began several education campaigns targeting food they saw as unhealthy and began with the book, *Nutrition Scoreboard*, which was published in 1973. Jacobson devised the scoring system that was the basis of the book, hoping that it would be easy to understand for the general public. They also began the Alcohol Policies Project to spread the word about the negative effects of alcohol, as well as ways to combat alcohol abuse and alcoholism. These publications helped inspire reform laws concerning alcohol advertising and increased alcohol taxes. Jacobson and the CSPI also put out a Fast-Food Guide that examined the nutrition content of popular fast-food items. Jacobson continued to publish books on his own and with the CSPI concerning diet and harmful foods, including *How Sodium Nitrite Can Affect Your Health*; *Marketing Disease to Hispanics: The Selling of Alcohol, Tobacco, and Junk Foods*; and *What Are We Feeding Our Kids?*.

These books and other campaigns for public health have helped lead to the mandatory nutrition labels found on all packaged foods, the banning of sulfite preservatives, a more stringent code for "organic" labeled food, and the government warning labels on alcoholic beverages. Continuing efforts to improve the accuracy on nutrition labels have led to the required trans-fat disclosure and warnings of potential harmful diseases on raw eggs and meat. The organization has also pushed fast-food companies and chain restaurants to provide nutrition information on their menu items and has helped New York City in its process of banning **trans fat** and excessive amounts of sodium in city restaurants.

The CSPI continues to pursue campaigns to eliminate junk food from schools, limit the amount of trans fat in products, get warning labels on nondiet soft drinks, and improve food safety laws. They would also like to see higher taxes on unhealthy food and increased lawsuits against corporations that insist on selling unhealthy food. Their success in these campaigns depends on the quality of their research as well as the effect of countering arguments by organizations such as Rick Berman's **Center for Consumer Freedom**.

The CSPI uses a variety of techniques including widespread advertising, free pamphlets, and a newsletter, *Nutrition Action Healthletter*. Jacobson gives a number of interviews and provides commentary on news stations to promote the organization's goals.

Jacobson is also well known for his personal habits, which follow his public campaigns for better food and healthier eating. He banned junk food in the CSPI offices, including soft drinks, and he keeps to a diet based on whole grains, fruit, vegetables, and occasionally fish. He hopes that his efforts and the work of the CSPI will lead to a healthier and more informed American public, and he hopes to see a reduction in childhood obesity as well as the general obesity. **Richard Berman** and his companies often lambaste Jacobson for his belief in the "nanny-state" of government, where the government can intrude on the personal freedom and choices of its people so as to keep them healthy. It is a continual battle in Washington and throughout the country to see who can gather more power and influence to convince the most people to support them. It is a battle that Jacobson seems content to fight as long as he can.

See also: Advertising of Alcohol; Labeling, Nutrition; Appendix 3A: *Pelman, et al. v. McDonald's Corporation*; Appendix 3B: *Pelman, et al. v. McDonald's Corporation*, Amended Complaint; Appendix 3C: *Pelman, et al. v. McDonald's Corporation.*

Kelsey Parris

K

KITCHEN APPLIANCES, SAFETY OF

The Consumer Product Safety Commission (CPSC) is the independent agency responsible for monitoring kitchen appliances. The CPSC was established by Congress through the Consumer Product Safety Act of 1972. The agency maintains statistics on injuries associated with household and kitchen appliances, including the age of the person sustaining the injury. The CPSC also monitors and reports on recalls. The CPSC also provides a Web site and telephone hotline for reporting hazards.

Certification of safety comes from various organizations. Electrical appliances are certified by Underwriters Laboratories (UL), which works with manufacturers through testing, certification, and continuing audits to ensure that its certification maintains it reputation. Underwriters Laboratories has been accredited by the Occupational Safety and Health Administration (OSHA) as well as other nongovernmental groups. Underwriters Laboratories is itself an independent nonprofit organization that has been determining safety standards and guidelines since 1894. It is considered the premiere certification for electrical appliances. Those that are certified are allowed to use the UL symbol on their labels or packaging. The Canadian Standards Association (CSA) is a governmental certification program.

The Energy Star Program of the **Environmental Protection Agency** (EPA) maintains an Appliances Rebate program that is administered by each state. The program allows for the upgrade of appliances to Energy Star appliances, which are energy efficient. A secondary benefit of the program is to ensure that newer, safer appliances are finding their way into the kitchens of consumers.

In addition, the National Center for Standards and Certification Information, a subgroup of the Standards Division of National Institute of Standards and Technology, also sets U.S. standards and coordinates with international organizations. This ensures that imported appliances comply with U.S. standards and that U.S. appliances can be exported successfully to other countries. The American National Standards Institute is another private organization, made up of other standards organizations, that protects the products available to consumers.

In addition to the intrinsic safety of the appliance, both UL and the CPSC have recommended use guidelines that, when followed, ensure the safe use of the appliances.

Further Reading Consumer Product Safety Commission. www.cpsc.gov; Underwriters Laboratories. www.ul.com.

Elizabeth M. Williams

KOSHER AND HALAL LABELS

Kosher and halal labels are unregulated by the U.S. government. Most kosher and halal symbols seen on food labels are registered **trademarks** of their respective certification organizations. According to the Fact Sheet on the Web site of the Food Safety and Inspection Service (FSIS) of the **U.S. Department of Agriculture** (USDA), "products prepared by federally inspected meat packaging plants identified with labels bearing references to "Halal" or "Zabiah Halal" must be handled according to Islamic law and under Islamic authority." The label "kosher" is authorized when meat and poultry have been processed and handled under the supervision of approved rabbis.

Kosher certification organizations are comprised of rabbis and field supervision specialists. They ensure that the food products are produced in accordance with Jewish law by inspecting slaughterhouses, processing facilities, and food ingredients. Meat and dairy must be kept separate in the kosher diet, so food products are indicated as fleishig (meat), milchig (dairy), or pareve (meat-free and dairy-free) by certifying organizations. The symbols placed on foods by kosher certification agencies are usually registered trademarks and cannot be used without the certifying agency's permission.

Kashrut refers to Jewish dietary laws. According to these religious laws, certain animals and their products may not be eaten. Those animals that Jews may eat in accordance with the kashrut must be slaughtered under the provision of Jewish law. Processors must drain all of the blood from the meat, or cook it out, before the meat can be eaten. Of the types of meat that are permitted for consumption, eating of certain parts is still prohibited. Meat and dairy may not be eaten together and must not be on the same plate. They must not be consumed using the same utensils either. Utensils used or even coming into contact with nonkosher food must not be used on kosher food if the touching took place while the food was hot. Fruits and vegetables must be free of insects. Grape products that are not produced by Jews may not be eaten. A mark referred to as a hekhsher usually identifies the rabbi or the certifying organization that certified the food product. There are several kosher certification organizations, though not all of them are equally strict. A commonly used kosher symbol is the letter k in a circle, a symbol used by the OK Kosher Certification Company. The Orthodox Union (OU) is the largest agency in the United States that certifies kosher food. The fee they charge companies for their certification ranges Based on a company's size the fees charged by certification organizations range from range from $4,000 to$10,000. They generate millions of dollars in profit each year. In fact, the certification companies have become a $12.5 billion a year industry.

Halal is an Arabic word meaning lawful or permitted. Halal labels certify that the labeled food is permissible under Islamic law because it has been produced and handled properly under Islamic authority. A Halal certification agency inspects ingredients, how the food was prepared, and where and how it was processed to see that it meets Halal standards.

The opposite of halal, or lawful, is haram, which means unlawful or not permitted under Islamic law. Haram foods include pork and pork by-products. In addition, animals not slaughtered in accordance with the law or those dead before killing, and animals not killed in the name of Allah (God) are haram. Alcohol and any beverages that can cause intoxication or drinks that are hazardous are also haram. Carnivorous animals, birds of prey, and animals without external ears are not allowed to be eaten. Animals considered pests are not permitted. There are also lists of animals that may not be killed in Islam. Some of these animals are considered beneficial, such as bees, and others that eat pests such as ants, spiders, and woodpeckers. Animals considered "generally repulsive" are forbidden. These include lice, flies, and maggots. Animals, such as frogs, that live both in the water and on the land are considered haram. Blood and by-products of blood are also forbidden.

There are a few controversies regarding the certifications. One is that the certification agencies may differ in levels of strictness, making it difficult for consumers. Another issue is the fee involved for certification. Some critics believe that it escalates the cost of a product, which is unfair to people who do not require kosher and halal labels. More than 70 percent of kosher-food consumers in the United States. are not observant Jews, according to the *New York Times*. However, people who support the certification fees say that the cost of the certification is negligible. Moreover, they say the fee goes toward researching ingredients and inspecting facilities. Those who keep kosher say that the kosher certification symbol, K, is highly controversial. Since a letter of the alphabet cannot be trademarked, any food manufacturer can legally, though not ethically, use the letter K. Jell-O labels its product with a K. This symbol is placed on the product by the product manufacturers, not by a kosher certification organization. Many Jews believe that Jell-O is not satisfactory for a kosher diet, and further question why the Jell-O Company has not had its product certified by a kosher certification agency. Another issue with halal and kosher labels is that, although they indicate whether the food product is acceptable for these diets, consumers often believe that they are indicative of more. The labels do not indicate how the animals were treated prior to slaughter, just that they were slaughtered in accordance with Jewish or Islamic law. The meaning of kosher gained attention in 2004 with legal

and ethical violations at the largest independent kosher slaughtering facility, Agriprocessors. People for the Ethical Treatment of Animals (PETA) obtained video footage of workers "ripping the trachea out of live cows after their throats had been cut" (*New York Times*, October 9, 2008). In addition to unethical animal treatment, Agriprocessors became the site of the single largest violation of immigration laws taken by the Immigration and Naturalization Service (INS) in U.S. history with the arrest of 389 employees. Over 9,000

Islamic Food and Nutrition Council of America

The Islamic Food and Nutrition Council of America (IFANCA) certifies food as Halal and grants those products that have passed its inspection the use of its symbol, a crescent M. The INFANCA is a nonprofit organization that operates independently of government, although it is recognized by the USDA, with headquarters in Chicago. The organization has offices in several countries including Canada, China, Malaysia, and several European countries. It certifies food in more than 50 countries. It is essentially licensing its trademarked symbol to those who qualify through its application process.

counts of various violations of child-labor laws were filed against the company by the Office of the Attorney General in Iowa. Many people questioned what kosher meant when respect for life was excluded from kosher slaughter. As a result, many groups have begun to create kosher meat companies that embrace these values. In addition, the fact that people rely on kosher and halal labels marks a trend away from previous practices. People used to know a food was kosher or halal because they knew the person who slaughtered it. That no one knows who slaughters his or her meat and the reliance on labels for assurance marks the trend from small, family-run farms to corporate farms.

See also: Farms, Corporate; Farms, Family; Humane Slaughtering Practices; Appendix 2: *Commack Self-Service Kosher Meats, Inc. v. Weiss.*

Further Reading FSIS Factsheet, http://www.fsis.usda.gov/factsheets/Meat_&_Poultry_Labeling_ Terms/index.asp

Stephanie Jane Carter

LABELING DEFINITIONS

The **Fair Packaging and Labeling Act** (FPLA) of 1966 requires labeling and packaging to give consumers the information that they need to compare brands and make intelligent choices. That means that the consumer must be able to ascertain the name of the manufacturer and the quantity contained in the package. The regulations that were promulgated in the implementation of the FPLA contain the definitions of the terms such as "light" or "organic." These words describe attributes of food. There are also definitions that actually define the food itself.

Besides the FPLA requirements, there have been established definitions for foods that are processed. What the food is may not be immediately apparent to the consumer; the generic name of the item may be loosely defined, and if used in a particular way, will be confusing, if not deceptive to the consumer. For example, the term "ice cream" is used in common speech to describe a frozen dessert made from milk or cream. But the industry developed something called ice milk that was a similar dessert made from milk. In common use, however, it might still be called ice cream. A question arises about whether a frozen product made of tofu without any cream or even milk, which resembles ice cream, might be called ice cream. There is also the question of whether the milk or cream has to be cow's milk or whether it can be goat's milk or another kind. To ensure that the fat count and richness of a product called ice cream would meet the consumer's expectations and to avoid deception and confusion, the **Code of Federal Regulations** (CFR), Title 21, Part 135, Section 135.110 entitled Ice Cream and Frozen Custard, defines the rules. Section 135.115 defines goat's milk ice cream.

To be called ice cream, the product is defined as generally a food created by freezing while stirring a mixture that contains certain dairy ingredients. The provision goes on to specify the minimum level of milk fat that the product must contain, as well as other aspects of the food. If the food does not meet these requirements, it may be perfectly tasty and healthful; however, it cannot be labeled "ice cream." The provision also includes the definition of frozen custard.

The CFR contains the definitions of food that are not single product foods. As food processors develop new foods that mix unusual ingredients to form a product similar to traditional foods or they develop different forms of traditional foods, the definition of the traditional foods becomes imperative. Many of these definitions have been formulated and are found in the CFR.

Examples of foods that have been defined are frankfurters, bologna, knockwurst, cheese, and pizza. Cheese for example is also defined in Title 21 of the CFR. The title of the section is Food for Human Consumption. This section not only contains definitions, but also lists colorants, preservatives, maximum levels of foreign objects, and other considerations that must be referenced in providing food for humans. The provisions are not designed in the whole as consumer protection regulations, but as health regulations. But assuming that food is being prepared in a healthful way, the definitions make it possible for consumers to know what they are buying and eating. In addition it is an assurance to manufacturers that they are properly labeling and identifying the food.

The CFR also provides definitions for milk, curds, and other milk products. It defines methods like pasteurization and provides definitions of other food products such as "cheese food." Many kinds of cheese are defined.

The regulations also define a methodology for processing foods. This means that if a manufacturer wishes to make cheese, the method is defined by regulation. These regulations allow some flexibility. They would apply to cheese made in mass quantities by a large manufacturer as well as on a small basis by an artisanal cheese maker and affineur. An important aspect of the regulations is that cheese of various types is defined as cheese and actually becomes cheese when it meets the requirements of the definition of cheese. What looks like cheese and might be called cheese in common speech cannot be labeled and sold as cheese except by the smallest of producers if it does not conform to the definition.

And the CFR also provides definitions for the methodology needed for the proper analysis for conforming to the definitions. These definitions not only provide the analytical methodologies for manufacturing and testing, but also for testing by the **Food and Drug Administration** (FDA) if there is a question about conformance to the minimum standards set in the definitions.

There are regulations that define ingredients and nutrients that are used in food, such as fiber, cholesterol, and fat. And there are definitions that explain how to label. In 1993 the FDA and the **U.S. Department of Agriculture** promulgated regulations that specified how and when certain claims could be made on a label. There are certain words that have been identified as allowable words that can refer to certain health claims. The way that these words can be used is also regulated. These words are "free," "low," "lean," "extra lean," "high," "good source," "reduced," "less," "light," "fewer," and "more."

See also: Kosher and Halal Labeling; Labeling, Nutrition; Lite Labeling; "Natural" Labeling; Appendix 12: Excerpts from 21 United States Code Sections 341 and Others; Appendix 13: Excerpts from the Code of Federal Regulations Regarding Cheese and Cheese Food.

Elizabeth M. Williams

LABELING, INTERNATIONAL

International labeling is the generic reference to labeling laws that apply to products that are imported into the United States, and to labeling laws that must be complied with to export domestic goods. These laws are based on the requirements and regulations of the United States, as they apply to international food imports, and on the requirements of other countries, as they apply to U.S. food exports.

Imports

Imports must generally comply with all labeling applicable to domestically produced and manufactured goods. However, there are a few additional components for imported goods. These goods must also include the nutritional label in English. The label must show the country of origin of the product or the place where it was manufactured.

Exports

Labeling for export is a complex matter that depends on the country or area into which the product is being imported. Thus, if a product is being exported for sale to the European Union (EU), the product must comply with the EU's requirements. This is also true with regard to exports to any country with import and labeling requirements. The requirements for labeling, as opposed to other types of compliance, can include language requirements, quantity labeling, ingredient labeling, nutritional labeling, naming issues related to **geographic indicators**, and certain limitations of graphic design of labels.

In addition to labeling requirements there may be limitations based on health bans, limitations on genetically modified foods, and many other issues that spring from health and religious beliefs.

See also: European Union Regulations; Labeling, Nutrition; Labeling, Quantity.

Elizabeth M. Williams

LABELING, NON-NUTRITIONAL RESTAURANT

Descriptions on restaurant menus and those communicated by waiters are typically designed to entice and inspire a guest to order a particular item, but they must also *accurately* portray the menu item and its associated price. The concept, laws, and regulations that govern and describe accuracy in wording for restaurant menu items are generally known as truth-in-menus or accuracy-in-menus. The laws and regulations associated with truth-in-menus are typically overseen by a variety of government agencies and fall into several different legal categories. Generally, the term "truth-in-menu" is used within the restaurant industry to describe this loose body of laws that exist at the local, state, and national level. Violators can incur fines and lawsuits based on emotional distress, breach of warranty, false advertising, and violation of consumer protection laws. For example, a warranty that the product described is the product that will be served is created when a restaurant describes an item on the menu. At the most basic level, truth-in-menu laws require a restaurant to serve what it advertises.

In the 1970s, the idea that menus were misrepresenting food became a popular topic for publications such as magazines, newspapers, and trade journals, as well as sources of debate and legislation in state and local governments. The main focus of this legislation was to make it illegal for restaurants to misrepresent quality, quantity, or the place of origin of the food served. On September 8, 1977, the *St. Petersburg Times,* a Florida newspaper, reported that fried scallops were not scallops at many restaurants, but "neatly shaped chunks of shark meat." Florida's truth-in-menu laws make it illegal for fish to be misrepresented as another kind of fish. Each violation carries a $1,000 fine and restaurants are held strictly liable. In 2006 and 2007, the Florida Department of Agriculture and Consumer Affairs investigated and prosecuted those they found to be in violation of these laws using DNA testing. In 1976, Los Angeles enacted a truth-in-menu policy that carried a fine up to a $2,500. The most common violations were related to the re-use of food. Other violations included restaurants labeling frozen orange juice as freshly squeezed and referring to table syrup as maple syrup. The Los Angeles County Department of Health Services still regulates and enforces its truth-in-menu laws. While Los Angeles' truth-in-menu regulation received a great deal press because of the large fine associated with it, other states and cities considered or passed regulations as well. In 1976, noted food writer Mimi Sheraton of the New York Times reported that Connecticut had an "unfair trade practices act that [prohibited] misrepresentation in advertising, which is interpreted as including restaurant menus." In the late 1970s, the Washington, D.C., Department of Environmental Services sent agents to restaurants in an effort to enforce truth-in-menu regulations. According to reports, 75 percent of the chicken salads examined were made with turkey, which was less expensive. All of the "fresh" shrimp examined had been previously frozen. Although the federal government has specific definitions of dairy products, 90 percent of the "cream" examined was actually half-and-half. All of the "maple" syrup was just table syrup. In 1981, New Jersey put truth-in-menu legislation into effect. New York City proposed truth-in-menu legislation several times since the 1970s. Proposed by Councilwoman Carol Greitzer in 1974, 1985, and 1990, the bills were unpopular with the New York City restaurant industry. The restaurant industry complained about several aspects of the bill, including one that required that "the description of all beverages on the menu shall mention the serving size in ounces and metric measurement." Greitzer's unsuccessful 1990 bill was considered simpler, forbidding misrepresentation on menus, requiring menus to be posted in public view, and that prices be quoted with specials. Still, the restaurant industry rejected the bill. Menu descriptions fall to the legislation and enforcement of local and state governments, but the federal government became involved in health and nutrient claims on menus in the 1990s. Congress passed the Nutrition Labeling and Education Act (NLEA) in 1990, requiring nutritional information and labeling for many foods. With this act, the **Food and Drug Administration** (FDA) created specific regulations for these claims. However, the NLEA did not apply to restaurant menus. In July 1996, the Federal District Court in Washington, D.C., mandated that FDA regulate these types of claims on menus. In 1997, the government extended the NLEA of 1990 to include restaurant menus. Since then, claims such as low-sodium, low-fat, light and **lite**, cholesterol-free, and others must meet the FDA standards for those definitions. Even though the federal requirements apply to everyone, the requirements of the state and local governments vary according to the location of the restaurant.

There are several common issues in truth-in-menu legislation. Restaurants normally oppose them because it makes menu-writing more difficult. One common issue in truth-in-menu legislation is whether it is necessary. Many states have laws that cover truth-in-menus. For example, even though truth-in-menu legislation was regularly proposed, the New York State Department of Agriculture and Markets had some form of the legislation relating to this since 1920, known as Article 17. However, many people did not know of the legislation because it was rarely enforced, except in cases of misusing the word "kosher." Some states reported that once enacted, they had few consumer reports of violations. Although this could be interpreted as an indication that the legislation was useless, it could also be interpreted as the restaurant industry responding to the issues that the legislation regulated. Generally, restaurant associations have proposed their own guidelines and have published educational materials for restaurants. These help restaurants understand and comply with current laws and attempt to avoid future legislation.

The following are some categories of menu description that entail legal issues.

Size
The federal government has established specific definitions of the sizes of certain products. For example, the **U.S. Department of Agriculture** (USDA) grades eggs according to size, and the sizes are clearly defined. Whether or not there is a specific definition of a product, the restaurant may be held to a relevant industry standard. Another size issue is related to **portion sizes**. For example, if the restaurant advertises an 8-ounce steak, the restaurant has an obligation to serve an 8-ounce steak. When a restaurant orders a 8-ounce steak from a distributor, the product may purge liquids that yield a 6-ounce steak on arrival at the restaurant. Usually, "purge" is covered in a contract between the restaurant and the purveyor. However, the customer is not part of that contract and the restaurant must be careful to serve the product that has been advertised to the consumer. Size is particularly important to consumers, who often base how much they are willing to pay for an item on advertised sizes.

Quality
The federal government has also created specific quality definitions of certain products. The Prime, Choice, and Select grades of beef have specific meanings under USDA guidelines.

Price
Restaurants are encouraged and sometimes required to make prices of items clear to customers. For example, if an item is advertised at $6, it must be sold at $6. Restaurant industry experts often encourage restaurants to make it clear to customers when they will be charged for refills, substitutions, and/or service charges.

Ingredients
Ingredient lists should be accurate and not misleading. For example, they must not refer to half-and-half as cream in breach of USDA guidelines. Misleading customers

about ingredients may cause bigger issues for the restaurant if consumers rely on an ingredient list to their detriment. Many consumers have allergies, religious beliefs, and other issues that prohibit them from eating certain foods. In 1990, McDonald's was criticized for leading customers to believe that its French fries and hash browns were vegetarian. McDonald's responded by saying that it never claimed that the French fries it sold in the United States were vegetarian. However, consumers found McDonald's ingredient list misleading. The ingredient list mentioned no animal products but did include "natural flavors." The natural flavor was beef extract. Using natural flavors as a synonym for beef extract was within FDA guidelines. Many vegetarians consumed the French fries and hash browns, including Hindus in the United States, who are vegetarian for religious reasons and consider the cow sacred. Lawsuits were filed on behalf of any vegetarian who ate these products before 1990, when McDonald's announced it would stop using animal products in the French fries and hash browns. The 11 plaintiffs, who claimed emotional distress, were each awarded $4,000 and McDonald's agreed to donate $10 million to Hindu organizations closely linked with the concerns of the lawsuit in an agreement to settle the lawsuit.

Brand Name Usage

Words like Coke and Jell-o are brand names. Misuse of these names creates a trademark infringement. For example, a restaurant cannot advertise that it sells Coke when it is using a substitute. It cannot refer to a dessert as a Coca-Cola Cake unless that cake actually contains Coca-Cola.

Product Identification

The FDA has established standards of identity for certain products, such as maple syrup.

Point of Origin

It is fraudulent to misrepresent from where an item originates. In some cases, state law creates specific regulation dealing with this issue.

Preparation Style

Several preparation styles have been defined by the government. Items that are "grilled" must be grilled rather than steamed with grill-marks added mechanically. Items called "**kosher**" must meet the requirements of Orthodox Judaism. "Baked ham" must be baked in an oven for a certain amount of time.

Merchandising Terms

Merchandising terms such as "home-made" and "fresh" have been defined by the government. An item cannot be called "fresh" if it has been frozen, dried, canned, or processed.

Illustration/Graphics
Illustrations and graphics are a visual way of describing a menu item to a customer. Many experts recommend adding a qualifier such as, "not actual size," to avoid misrepresentations.

Nutrition and Health Claims
The federal government regulates health and nutrition claims on menus under the 1997 amendment to the NLEA of 1990. Additionally, more health information is required under the health care reform of 2010.

Menu Caution Statements
Certain foods require caution statements. Raw and undercooked foods require a disclaimer of a certain size that explains that consuming these foods increases the risk of food-borne illness.

See also: Diet Foods; Dietary Supplements; Food Laws, Enforcement of; Geographic Indicators; Imitation Foods; Kosher and Halal Labels; Labeling Definitions; Lite Labeling; Milk, Organic; National Organics Standards Board; "Natural" Labeling; Portion Sizes; Pricing; Labeling, Nutrition; Appendix 3A: *Pelman, et al. v. McDonald's Corporation*; Appendix 3B: *Pelman, et al. v. McDonald's Corporation*, Amended Complaint; Appendix 3C: *Pelman, et al. v. McDonald's Corporation*.

Further Reading Barth, Stephen, and David K. Hayes. *Hospitality Law Managing Legal Issues in the Hospitality Industry.* 2nd ed. Hoboken, NJ: John Wiley and Sons, 2006; Denney, David T. "What You Say Is What You Get: Understanding Truth-in-Menu and Labeling Laws." *Restaurant Start-up and Growth* (October 2009): 24–31; Sheraton, Mimi. "When the Menu Misleads You." *New York Times*, June 29, 1977, 46; Sherry, John, E.H. "Truth-in-Menu Legislation: Do the Benefits Outweigh the Costs?" *Cornell Hotel and Restaurant Quarterly* 18. no. 3 (1977): 4–5

Stephanie Jane Carter

LABELING, NUTRITION
In 1990, the Nutrition Labeling and Education Act (NLEA) became a law under President George H.W. Bush. It greatly expanded what the information manufacturers had to include on labels. It requires processors of food to determine certain nutrition and component quantities of the food that is produced and state that information in particular format on the food label. The information that must be included is the saturated and unsaturated fat, cholesterol, sodium, sugar, fiber, protein, and carbohydrate content. This information must also be provided for the 20 most popular fruits, vegetables, fish, and shellfish. Retailers are allowed to post a sign or placard in their store that includes all of the applicable nutritional information. The law also includes exemptions. The exemptions includes "meat, poultry, and egg products, food sold in restaurants and at prepared food counters in grocery stores, infant formula, foods sold in bulk, foods with insignificant amounts of nutrients, and foods sold by retailers with total sales of less than $500,000."

The NLEA places responsibility on the **Food and Drug Administration** (FDA) to promulgate and set minimum standards and create definitions for popular adjectives that are used to describe food such as "low," "lean," "lite," "reduced." The FDA is also mandated to create and promulgate minimum standards for approving health claims that appear on food labels where there is sound science behind the claims. The claims asserted need be based on solid evidence, be accurate, truthful, and not be misleading. Finally, the health claims should have a provision to allow endorsements or some form of third-party comment.

The FDA and the **U.S. Department of Agriculture** (USDA), acting in cooperation, issued regulations that stipulated the format and content for the food labels. These regulations included processed meats and poultry products. The purpose of the law and the entire labeling format is to provide consumers with pertinent information in an easy-to-read format.

The USDA and the U.S. **Department of Health and Human Services** (HHS) issued new dietary guidelines in 2000. The USDA will now require that meat and poultry products contain nutrition labels. In concern for the health of Americans, the USDA's required nutrition labeling now coordinates with the new dietary guidelines in terms of portion and other components. The new guidelines also contain admonitions to engage in physical activity. In 2006, the FDA required that the nutrition facts labels on packaged food products list information about the amount of **trans fat** per serving.

Labels

The labels on food packages are designed to help consumers make intelligent decisions about the kinds and selection of foods they choose to eat. The nutrition facts label first states the standard serving size followed by the number of calories contained in a serving. Following this initial information is an analysis of the components that the law requires to be reported. Fat, sodium, carbohydrates, and protein are always listed. There are 15 nutrients or components that are almost always listed. They are calories, calories from fat (saturated, unsaturated, and trans fat), cholesterol, sodium, carbohydrates, dietary fiber, sugars, protein, vitamins A and C, calcium, and iron.

The regulations provide that if a product contains less than 5 grams of fat, the amount shown can be rounded to the nearest .5 grams. When the product contains less than .5 grams of fat, the report can be rounded to 0 grams. For example, when a product contains .35 grams of trans fat per serving (where the package contains 30 servings), the label could show 0 grams of trans fat, because .35 is less than .5. This is the case despite the fact that the total amount the food contains is 10.5 g of trans fat.

Child Nutrition Labeling

The USDA's Child Nutrition (CN) Labeling Program allows food manufacturers to include a standardized food crediting statement on their labels if they choose. However, the USDA Food Nutrition Service (FNS) has to approve the labels before they are applied to the products, and manufacturers have to follow FNS quality control procedures and submit to inspection. The CN Labeling Program typically is applied to products that are sold to food service providers who offer FNS meal programs.

The program is operated by FNS in partnership with the industry. This program is voluntary, so there is no enforcement or regulation of CN labeling. The industry is anxious to test voluntary programs to avoid stringent regulation. The program requires an evaluation of a product's formulation by FNS to participate. The purpose of the FNS evaluation is to determine the contribution of the product to meeting requirements of each meal. Food manufacturers are permitted to provide the FNS statement of this contribution on their labels.

See also: Labeling, International; Labeling, Quantity; Appendix 3A: *Pelman, et al. v. McDonald's Corporation*; Appendix 3B: *Pelman, et al. v. McDonald's Corporation*, Amended Complaint; Appendix 3C: *Pelman, et al. v. McDonald's Corporation*.

William C. Smith and Elizabeth M. Williams

LABELING, NUTRITIONAL RESTAURANT

Americans are eating in restaurants and buying take-out from restaurants at an ever-increasing rate; however, most restaurants do not post nutrition information for consumers in menus or anywhere in the restaurant. Because consumers usually do not know how many calories they are getting in their order and have no idea how much fat and salt they are consuming, they are probably eating more than they think they are. Some consumer advocates believe that restaurant patrons should have point-of-purchase nutritional information. They claim that without this information consumers have tremendous difficulty making informed choices at restaurants. In a growing trend, there is more and more demand that chain restaurants, at least, should be required to give nutritional information in the restaurants, either on the menu or on or near a posted menu.

Restaurants, in an effort to preempt any legislative action and because of a desire to give consumers what they want, have begun giving consumers nutritional information on their Web sites and in brochures. Some have posted the information inside the restaurant, even in the rest room. Consumer groups believe that this information will help consumers make better choices or at least informed choices, when making purchases in their restaurants. They want restaurants to provide information that is equivalent to packaged and processed foods.

In Seattle, the King County Board of Health adopted a law in 2007 that mandated nutritional information be placed on menus and menu boards in chain restaurants, including fast food restaurants in the county. The legislation is applicable to any chain that has 10 locations, including nationwide, and $1 million in sales per year. These restaurants are required to give nutritional information for foods that are sold there. The information required to be given includes caloric intact, fats, sodium, and carbohydrate content. When a menu board is used in the restaurant, calories must be listed by the name of the menu item. The rest of the information does not have to be on the board but needs to be easily readable at the order point. Specials that do not remain on the menu for 60 days are not subject to the law.

Regulations were adopted by the New York City Board of Health in 2008 requiring nutrition labeling in chain and fast-food restaurants in New York City. The information must be posted on menus and food tags and menu boards. The regulations are applicable when a chain has 15 restaurants or more, including nationwide. The restaurants are mandated to post on menu boards the caloric levels of the regular items. The information must be in the same font size as the name of the item and its price.

The National Restaurant Association claims that laws requiring that this information be displayed in restaurants are not good for restaurants. They also claim that it does not really help consumers and can actually be confusing. They claim that restaurants are serving healthier food and are trying to give consumers what they want.

Senator Tom Carper (D-Del.) and Senator Lisa Murkowski (R-Alaska) sponsored the Labeling Education and Nutrition (LEAN) Act of 2009. Mirror legislation was introduced by Representatives Jim Matheson (D-Utah) and Fred Upton (R-Mich.) in the House. The bills are designed to create a national nutritional label mandate that provides disclosure the same information as is required in processed food labeling, but that is applicable to chain restaurants. This law would establish a minimum nutritional standard that would be nationally applicable. The LEAN Act tries to provide some flexibility for the restaurants, but prescribes a method of calculation of nutritional levels with a single set of guidelines in how nutrition information is calculated. The LEAN Act would apply to those chains with at least 20 restaurants.

Still other consumer groups wish to apply the Nutrition Labeling and Education Act of 1990 not only to chain restaurants but also to food service organizations that process and distribute food to restaurants.

See also: Labeling, Nutrition; Appendix 3A: *Pelman, et al. v. McDonald's Corporation*; Appendix 3B: *Pelman, et al. v. McDonald's Corporation*, Amended Complaint; Appendix 3C: *Pelman, et al. v. McDonald's Corporation.*

William C. Smith and Elizabeth M. Williams

LABELING, QUANTITY

All food product packaging must list the ingredients, the amount of product, as well as the serving portion, in accordance with the **Fair Packaging and Labeling Act** administered by the U.S. **Food and Drug Administration** (FDA).

The statement of the amount of product in the package is called the net quantity statement and informs the consumer of the quantity of the food. This statement must be placed within the principal display panel—the bottom third of the main area of the label that contains information. The quantity statement must be written in a way that is obvious and parallel with the bottom of the package as it sits during normal display.

Packages must provide quantity information in both U.S. Customary System measures, such as ounces and pounds, and in metric units, such as grams and liters. The units selected must be straightforward and written in a conventional manner. The rule does not specify whether quantity shown as either metric units or the U.S. Customary Units should come first, be next to, below, or above each other. Numerous examples of acceptable methods of stating quantity are found in the regulations.

The regulation sets type and font sizes for different-sized labels. There is a minimum size for various types of information. Quantity statements may not be smaller than the minimum size for the label.

The net quantity statement refers to the amount of food in the package and not other materials. For example, the weight of the package and any wrapping materials should not be added into the quantity statement. Because each package might not be individually weighed or measured, the producer can use the following rules to find the net weight. It may begin with the average weight of the empty package and any wrapping or packaging materials, the top or lid, and then subtract that figure from the average weight of the same package with wrapping materials and tops or lids when the package contains food.

If the food product contains liquid, whether water or another liquid, the net quantity should contain the weight of the liquid. However, when the liquid is not eaten, and would be drained and thrown away, such as the brine of pickles, the net weight would be given without the weight of the liquid. When the product is contained in a container that is pressurized, like whipped cream or oil spray, the net weight statement will state the amount of product that can be obtained from the can and the weight of the propellant or its volume.

Food weight must be described in a straightforward manner without exaggeration of words that are imprecise and overly descriptive.

Serving Size

Describing serving size is based on the nutrient content. The package describes the nutrient content that each serving contains. It allows the person who eats in accordance with the serving size to know how many nutrients have been consumed. Consumers are expected to consume a portion or serving size. The number of servings in a package has been criticized by those concerned about overeating. They claim that regardless of what the label states, consumers expect an even number of portions in a package. Packaging for one-and-a-fraction servings are usually eaten by the consumer as one portion, thus selling more products and causing consumers to over eat.

See also: Portion Sizes.

Williams C. Smith and Elizabeth M. Williams

LAWS, ENFORCEMENT OF FOOD

The enforcement of food laws on a federal level can be undertaken by the **Food and Drug Administration** (FDA), the **U.S. Department of Agriculture** (USDA), and other agencies granted enforcement powers by Congress through their enabling **legislation**. Similarly, state and local governments have the authority to enforce the laws within their jurisdiction. This is all in the normal course of the regulation of its jurisdiction by government.

When laws are adopted by Congress or a state or local legislative body that requires the promulgation of further regulations, the law usually contains the authorization to create an agency to write the regulations and to enforce them. Occasionally the authority of an existing agency is expanded to include additional powers, as has been seen with the FDA. When an agency is created, not only will it promulgate regulations that help it carry out its mission, but it will promulgate regulations regarding definitions, methodologies, standards, and enforcement. The agency may create an enforcement branch to investigate, enforce, and prosecute violations. It may also apply to the courts for enforcement such as an injunction, or the agency may work with other enforcement agencies such as the FBI.

Corporate Enforcement

If a consumer or health rights advocate group uses its political influence to encourage certain laws to be passed that are not favored by industry, an industry organization may challenge the law for being unconstitutional. In determining the constitutionality of a legally mandated restriction, a court will first identify the constitutionally protected right. The personal right will be viewed in the light of precedent, that is, whether this right has been previously restricted and by what justification. It will be examined in light of other rights, both constitutional and legislative, and a priority of rights will be established. The public good to be obtained by the restriction will be balanced against the harm that the restriction causes to personal and public rights. This assessment is very similar to the assessment of personal rights espoused by John Stuart Mill in his treatise, *On Liberty in 1869*. This assessment includes the right to make a decision that causes personal harm, as long it does not harm others. A court may have applied this analysis to the action of the Chicago City Council in passing the ordinance that banned the sale of **foie gras** in April 2006. The argument would have been that the right to eat the product was of higher constitutional protection than the protection of the city's reputation.

In applying this analysis a court, ultimately the U.S. Supreme Court, the ultimate arbiter of constitutionality, is figuratively determining where to place a phantom fulcrum on a balance. Deciding which rights to protect and how to protect them is a process in constant flux. Today, reasonable people can differ as to the need to protect the public from its own actions and the need to protect the right of the public to make personal choices.

In determining which justifications provide a moral or constitutional basis for the restriction of the consumer's access to food stuffs, they do not fall neatly into categories, but overlap messily.

Citizen Enforcement

Citizen enforcement usually refers to citizens who individually or through an organization think that an existing law or regulation is not being properly or vigorously enforced. Citizens have the option of suing the agency that is not being vigorous and asking the court to issue a mandamus ordering the agency to perform its duty. A second option is for the citizen or organization to directly sue the offending party.

It is also possible that individuals or special interest groups with a particular agenda may bring cases to court or find willing plaintiffs to go to court, whose cases they financially support, to litigate the enforcement of existing laws or to have the court recognize a new interpretation of the law or a new duty, creating a new tort.

On one hand, today there are those who wish to impose right-eating on the population by operation of law. These are the consumer groups that advocate that the society eats too much fat, sugar, protein, salt, refined carbohydrates, and overly processed foods. They are also concerned about portion control. They advocate eating more vegetables and eating fewer engineered foods such as low-fat cheese food, soy cheese, fat-free mayonnaise, and textured soy protein.

Legislators are influenced by lobbyists, thus Congress continues corporate subsidies that distort the market and create the lowest food safety threshold instead of aiming higher. In other words, the law is used to support the industrial food industry as well as to enforce the position of consumer advocates.

In addition to bans created by legislation, a trend in the United States has been to use the courts as a means to enforce a ban. A lawsuit against McDonald's claiming that its food caused a person to become fat, a lawsuit against Kentucky Fried Chicken because its product contained trans fat, and a threatened lawsuit against Kellogg's because it markets sugary cereal to children are examples of the use of the courts to advance the agenda of right-eaters. The existence of these lawsuits shows the degree of fervor of belief held by the health advocates, as well as the interesting position of the corporations re-inventing themselves in the court of public opinion.

Consumer advocates have also used legally imposed bans on foods that are considered most unhealthful. The constitutionality of these bans remains questionable, when the health science that is used to support them is not well established. The courts also must balance the rights of individuals to make bad food choices.

Court of Public Opinion

The trans fat transformation is a recent example of using marketing and the threat of legal action to influence the marketplace. As the threat of a trans fat ban loomed after 2006 when trans fat was required to be identified in nutritional food labels, and as information about the negative impact of trans fat on health proliferated, the food industry immediately began to prominently label products without trans fat and tout them with celebrity endorsements. In a short time, products were reformulated without trans fat and once again advertised for their healthfulness. Producers know that if a fad takes hold, the marketplace reflects it. The very recent low carbohydrate fad had a strong negative impact on the bread and pasta industries. There was fear of a similar reaction to products containing trans fat.

An excellent example of marketing as the way to change producer behavior before resorting to legal action is the **Center for Science in the Public Interest** (CSPI). The CSPI was able to influence movie theaters across the United States to stop using palm oil and to switch to other oils in making popcorn. The question is not whether in fact the alternate oil was healthier. The point is that consumers will demand what they are educated to demand, whether it is a right-eating choice such as no trans fats or a nonhealthy choice such as supersizing.

Courts are mindful of the power of consumer demand. When balancing constitutional issues—the right of consumers to eat something, even if it is not healthy; the rights of the food producers to produce, market, and sell the product; the rights of the public to be protected from harmful products—must all be balanced. Part of that balance is the consideration of demand for the product versus the harm done by legally changing it or banning it rather than voluntarily changing it. The analysis applied by the courts to these issues is multifaceted and complex. Currently these issues are in development and have not been finally resolved.

See also: Foie Gras, Bans on; Litigation; *Pelman v. McDonald's Corporation*; Torts.

Elizabeth M. Williams

LEGISLATION

Legislation is a generic word that refers to any rules, regulations, or laws passed or adopted by a legislative body. Legislative bodies are a part of the three-branch system of government that is established in the U.S. Constitution and is mirrored in state and local governments. The three-branch system consists of the executive, legislative, and judicial branches. Each branch has different powers. The three-branch system ensures that no one branch of government becomes too powerful by limiting powers and creating a system of checks and balances with each branch being able to check the other two.

The legislative branch of government is an elected branch. Members are elected to represent groups of people usually defined by geographic areas. On behalf of the electorate the legislature passes laws that operate as rules to live by, create order, and punish wrongdoing. In the field of food and beverage, laws affect every aspect of the process of raising food through putting it on the table.

Congress

Congress is the two-chamber (the House of Representatives and the Senate) legislative body that makes laws that affect the entire country. After Congress has passed a bill, it either becomes law because it is signed by the president or because it automatically becomes law by the passage of time. Congress has the authority to pass these laws because of the direct authority given it by the Constitution with jurisdiction over certain subjects granted through various clauses found in the Constitution, most notably the commerce clause. The **U.S. Department of Agriculture** was created by Congress by legislation. The mandate to create organic standards was passed by Congress. The **Food and Drug Administration** and all of its programs were established by legislation passed by Congress. Other laws include the Clean Air Act, the **Clean Water Act,** the establishment of the **Environmental Protection Agency**, the Lanham Act, and the **Fair Packaging and Labeling Act.**

Rulo Making

Congress passes laws that create a mandate and describe a purpose. Some laws need further details for the laws to have meaning and to be put into practice. Often the rules require special expertise in the field. When Congress passes a law such as the Fair Packaging and Labeling Act, it mandates an agency to develop rules under the **Administrative Procedures Act**. The agency is a part of the **executive branch**, which is part of the checks and balances of government. The agency and boards and commissions are not elected, but appointed through the executive branch, thus the need for comment and input from the people. The rules and regulations promulgated by the various agencies have the force of law and are a form of **legislation**.

State Legislatures

Each state in the United States has a legislature that is a part of the state's three-branch system. It is made up of persons elected to serve in the legislature. The jurisdiction of the state legislative body is limited to the geographic limits of that state. As with the laws passed by Congress, laws take affect with the signature of the governor or with the passage of time. State legislatures can regulate such things as food markets, local environmental practices, create licensing standards for operating businesses like restaurants, groceries, manufacturing facilities operating within the state like bakeries and soft drink bottling plants, and special labeling laws for recycling, and other purposes. Any authority not specifically granted to the federal government is reserved to the states, so the authority of the states over its citizens remains very broad.

States also have rule-making bodies that are agencies similar to those on the federal level. These agencies are part of the executive branch. The documentation needed for licensing, the inspection rules, and the application process are all created by rule making. These rules have the force of law even though they are promulgated by the executive branch.

Federal laws preempt state and local legislation when there is a conflict, unless the federal law creates an exception. For example, if state law contains a more stringent environmental requirement than the federal law, for example, in the area of agricultural run-off, the state law can be enforced within the state. But where state law is in conflict with federal law and state law sets a lower standard, federal law will prevail in those areas where the federal government has jurisdiction.

Local Government Legislation

The different states have different types of local governments often depending of their size. Some states have several types of local governments, one for rural areas and another for urban areas.

Cities like Chicago have city councils that pass laws, known as ordinances. The jurisdiction of city councils is limited to the geographic area of the city. The city council in Chicago, in its concern for the reputation of the city, passed a ban on serving foie gras in restaurants. The Illinois Restaurant Association challenged the ordinance in court. This court challenge is a part of the checks and balance system of government. The trial court ruled that the city council had the authority to pass the ordinance. Before an appeal on the matter could be heard, the city council repealed the ordinance. Other types of local legislative bodies are based not on city limits but on the county (parish in Louisiana) limits.

As in the relationship between federal legislation and state legislation, state legislation generally preempts local legislation. The exception to this is something called "home rule." When a state constitution grants home rule to a municipality, the city has the authority to pass certain laws even when in conflict with state law.

Sometimes state constitutions reserve certain authority to each county and counties vote on these matters. An important example of this county-by-county authority deals with the sale of alcohol. Many states still reserve this power to each county, and in these states there are dry (alcohol-free) counties where alcohol cannot be purchased and wet counties where alcohol is available.

See also: Executive Branch and Executive Orders; Appendix 7: *In the Matter of McCormick & Company, Inc.*; Appendix 9: Twenty-Eight Hour Law of 1873 as Amended in 1994; Appendix 10: Senate Bill Introduced into the 111th Congress, Amending the Food, Drug, and Cosmetic Act; Appendix 11: Bill AB1437 Introduced into the California Legislature Dealing with Shelled Eggs; Appendix 12: Excerpts from 21 United States Code Sections 341 and Others.

Elizabeth M. Williams

LIABILITY

In tort (civil) cases, liability refers to the responsibility for damages when through negligence or intention the defendant has caused harm. This might happen when, for example, a restaurant does not follow its own procedures in thawing food and allows the bacteria level to rise to a toxic level. Patrons who become sick are potential plaintiffs in a lawsuit. The liability is the level of monetary exposure the restaurant has. Not all liability is based in tort law. The requirement to pay money under a contract or mortgage is also called a liability. It is a legally recognized obligation.

In cases of consumer protection the law can require certain disclosures about a product, for example, the country of origin. Failure to comply with regulations regarding such disclosure can give rise to a liability. Closely related to consumer protection, regulations to protect health are generally considered to be an acceptable basis for certain requirements. They put an obligation on the manufacturer to provide information and to provide safe food. As with consumer protection arguments, the more processed a food is, the more citizens need to rely on the government to protect them. The label, which discloses ingredients, is a proper use of the law and regulation to protect consumer health. If the manufacturer fails to provide the labeling in spite of the legal requirement, there is liability.

When there is a special law, like a consumer protection law or a labeling law, the failure to obey the law creates a financial and legal liability that can amount to a criminal action, especially if the failure is intentional. This liability is based on the requirement that the law is obeyed. The liability is defined by law as a monetary fine or a period spent in jail or both. There is, however, an additional potential liability. If a person is injured by the failure to comply with the law, the manufacturer may also face a tort liability. That liability is determined in relation to the actual damages suffered by the injured party.

In individual cases, liability may be ended by the paying of damages. The injured party has been made whole. However, liability in consumer and health cases involving a failure to comply with legally mandated actions like labeling, proper use of preservatives or colorants, or proper handling of food liability may be greater and more wide-spread. In addition to any criminal liability and any individual tort liability, the manufacturer or producer may have the liability to bear the cost of the recall of products and bear the burden of loss of goodwill with consumers. The cost of correcting wrong practices and developing proper procedures are additional liabilities that are established by law and regulation.

In consumer protection law when there is a manufacturer's defect such as tainted food, the liability for selling the goods that do harm may lie not only with the manufacturer but also with the wholesaler, distributor, and retailer. Celebrities who make or have made endorsements of products that are held to have defects have also been sued on occasion. Thus, it behooves the entire chain of sellers to pressure manufacturers to comply with the rules and sell safe products.

See also: Litigation; Appendix 3A: *Pelman, et al. v. McDonald's Corporation*; Appendix 3B: *Pelman, et al. v. McDonald's Corporation*, Amended Complaint; Appendix 3C: *Pelman, et al. v. McDonald's Corporation.*

Elizabeth M. Williams

LITE LABELING

Lite labeling refers to the practice of food manufacturers implying that certain health qualities exist in their products. Lite—being a corruption of the word *light*—could imply several things: low fat, low calories, low sugar, low sodium, or even low cholesterol. When found on a label, the person who is reading the label cannot know exactly what aspect of the product is "lite"

In 1993 the **Food and Drug Administration** (FDA) and the **U.S. Department of Agriculture** (USDA) promulgated regulations that specified how and when certain claims could be made on a label. Certain words are allowed that can refer to certain health claims. The way that these words can be used is also regulated. These words are "free," "low," "lean," "extra lean," "high," "good source," "reduced," "less," "light," "fewer," and "more."

"Free" can be used when the food contains none of the ingredients labeled "free." In some instances it is impossible to measure to zero, so some dietarily insignificant level is allowed when the free label is used. Thus, fat-free milk may contain an insignificant level of fat. When a food naturally does not contain a certain ingredient or nutrient, the "free" reference must be generic, as in lemon juice, a naturally fat-free food. No claim can be made that this lemon juice is fat free. "Zero," "no," "without," and a few other phrases can be used interchangeably with "free."

"Low," as well as "little," a "low source of," or "few," refers to a food that contains a small amount of something, such as calories or cholesterol, so that even if multiple servings are eaten, an insignificant portion of the daily limits are consumed.

"Lean" and "extra lean" are references to fat content. The FDA regulates seafood and game. The USDA, through its Food Safety and Inspection Service (FSIS) regulates meat and poultry. The regulations list the maximum levels of fat in the various foods that qualify for the "lean" and "extra lean" attributes.

In contrast to "free," the term "high" and the phrase "good source of" refer to nutrients that are deemed desirable by consumers. For example, fiber is something that consumers value in a food product. To use the word "high" the food must contain at least 20 percent of the daily requirement in a serving. The phrase "good source of" can be used when the food product contains between 10 and 19 percent of the daily requirement in a serving. "Rich in" and "excellent source" are also terms that may be used instead of "high."

Another way that a manufacturer may wish to distinguish its product from another more standard product is by making a comparison claim. This means that the new product might contain "more," "less," "fewer," "reduced" or be "light." The regulations define these terms and contain the requirements for their use. The standard may be a naturally occurring food. But if the food is processed, then the standard may be determined by creating an average of industry leaders. An example of a processed food might be standard peanut butter.

The regulations about comparison claims prohibit making a comparison claim of "low" when the standard product is already within the percentage for the particular claim. The standard product must be clearly identified and be similar to the special product when using "reduced" and "light" claims. In other words cottage cheese must be compared with cottage cheese and not ice cream. The use of "less" or "fewer" can be used to compare products that are not alike, when the implication is that the product with "less" or "fewer" is a better or healthier choice. However, the percentage of "less" or "fewer" must be accurate. When the comparison claim is for "more," it must contain at least 10 percent more of the nutrient than the daily value of the food being used as a standard. Once again the standard may be an average of processed food, such as the fiber content of certain bread.

"Lite" or "light" may refer to a reduction in fat in a nutritionally modified food, such as mayonnaise. "Lite" or "light" may also refer to a reduction in calories in a nutritionally modified food. In either case, the reduction is in comparison to a standard, nonmodified product. "Light" or "lite" may also refer to a nutritionally modified food that has a lower than standard sodium content. This can be confusing because the product may qualify for a label that says light in sodium, but still not qualify to be low in sodium. If this is the case it must be further labeled, "Does not qualify as a low-sodium food." "Lite" or "light" can be so confusing that reading the entire label may be the only way to be sure what one is eating. Something may be light because it is lower in fat, but be higher in sugar. Foods that have been traditionally referred to as "light" because of its color, such as light brown sugar, may continue to use that name.

Both the FDA and the FSIS have regulations regarding what they consider implications when certain ingredients are identified. For example, when oat bran is identified as an ingredient, there is a presumption that the product is high in fiber. Therefore, the product cannot be labeled "made with oat bran" unless it also qualifies to be labeled high fiber. These rules also refer to labels on foods made with certain oils, such as "made with canola oil."

Other claims that do not refer to nutrients or that are about the origin of the product are allowed. For example a claim that a food does not contain preservatives is allowed as long as it is true. If the term "free" is used to help a consumer who is concerned about religious dietary practices, that is allowed. It is not a health claim.

See also: Food and Drug Administration, U.S. Department of Agriculture Appendix 12: Excerpts from 21 United States Code Sections 341 and Others.

Elizabeth M. Williams

LITIGATION

Litigation is the generic reference to the form of dispute resolution that resolves controversies in the courts. The term is used to cover all of the aspects of a trial, including pretrial activities, post-trial activities, and appeals. The term may be used to refer to lawsuits brought in state courts as well as federal courts.

To bring a lawsuit, the plaintiff or petitioner must have a case or controversy that is actionable at law. The controversy must be one that involves duties created by law or by contract. Not all disagreements or wrongful acts are actionable. Examples of actionable disputes are breach of the terms of a contract or a tort, which is a civil wrong caused by negligence or intentional act. If there is mere disagreement over the contract terms, but not yet an actual breach, the matter is not actionable.

Along with a case or controversy and an actionable issue, there must be jurisdiction over the person and subject matter. Personal jurisdiction refers to the authority of a court to hear a case involving the people, including businesses, in the matter. The plaintiff may merely submit to the jurisdiction of the court, but a defendant may assert a lack of jurisdiction. Usually this means that the business is not sufficiently associated with the state or the person is not in the state and has little or no association with the state. Personal jurisdiction can be had by being served with the petition in the state.

Subject matter jurisdiction is either defined by legislation or the application of the rules of Conflicts of Laws. For example, a state legislature may create a Domestic Court that only hears domestic matters, whether divorce or adoption. That court would not have jurisdiction to hear a tort case brought for food poisoning. Sometimes subject matter jurisdiction is defined by the dollar value in controversy. States have created small claims courts where the amount in controversy is limited to a stated dollar value. These courts lack the jurisdiction to hear matters of a higher value.

It is possible that an event that forms the basis for suit may occur in a particular state. One or more parties may be from another state. Or a product may be manufactured in one state and cause injury in another, not because it was in interstate commerce, but because a person was on a trip and brought the product home. The guiding principle of law is to find jurisdiction that is most logical and that is based on reasonable expectations of the matter. But sometimes Conflicts of Laws find an arbitrary rule to determine if a state has jurisdiction over the person or subject matter. This problem is often resolved in contracts by simply agreeing to the applicable law that would govern in case of a dispute.

The petitioner must have standing to bring the lawsuit. This means that the petitioner either is the person who claims to have been wronged or legally represents such a person. An example of legally representing another is a parent filing a lawsuit on behalf of his or her child or an officer of a corporation filing suit on behalf of the corporation.

In the federal system all of the requirements of civil procedure apply—a case or controversy, an actionable matter, and jurisdiction. But the federal system is more limited in that there must either be a law that allows the litigation or there is a dispute that is recognized by common law involving parties from more than one state. This is called "diversity jurisdiction." Traditionally the federal system has left many matters to the exclusive jurisdiction of the states—most criminal matters, domestic matters, matters of education, among others. When the federal system creates jurisdiction, it has done so either through the Constitution or through legislation. Diversity jurisdiction is based on diversity of the parties and the amount in controversy. The lawsuit must meet both criteria to have diversity jurisdiction where there is no other basis for federal jurisdiction.

To initiate litigation, a party files a claim or a petition with the clerk of court of the appropriate court. The petition establishes that the petitioner or plaintiff has an actionable claim, has standing, and that the court has jurisdiction. The petition also states the facts of the action and the controversy, names the defendant or defendants, and explains how and why they are responsible. Finally, the petition prays to the courts for the remedy that it seeks to rectify the damage outlined.

Remedies in private disputes (between persons or businesses) usually are money damages. Some states require that damages sought be stated in the petition. Other states allow only the claim that money damages will be sought with the amount to be proven in court. Damages can be quantifiable, such as loss of wages or medical expenses, or more subjective, such as pain and suffering.

In addition to money damages a plaintiff may sue to ask the court for an injunction to stop certain activity. This extraordinary form of litigation is initiated by a petition or claim asking for a temporary restraining order (TRO), which can be signed by the judge without a hearing (ex parte). The plaintiff must convince a court that the blocked action will cause irreparable harm and that the plaintiff has a likelihood of success in the matter. Often the plaintiff must post a bond in the amount of damages claimed in case the plaintiff is unsuccessful. The TRO is issued to prevent the activity in question until a hearing on the matter can be had. The time frame for a hearing is set by law in each jurisdiction. After the hearing the court may issue an injunction that will permanently prevent the activity or dismiss the TRO.

After the petition or claim is filed, it must be served on the defendant. This gives official notice to the defendant that he has been sued. This may be done by a sheriff or marshal, a private process server, or by mail depending on the jurisdiction. The defendant then has a prescribed number of days in which to file an answer with the court. The answer sets out the defense and denies the claim. If there are any counterclaims or other parties who should be brought into the litigation, the defendant must do so with the filing of the answer.

The discovery period is the period after the filing of the petition and answer during which the parties may question each other and acquire documents and other evidence. Forms of discovery include the deposition, which is a formal questioning of a witness under oath, usually made with a record made by verbatim transcript by a court reporter. The deposition may also be recorded visually. The subpoena duces tacem is the request for production of documents or other evidence. A request for examination by experts of certain evidence or the physical examination of the plaintiff may also be requested. The results of this discovery may be used at trial.

Another phase of the litigation process is the filing of motions to limit discovery, limit jurisdiction, dismiss the case, limit the use of evidence, or force the parties to more fully cooperate. These motions are heard by the judge sitting as a trier of law and the motions themselves are not shared with the jury.

Finally, after all discovery is complete and the motions are resolved, the trial begins. The trial is that portion of the proceedings where evidence is presented and argument is made. This is what may be called "one's day in court." It includes opening statements, testimony, presentation of other evidence, and closing arguments. Most trials are public proceedings and may be attended by anyone except potential witnesses. In some jurisdictions television cameras are permitted in the courtrooms.

There is great disparity among the various jurisdictions regarding juries in civil, that is, noncriminal, litigation. There are two parallel trials being attended to during litigation, one involving the legal decisions that must be made during the case, such as ruling on the objections made by counsel. These decisions are always made by the judge, who is the trier of law. When there is a jury, the jury is the trier of facts—making decisions about whom and what to believe and assigning weight to this or that evidence. When there is no jury, the judge is the trier of law and fact. When the case is decided by a judge, the decision is called a judgment. When the outcome is decided by a jury, the decision is called a verdict.

After a case has been decided the losing party has the right to file an appeal. This must be done within the prescribed time or the opportunity is lost. In some matters there is an appeal on several tiers.

Litigation is a useful tool in bringing public attention to matters that a party may find objectionable. The government may be called to task for not properly enforcing its own laws. It may be used when an interpretation being applied by the government does not coincide with an interpretation considered proper by a potential plaintiff. Federal agencies, such as the **Food and Drug Administration**, have been called to task by watch dog groups who have thought that the government was not enforcing laws with sufficient vigor.

See also: Torts; Appendix 1: *United States v. Fior D'Italia, Inc.*; Appendix 2: *Commack Self-Service Kosher Meats, Inc. v. Weiss*; Appendix 3A: *Pelman, et al. v. McDonald's Corporation*; Appendix 3B: *Pelman, et al. v. McDonald's Corporation*, Amended Complaint; Appendix 3C: *Pelman, et al. v. McDonald's Corporation*; Appendix 4: *Arnett, et al. v. Snyder*; Appendix 5: *North American Cold Storage Co. v. City of Chicago*; Appendix 6: *United States v. Park*.

Elizabeth M. Williams

LOANS AND BANKING, AGRICULTURAL

Farmers and ranchers can choose between commercial and noncommercial loans to finance their agricultural endeavors. The federal government offers direct and guaranteed operating and farm ownership loans through the Farm Service Agency (FSA) of the **U.S. Department of Agriculture** (USDA). A loan can be secured through a guarantee from a commercial lender, which the FSA guarantees it against loss up to 95 percent. If a farmer or rancher does not qualify for a commercial loan, the FSA can provide a direct loan. The USDA views these loans as way to help farmers and ranchers that may not qualify for commercial loans. Once the farmer or rancher is able to qualify for commercial credit, the FSA is no longer needed by that individual. Operating loans finance materials used in agricultural production, such as feed, seed, livestock, and equipment. Farm ownership loans finance items, such as land and the materials needed to improve the land. Guaranteed loans of both types may be used to refinance debt. The USDA also provides emergency loans to farmers and ranchers. The USDA offers loans through various services.

The loans that the USDA can make to farmers and ranchers were shaped by a number of legislative developments. The Federal Farm Loan Act of 1916 established regional Farm Loan Banks. Direct operating loans were authorized under the Consolidated Farm and Rural Development Act of 1961 (CONACT). Guaranteed operating loans were authorized under the Rural Development Act of 1972, which amended CONACT. The Rural Development Act of 1972 also allowed the USDA to make ownership, emergency, and youth loans. The legislation of the late 1980s and early 1990s focused a portion of the loans to fund Socially Disadvantaged Applicants (SDAs). The USDA defines SDAs as African Americans, natives of Alaska, Hispanics, Asians, American Indians, Pacific Islanders, and women. The Agricultural Credit Act of 1987 developed ownership loans for these applicants, while the 1990 farm bill developed operating loans for these applicants. The Federal Agricultural Mortgage Corporation (Farmer Mac) was established as part of the Agricultural Credit Act of 1987. Farmer Mac was created in response to the farm crisis of the 1980s, which threatened the success of the FCS. As a secondary mortgage market, it operates with two programs. Farmer Mac I purchases or promises to purchase loans. Farmer Mac II purchases loans guaranteed by the USDA. The Farm Credit Administration's Office of Secondary Oversight oversees the function of Farmer Mac programs. The Farm Credit System (FCS) is the largest agricultural lender in the United States. Although it is a federal agency, it does not operate with federal finances. Instead, it is funded by assessments from FCS institutions and the Federal Agricultural Mortgage Corporation. Beginning farmers and ranchers receive a portion of the funding through the Agricultural Credit Improvement Act of 1992. The

Direct Farm Ownership Down Payment Loan Program is designed to aid beginning farmers. The USDA provides some very specific loans. For example, it offers a Farm Storage Facility Loan.

The USDA's FCS loan programs are not without criticism. In 1997, a class-action lawsuit was filed claiming that the USDA discriminated against African American farmers. In a 1999 settlement, the government paid $1 billion to 16,000 African American farmers. In 2010, the government agreed to a settlement that would require it to pay $1.25 billion. Some critics claim that the FCS does not serve beginning farmers as it was required to do under the Farm Credit Act of 1980. The Government Accountability Office (GAO) agreed in 2002 that oversight of this requirement is needed.

Stephanie Jane Carter

M

MEDICAL PATENTS AND OBESITY

Although obesity has many contributing causes, eating or overeating is considered at least one of them. But people cannot just stop eating, so finding a method that allows them to continue to eat, but have less food available to the body, has been a source of experiment. People have been so willing to lose weight and obesity can be so dangerous a health risk, that extreme measures have been seen as medically acceptable. Thus, scientists have invented and created devices and drugs that stop patients from eating, reduce the amount of food absorbed by the body, or actually mechanically limit food intake. Patents are special licenses granted by the federal government or the governments of other countries that allow the patent holder the exclusive right to exploit the patented item during the life of the patent.

Because patented items that help fight or treat obesity are implanted in or ingested by human beings, the **Food and Drug Administration** (FDA) must approve them before they are allowed to be sold to the public. The approval process by the FDA includes medical trials that ensure effectiveness as well as safety. The FDA approval is independent of the patent process. Both are required if the product is to be protected and allowed to be used by the public.

Some patented devices are used to interfere with the eating process and are intended to help obese people to lose weight. These devices and the medical procedures to install or implant them are often not covered by medical insurance, especially when obesity is not accompanied by corresponding health problems like arthritis or Type 2 diabetes. Unlike diet and exercise programs adopted by an obese patient, patented devices and drugs are proprietary and are developed by businesses to take advantage of the booming anti-obesity business.

There are several patented devices used inside of the body that mechanically restrict the amount of food that can be swallowed. These devices can be rings or bands that fit around various parts of the stomach or esophagus. With these devices the patient must eat slowly, chew very well, and take small bites or the food cannot pass through the small opening. The device may be inserted by laparoscopic surgery or by regular incision. The type of device is determined by the patient's physician.

A second type of device that restricts the amount of food that can be eaten is a type of balloon that is inserted into the stomach and inflated. The balloon serves to displace the area in the stomach so that the patient simply cannot hold as much in the stomach. The purpose is to make the patient eat less but feel full. Other types of medical devices may be tubes that bring the food directly into the small intestines, by-passing the stomach or part of the stomach so that food is not in the digestive tract as long. If the food passes through without being absorbed, the patient should lose weight.

There are patents that test the metabolism and measure substrate utilization in the obese. It is believed that obese people metabolize food and nutrients differently from lean people, especially during exercise. To properly measure the metabolism of obese people, some specialized patented devices provide information and analysis of data quickly, allowing physicians to make assessments, measuring such things as lipid and carbohydrate oxidation, and diagnoses within a shorter period of time. Some patents are for drugs that are being developed to curb or lessen obesity. Some drugs, being tested on animals, block the deposits of fat in the body. Other patented drugs interfere with the absorption or metabolizing of fats in humans. An example of a patented drug that is available to fight obesity is Alli, the brand name of the drug orlistat. This drug has been approved by the FDA for over-the-counter sale to adults. Orlistat partially interferes with the absorption of fat by the body, thereby reducing the number of calories that the body absorbs. The drug partially stops lipase, an enzyme that digests fats, from functioning in the body. Undigested fat is eliminated through the bowels.

Other drugs, not as widely publicized as Alli, are also being used to fight obesity. There is a drug in the patent process that blocks the patient's ability to smell and thus taste food. It is believed that the result of loss of smell and taste will be that the patient eats less. Other drugs, called anorectics, reduce appetite. Sibutramine is the generic name of the drug marketed under the brand names Meridia and Reductil. The brand names are registered trademarks.

Redux and Fen-phen are drugs that were prescribed for obesity that caused side effects such as damage to the heart valves. Redux, also known as Fen-phen, had been approved by the FDA prior to being made available to the general public through prescription. It was widely available as an anorectic during the mid-1990s. The actual generic name of the drug was dexfenfluramine. Because of the concerns over the side effects, the FDA revoked approval of the drug. American Home Products, now Wyeth, sold Redux and has been the source of lawsuits for damages caused by the side effects. There have been reports of over 50,000 lawsuits with 63,000 plaintiffs being filed by parties who have claimed some harm from the product with a potential **tort** liability of over $10 billion. Despite having been through the FDA approval process, drugs can have side effects that outweigh the risk of the disease.

Other drugs being explored mimic the work of certain hormones that are part of the digestive process. People with certain conditions like Type 2 diabetes who are also obese do not properly produce those hormones. It is hoped that use of the synthetic hormones would aid in the proper metabolism of food and lead to weight loss.

See also: Court System; Litigation; Obesity as a Disability; Torts.

Further Reading "Fen-Phen Case Lawyers Say They'll Reject Wyeth Offer," *New York Times*, February 17, 2005, http://query.nytimes.com/gst/fullpage.html?res=9505E7D6133AF934A2 5751C0A9639C8B6.

Elizabeth M. Williams

MILK, ORGANIC

Organic milk is milk from cows that are free from antibiotics, growth hormones, and pesticides. There is consideration now by the **U.S. Department of Agriculture** (USDA) to require that dairy cattle spend a certain part of their day in a pasture grazing on grass. Currently, the requirement that dairy cattle graze does not exist.

Federal organic rules are found in the Organic Foods Production Act (OFPA), which was part of the 1990 Farm Bill. The bill authorized the National Organic Program under the USDA to promulgate regulations defining what is organic in all areas including the production of milk. To be organic under federal regulations, the food, including milk, must be produced in accordance with the OFPA.

The question of pastured dairy cattle versus those that live their entire lives on concrete and are fed as opposed to grazed is an important economic question. Many large producers who feed their cattle organic feed, and do not use hormones or antibiotics, have a large stake in the question. If they are required to pasture their animals, the cost of their milk will increase, because the cows will not always be available for milking. Small farmers who pasture their cows believe that the large producers who do not pasture are given an unfair advantage by being able to label their milk organic.

Consumers who want milk from pastured cows say that the milk is more healthful both because of the exercise that the cows get and because of the variety of grasses eaten by the cows. This health claim is refuted by the dairy industry.

See also: Free-Range Farming; Growth Hormones.

Elizabeth M. Williams

MILK, RAW

Raw milk is milk that has not undergone pasteurization, a heating process that kills bacteria. Historically, most milk consumed by humans was raw milk, but the unsanitary conditions and pooling of large quantities of milk that occurred during industrialization heightened the dangers of food-borne illness. Pasteurization, which was originally developed to prevent spoilage in wine and beer, was adapted for dairy to eliminate harmful bacteria. This resulted in a much safer supply of milk and the passage of state laws requiring pasteurization for milk intended for sale. Today, there is renewed interest in raw milk and raw milk products among consumers who view it as a healthier "whole food" than the milk typically found in grocery stores. Sales of raw milk are legal in only about half of states and in those it is often very restricted. Sale of raw milk across state lines is prohibited by federal regulations, and the **Food and Drug Administration** (FDA) requires aging for at least 60 days for raw milk cheeses. State regulation of milk is usually based on the Pasteurized Milk Ordinance, a model regulation that was developed by the FDA in 1924. Where raw milk is not legally sold, there is often a black or unregulated market.

Widespread problems with unpasteurized milk came along with urbanization during the Industrial Revolution. As people moved into cities, large dairy operations moved with them. Cows were kept in cities in packed, unsanitary conditions, fed the nutrient-poor grains leftover from brewing and distillation. The invention of the refrigerated rail car allowed fresh milk to be brought in from the country, but this necessitated pooling of milk from many sources, creating opportunities for bacteria to spread. During this time, milk was a source of typhoid fever, undulant fever, bovine tuberculosis, diphtheria, and food poisoning. Pasteurization was a boon to urban milk drinkers; from 1906 to 1916, the death rate of children under 1 year of age fell from 160 per 100,000 to 90 per 100,000. In the 1940s, the first state to require that milk be pasteurized was Michigan and many states followed suit.

Many of the aforementioned diseases are no longer a significant concern. Contemporary dangers in raw milk are typical food-borne bacteria such as *Listeria, E. coli, Salmonella*, and *Campylobacter*. These diseases are especially dangerous to young children, the elderly, pregnant women, and those with weakened immune systems. Consumption of contaminated milk can lead to miscarriage, hemolytic-uremic syndrome, and death.

Advocates of raw milk counter that these dangers are overstated by government authorities, that contamination can be prevented by careful handling, and that pasteurization kills bacteria that are beneficial to human health, known as probiotics. It is difficult to determine how many illnesses are caused by raw milk produced and distributed in ideal circumstances because so much of raw milk sales occurs in unregulated markets. Therefore, government statistics may overstate the risks of drinking milk produced by dairies that specialize in raw milk and take careful precautions. Nonetheless, a few illnesses have been linked to regulated dairies that produce raw milk, and few would deny that consumption of raw milk carries some risk even in ideal conditions. Advocates point out that pasteurized milk is not 100 percent safe either, given the possibility of contamination after heating.

The benefits of probiotics are a matter of debate. The most common claim on behalf of raw milk is that it contains bacteria that make milk easier to digest for those who are lactose intolerant. Advocates of probiotics also claim that consuming the bacteria in raw milk leads to a wide variety of health improvements, from lessened allergic reactions to reduced effects from autism and attention-deficit hyperactivity disorder. This evidence is largely anecdotal and claims of probiotic benefits from drinking raw milk are rejected by the FDA.

Raw milk advocates also prefer the product for its superior taste. Pasteurization creates a "cooked" flavor in milk due to the creation of hydrogen sulfide. This flavor was initially considered a defect by consumers, but it has come to be accepted. Additionally, because raw milk is usually not homogenized, it tastes richer than mass-market milk. Connoisseurs of fresh cheeses also claim that the unpasteurized versions of these products, often consumed in Europe, are superior to those made with pasteurized milk.

Raw milk is available for sale in retail stores in only ten states. Many other states allow incidental sales of raw milk at the farm but not of other raw dairy products. In many areas, consumers and farmers circumvent bans on the sale of raw milk by forming cow shares or herd shares, arrangements in which consumers purchase shares in a herd and contract with a farmer to board and care for the animals. In exchange, the share owners receive a regular allotment of raw dairy products. Such arrangements are not always approved by local authorities and some farmers have faced prosecution for taking part in them.

Some of the most contentious issues surrounding raw milk deal with proposals to expand access to raw milk, making it less cumbersome for consumers to obtain it. Sales of raw dairy can be profitable for small dairy farmers, who can charge a much higher price selling directly to consumers than to processors who would buy their milk in bulk for pasteurization. Farmers and advocacy groups also seek freedom to produce and purchase other raw dairy products.

Where raw milk is legal there are also disagreements over the safety regulations that govern its sale. California recently revised its raw milk regulations to require dairies to meet a strict standard of 10 coliforms/mL in milk that is regularly tested. Coliforms are harmless bacteria on their own, but regulators claim their presence can serve as an indicator of more serious contamination. Dairy farmers claim the standard is too strict to be economical and view it as a backdoor to prohibition. They have pushed for an alternative standard and safety measures. As legal and extralegal markets for raw milk expand, debate over inspection standards will likely be a recurring issue.

See also: Code of Federal Regulations; Appendix 13: Excerpts from the Code of Federal Regulations Regarding Cheese and Cheese Food.

Further Reading 21 CFR 1240.61 and 21 CFR 133.124; Gumpert, David E. *The Raw Milk Revolution.* Chelsea Green Publishing. (2009); McGee, Harold. *On Food and Cooking.* Scribner. (2004); Farm-to-Consumer Legal Defense Fund Web site: http://ftcldf.org/raw _milk_map.htm

Jacob Grier

MINIMUM WAGE LAW AND RESTAURANT WORKERS

Employees of restaurants and fast-food establishments are protected by the rules and regulations of the Fair Labor Standards Act (FLSA). The restaurant/fast-food industry is defined as "establishments that are engaged primarily in selling and serving to purchasers prepared food and beverages for consumption on or off the premises." These principles also apply to other employees who receive tips, such as workers in a bar.

In 1938 the FLSA established a minimum wage that was applicable throughout the country. It stated that its mission was "the maintenance of the minimum standard of living necessary for health, efficiency, and general well-being of work-ers." This was the first such national legislation and was authorized under the provisions of the commerce clause.

Many states have enacted minimum wage statutes that set a higher minimum wage than the federal law. The minimum wage law is an attempt to ensure that no one who works lives in poverty; however, the business community has not always supported these laws, claiming that not all jobs are worth the minimum wage. Because of the influence of the restaurant industry, some states have enacted "tip credit" laws. These laws provide that the calculation of the minimum wage can be off-set by the amount of tips collected by workers. These laws apply predominantly to restaurant and bar workers, who are traditionally tipped by customers.

Coverage

The FLSA is applicable to those restaurants/fast-food businesses that have gross sales from one or more restaurants that total at least $500,000 per year. Those individuals who work in interstate commerce or who touch goods in interstate commerce are covered by the FLSA's minimum wage provisions, as well as overtime provisions. This may include preparing foods that have been in interstate commerce, selling food at a fast-food business on an interstate highway, or even processing a credit card in payment of a restaurant bill. Because of the interstate commerce provision, unless a restaurant is a small, cash-only operation, the FLSA is likely applicable.

Requirements

Currently those workers who are covered by the FLSA must be paid at least $7.25 per hour. The exception is exempt workers. This minimum wage was effective on July 24, 2009. Payment of wages must be made on a day scheduled for the appropriate payment period. Although deductions may be allowed in theory for certain conditions, such as failing to collect a tab when a customer walks out, they are not permitted if the deduction creates a wage for that pay period that is less than minimum wage or reduces the applicable overtime payment. Certain deductions may not be made during an overtime period. Additionally, employers may be allowed to pay less than minimum wage when employees work in a position that normally receives tips, like a member of the wait staff. The tip may be used in the wage calculation. However, there is a minimum direct wage amount of $2.13 per hour. That amount and the employee's tips may not be less than the standard minimum wage. By applying tips to determine the minimum wage of the worker, the law is allowing the patron to directly pay the worker, thus saving the restaurant the difference between the minimum direct hourly payment and the minimum wage amount.

Credits

If the restaurant provides food to restaurant workers, the restaurant may deduct the actual cost of the food from the worker's pay, usually as an hourly wage credit. The employer may not take credit for discounts off of menu prices. Some restaurants that do not have a family meal do provide discounted menu prices to their employees. They simply require that the employees pay the discounted price when they order and eat the food, thus eliminating the need to take wage credits.

Tips

When an employee receives more than $30 in tips in a month on a regular basis, that employee is considered a tipped employee. If the employer elects to take the tip credit, the worker must be told of this position in advance. The worker must be informed of the amount of the tip credit to be claimed by the employer. To qualify to use the tip credit, the employer must be able to establish that the employee is receiving at least the minimum wage when the minimum direct payment and the tips are added together. Tips may not be taken by the employer and must be retained by the employee. An exception is allowed for tip pooling agreements within an establishment. However, employers cannot benefit as a participant in the pooling. The Internal Revenue Service has ruled that restaurants are responsible for the deduction of taxes on behalf of the employee, based on tip income.

Overtime

The law requires that a per-hour payment of one and one-half of the regular hourly wage of the employee be paid when overtime payments are due. Generally, overtime is required when a worker has worked more than 40 hours in a week. Even those workers who are paid the $2.13 direct payment must be paid one and one-half of the minimum wage, not of the direct payment wage.

Youth Minimum Wage

To encourage employers to hire youth, the FLSA was amended in 1996 to create a youth minimum wage. This wage has been widely used by the fast-food industry. It allows an employer to pay a youth worker $4.25 an hour to workers during the first 90 days of initial employment when the worker is under 20 years old. The law is applicable to new employees and cannot be used to substitute the youth minimum wage workers for other workers. This law encourages employers to hire youth, especially during the summer.

Youth Employment

Youths are permitted to work when they are 14 and 15 years old. However, the hours that they may work is very limited. The first and most important limitation is that they may not work during school hours. They may only work 18 hours during a school week, only 3 hours each school day, either before school or after school. They may not work before 7:00 A.M. They may not work after 7:00 P.M., except that during summer break, which is defined as between June 1 and Labor Day, they may work until 9:00 P.M. They may only work eight hours on a day where there is no school. When school is out, they may work up to 40 hours per week. They may not work overtime. Youth workers may be cashiers and do office work, clean up, certain restaurant prep work, and bagging but not cooking and baking.

The 16- and 17-year-old youths are not limited in the number of hours that they may work. However, they are limited to the performance of nonhazardous jobs. What is hazardous, however, depends on age. In a restaurant, operating saws and slicing machines would be considered hazardous. Operating other heavy machinery, including grinders and large bakery machinery, is also probably hazardous for youths of this age. Until reaching the age of majority, youth workers may not even repair or clean large machinery in restaurants and other food service establishments. Minor workers are not allowed to drive or work as a helper on a public roadway. There are exceptions for certain 17-year-olds such as pizza delivery and other types of delivery jobs. However, even when otherwise under an exception, 17-year-olds cannot make pizza deliveries that are time sensitive or at night, because these conditions are considered hazardous.

See also: Appendix 1: *United States v. Fior D'Italia, Inc.*

William C. Smith and Elizabeth M. Williams

MOLECULAR GASTRONOMY

Molecular gastronomy refers to the use of science to better understand cooking processes. Hervé This and Nicholas Kurti first coined the term in 1988 in France, initially as molecular and physical gastronomy. This shortened to molecular gastronomy on Kurti's death in 1998. In a 2006 paper, this defined molecular gastronomy as "the chemistry and physics behind the preparation of any dish." His main goals were to use science to investigate the "old wives' tales" associated with many culinary practices and to better define recipes, while also paying attention to the artistic and social components of food. Molecular gastronomy thus specifically refers to the use of science, usually in a laboratory, to understand cooking processes. It has nothing to do with what then takes place in a restaurant kitchen, even if chefs there look at science to innovate in their cooking and develop new technologies, techniques, and dishes.

One of the most contentious points of molecular gastronomy is its actual name. Chefs decry the term as being meaningless and having no relation with what they are doing on a daily basis in their restaurants. They cook, they say, and do not pretend to be scientists. They experiment, but have their own way of doing so, as opposed to a scientific, lab-like methodology, which they would apply to the development of any dish. It just happens that they decide to use more technology, different cooking techniques, or additives that allow them to manipulate the structure of certain ingredients. Because the media widely use the term to describe any dish or technique that appears experimental to them, it also often carries negative connotations with the general public, with critics accusing it of not being "real food." Chefs and culinary professionals tend to prefer terms such as modern cooking, experimental cooking, and science-based cooking, which they think more accurately represent what they do.

Molecular gastronomy has few direct relations with laws and regulations. It uses ingredients and techniques that large-scale food companies have often been using for many years; in those industrial applications, ingredients and procedures are tightly regulated. In the restaurant kitchen, specific ingredients are not regulated as much as proper handling techniques are. The department of health of each city will inspect kitchens to ensure that the conditions are sanitary and that food is cooked, refrigerated, or stored at proper temperatures—regardless of the chef's selected cuisine. It requires minimum cooking temperatures for many foods, which in certain cities and at times can conflict with chefs' use of sous vide cooking. Sous vide is a cooking method in which food is placed in a plastic bag, the air is removed, and it is then cooked in a circulating water bath held at a constant temperature for a long time. It offers the advantage to keep food particularly moist, to flavor it with liquid or other ingredients contained in the bag, and to maintain it at constant temperature during service. The water bath's temperature is often lower than the Department of Health's requirements, and sous vide is a technique that is either banned or subject to tight regulations in many cities as a result. In New York City, for example, chefs wishing to serve food cooked with the sous vide method must file a **Hazard Analysis Critical Control Point** (HACCP) plan with the Department of Health and Mental Hygiene, following a 16-page procedure that establishes requirements such as temperature and record keeping.

Italy, however, has gone beyond regulating cooking techniques. The Italian Ministry of Health announced in spring 2010 that it would ban the use of additives in restaurant kitchens, while still allowing them in industrial food manufactures. These additives are typically plant-based and allow chefs to make hot gels or skinless ravioli, for example. They are widely used in industrial food products, so their food safety qualities are not at stake as much as Italy's desire to preserve traditional food culture. The Italian ministry also plans on banning liquid nitrogen from these same kitchens. Liquid nitrogen allows chefs to freeze foods in seconds, for both savory and sweet applications.

One of the key aspects of experimental cooking is its use of technologies that are new to the restaurant kitchen. Such technologies, such as sous vide cooking, often arrived in the kitchen via the scientific laboratory. Chefs began buying used lab equipment and repurposing it to create new dishes. Many such pieces of equipment purchased early on were manufactured by Polyscience, a family-run, Illinois-based company. Polyscience saw an opportunity for a new market and began inventing and building new equipment specifically for restaurant kitchens. These companies benefit from knowing how to go from prototype to final product and how to patent their product. Today, they work with chefs directly to create equipment based on specifications or requirements provided by the chef. Polyscience created the Anti-Griddle for Grant Achatz of Alinea in Chicago, for example—a griddle that freezes foods on contact rather than cooking them. Companies patent these appliances as they would any others. Homaro Cantu, of restaurant Moto and associated company Cantu Designs in Chicago, has also patented several techniques, such as the impression of food imagery onto paper, which allowed him to serve diners sushi that in reality was a photograph of sushi printed on edible paper and rolled to look like the Japanese dish.

Restaurant dishes are not copyrightable or protected by intellectual property laws. Cooks can take others' dishes and pass them off as their own—legally, at least, if not ethically. The U.S. Copyright Office states on its Web site that

> Mere listings of ingredients as in recipes, formulas, compounds, or prescriptions are not subject to copyright protection. However, when a recipe or formula is accompanied by substantial literary expression in the form of an explanation or directions, or when there is a combination of recipes, as in a cookbook, there may be a basis for copyright protection.

Cooks and chefs throughout the world spend time in others' kitchens to learn new techniques or improve their existing skills. This is particularly true of experimental cooking. Many of the leading chefs and restaurants (for example, Ferran Adrià at El Bulli in Spain; Heston Blumenthal at the The Fat Duck in England; Pierre Gagnaire in Paris; Wylie Dufresne at wd-50 in New York; and Achatz) have their own tools and aesthetics, they are frequently solicited. The great majority of chefs spending a few days in one of those kitchens will strictly use what they learn for inspiration; a very small number of them go on to plagiarize the original chef. This was the case in 2006 when an Australian chef worked at Alinea and wd-50 for a few days. He went on to recreate Alinea dishes "verbatim" in his own restaurant, copying not just the composition of the dishes but their presentation and color palettes. Because photos of meals at both restaurants were widely available online, the "plagiarism" was quickly discovered. Articles in traditional media followed, as did countless discussions of the possibility of chefs being able to copyright their dishes. To this day, no solution has been offered, the problem remaining small enough—and visible enough thanks to the Internet—that chefs are comfortable being creative around others in their profession. Some kitchens, particularly those that have an attached food lab or a strong research component, however, at times require staff to sign confidentiality agreements.

Science-based cooking is not regulated by laws in the traditional understanding of the word. However, chefs who practice experimental cooking seek to break—or at least rattle—some of the standard "laws" of their craft. Wylie Dufresne, chef-owner of wd-50 in New York City, serves an everything bagel with lox and cream cheese—but the bagel is a frozen hollowed-out disc, the cream cheese is flattened into a brittle sheet, and the lox is frozen and shaven into miniscule flakes. It tastes like the classic New York breakfast but reinvents it, challenging notions of what is classic.

Further Reading Barham, Peter, et al. "Molecular Gastronomy: A New Emerging Scientific Discipline." *Chemical Reviews* 110, no. 4 (February 2010): 2313–365, http://pubs.acs.org/doi/abs/10.1021/cr900105w; Buccafusco, Christopher J. "On the Legal Consequence of Sauces: Should Thomas Keller's Recipes Be Per Se Copyrightable." bepress Legal Series. Working Paper 1629 (August 25, 2006), http://law.bepress.com/expresso/eps/1629; McGee, Harold. *On Food and Cooking: The Science and Lore of the Kitchen*. Rev. ed. New York: Scribner, 2004; This, Hervé. *Molecular Gastronomy: Exploring the Science of Flavor*. New York: Columbia University Press, 2006; Vega, Cesar, and Job Ubbink. "Molecular Gastronomy: A Food Fad or Science Supporting Innovative Cuisine." *Trends in Food Science and Technology* 19, no. 17 (2008): 372–82.

Anne E. McBride

NAMES OF FOOD AND TRADEMARKS

A brand is a common feature of all forms of commerce, from consumer goods like a Snickers candy bar to a commercial kitchen's Frymaster deep-fryer. Brands serve to identify specific products to consumers and differentiate them from the competition. Individuals and businesses may protect themselves from the misuse of their brand by registering for a trademark that provides exclusive rights to use that brand to sell a product. Trademarks were originally protected by the courts under English and American common law, as a protection against unfair competition from counterfeit goods.

In the United States, trademarks are regulated under the Lanham Act, the successor to earlier federal laws dating back to the 19th century. Trademarks are a form of intellectual property, and if they are used in interstate commerce they are usually registered at the U.S. Patent and Trademark Office (USPTO). Trademarks used in intrastate commerce may also be registered with the Secretary of State in the state of business. Businesses, including a food and beverage business, may obtain a trademark by either being the first to use the trademark in the course of business or the first to register the trademark with the USPTO or the state. Registered trademarks may use the ® symbol and any trademark may use the™ marking to provide notice of their protection.

Trademarks may be a word, a phrase, or a symbol, such as Pepsi and the red, white, and blue circular Pepsi logo. Trademarks may also include packaging, such as the shape of the Coca-Cola bottle. The scope of the trademark is generally limited to the geographic area in which the business is conducted, so there may be two, separately originated Grandma's Diner's in two separate cities, for example. To qualify as a trademark, the proposed mark must be distinctive. The most distinctive trademarks are arbitrary and bear no obvious relation to the product or company in question, such as a term like Pepsi, and these are provided with the highest levels of protection under trademark law. Suggestive or descriptive terms like Rice Krispies or Whole Foods also qualify for full trademark protection, but purely descriptive trademarks must acquire secondary meaning, or a brand identity, to be fully protected. This requirement prevents competitors from obtaining exclusive rights to use terms that are necessary for a competitor to describe their product or service.

Generic terms, such as milk, cheese, or hamburger, cannot be protected by trademark law. Protection for generic terms would prevent competitors from describing their products. In addition, some trademarks may become generic over time due to popular use and may lose their trademark protection. For example, terms such as shredded wheat and thermos were originally trademarks but have been held by the courts to be generic in the minds of a substantial majority of the public. Trademarks that are abandoned and not used for three years also lose protection.

Food and beverage names present unique trademark issues and other labeling issues, especially in regard to the use of geographic names and associations. Geographic place names are generally not eligible for trademark protection under U.S. law, because other producers from that area may need to use that name for their product, or a producer could use it to mislead the consumer. Many food products gain characteristics, and value, from using their place of origin, such as Wisconsin cheddar cheese, or Napa Valley wine. The Federal Food, Drug, and Cosmetic Act and various state laws prohibit the false or misleading food labels, which includes geographic origin indicators. However, the federal regulations provide two exceptions when geographic names are either part of the prescribed identity of the product name, such as French dressing, or by reason of long usage as the type or style of the food product, such as New England clam chowder or Buffalo wings. The federal **Food and Drug Administration** (FDA) has many other public health priorities and complaints exist about the lack of enforcement regarding place names on items such as Vermont maple syrup and Omaha steaks.

Although federal trademark law generally resists protecting geographic names, the Lanham Act provides for certification marks that indicate origin in a particular region. Like trademarks, certification marks may be a word, name, symbol, or other device, but unlike a trademark they are not exclusive to one producer, but rather to a third party that applies the certification. For example, the state of Idaho and the Idaho Potato Commission have registered certification marks with the USPTO for Grown in Idaho and Famous Idaho Potatoes. Certifications may also be for quality indicators or union labeling, and collective trademarks are available for producers from the association, such as an agricultural cooperative. States may also provide intrastate protection for geographic names, such as the Vidalia onions from the specific growing area in Georgia. In addition, a place name may be included in a federal trademark if it takes on secondary meaning, as in Rice-a-Roni's "San Francisco Treat."

Food and geographic name regulation adds an extra layer of complexity in the international arena. The 1995 **World Trade Organization** (WTO) Agreement on Trade-Related Aspects of Intellectual Property Rights (TRIPS) creates a classification known as geographic indicators (GIs) for protection. The GIs are generally equivalent to the U.S. trademark treatment of geographic certifications, and international producers from foreign geographic locations can also obtain protection in the United States. Under the international agreement, nations are intended to give reciprocal protections to GIs from other nations.

The European Union (EU) and many of its member nations have created a relatively strict GI system that gives GI protection to a variety of geographic names that have fallen under the long usage exception in the United States, such as Parmesan cheese, Roquefort, Cognac, Chianti, and Champagne. Even within the EU, some of these terms were used generically but have since been ruled to be GIs, such as feta cheese for Greece. Disputes over various European GIs continue within the EU for rights to a name and the debate continues in the context of broader negotiations of WTO agricultural trade agreements.

The TRIPS included a provision requiring continuing negotiations and in 2003, the EU proposed numerous names for GI protection, including Asiago, Manchego, Prosciutto di Parma, and Pecorino Romano. Translations and word variations are also an issue in several of these disputes. In 2005, for example, the WTO ruled in a dispute that Budweiser was not prevented from marketing its product that traced its name back to Budvar, a beer from the Czech Republic. The U.S. government has generally opposed the broadening of GI protection to common usage names, whereas the EU governments and nations have supported them at the WTO. For wines and spirits, the EU systems regulating names and appellations are also complex, and in the United States these GIs and names are regulated by the Bureau of Alcohol, Tobacco, Firearms, and Explosives within the Department of Treasury.

See also: Food and Drug Administration, Trademarks, World Trade Organization.

Andrew G. Wallace

NATIONAL ORGANIC STANDARDS BOARD

The National Organic Standards Board (NOSB) is an agency created by the Organic Foods Production Act of 1990, which was a part of the 1990 Farm Bill. Under the act the Secretary of Agriculture appointed a 15-member board to make rules and recommendations regarding organic standards. Until the founding of the NOSB there were no federal organic standards and no definition of organic. Any standards and definitions were established under various state laws. The standards were inconsistent and made interstate compliance with laws difficult.

The composition of the board is varied by occupation and by geographic region. It consists of farmers, processors, a retailer, a scientist, environmentalists, and a **U.S. Department of Agriculture** certifying agent. It is the intention of this diversity to provide a board that represents all interests attendant to the concept of organics.

The NOSB has defined organic food as a method of protection in a broad and philosophical manner. It describes an ecologically balanced method of production that is sustainable and that promotes biodiversity and soil health. Soil is the very core of the agricultural system. It forms the center of the ecological balance and promotes the health of the earth. The philosophy recognizes that farming is not inherently natural but strives for a system that melds farming into natural cycles.

Handling of organic products reflects and respects this philosophy. Farmers and processors must handle organic products in a manner that is environmentally sound and that does not compromise the organic nature of the products.

These standards are independent of the size of the farm or agricultural concern. Some organics advocates also include in their concept of organics the idea of small **family-owned farms.** To them organic farming is a way of life. When large agribusiness qualifies to use the organic mark, even though these businesses comply with organic standards, they argue that the standards are wrong, because they do not explicitly recognize the small, family-owned farms. For them organic farming is a way of life and not just a business.

These same advocates argue that when organics is a way of life, the farmer always makes the right decision in favor of organics. On the other hand, they say that large agri-businesses will always do the minimum to comply with the National Organics Program (NOP). The agri-businesses are not really interested in organic principles, but rather in the added value that the organic mark might add in the marketplace. Because it is only about money, they are willing to push the envelope to do less and less without losing the right to use the mark.

The products covered by the NOSB must meet the standards set by the Board, which reflect not only products from organic soil, grown without nonorganic pesticides, and animals raised without being dosed with antibiotics and hormones, but also other expectations that consumers who want organic products have. This means that environmental concerns and practices must be consistent with standards.

National Organics Program

The NOP is the agency that develops standards of organics for production, handling, and labeling of agricultural products. In addition, the NOP has the responsibility for accrediting certifying agents. These agents certify production and handling by inspecting to ensure that these are in accordance with organic standards. These standards are applicable to processed products that are made from organic agricultural ingredients as well as uncooked and fresh products. The exception to the NOP standards applies to those whose sales of organic products are less than $5,000 per year.

Those products that claim to be 100 percent organic must be made entirely of organic ingredients, except for water and salt. Nonagricultural products must be from an approved list. Certain agricultural products are approved even though they come from nonorganic farms. This list is made up of products that are not available as organic. This list may change and must be checked to ensure that the products labeled as 100 percent contain up-to-date approved ingredients.

The NOP has a special organic mark than can be used in labeling when the product meets the appropriate standards. The seal may be used directly on organic vegetables or fruit, or alternatively, the mark can be used on a sign positioned above the fruit or vegetables. The key is single-ingredient foods, so the seal may be used on organic eggs or beef packaging.

When the seal is used on multi-ingredient food packaging, it signifies to consumers that the product is at least 95 percent organic. The full-color seal is green and brown. The seal may appear in black and white or in black on a clear label.

The critics of these standards argue that the certifying agents do not have the necessary authority, and when much of the inspection is based on the maintenance of records, it is then record keeping rather than organic standards that is being measured. The exception to the use of only biologic pesticides or fertilizer may be that such products are not available or not reasonably priced. Thus, a farmer or producer could actually be using products that are nonorganic but that qualify as organic based on lack of availability.

The growth of popularity of organic foods is luring more farmers and farm companies into the marketplace. Organic food usually costs more than nonorganic food. If it is shown that consumers will pay a premium price for a product that qualifies for the organic mark, more companies wish to furnish those products. If those producers are not committed to the organic philosophy, then the standards for organics must be unambiguous and specific without discretionary decision making. If the standards are as objective as possible, the motivation of the producers will not be important and consumers can trust the organic mark, not because of the philosophy of the producers, but because of the high standards.

See also: Farms, Family; Labeling Definitions; Milk, Organic.

Elizabeth M. Williams

"NATURAL" LABELING

The Food Safety and Inspection Service (FSIS) of the **U.S. Department of Agriculture** (USDA) defines a natural product as a product that "does not contain any artificial ingredients or added color and is only minimally processed." "Minimal processing" is defined as not altering the raw product in any basic way. The USDA elaborates on "natural flavors" on meat and poultry labels as ingredients used chiefly for their flavor, such as black pepper and ginger. "Natural flavors" are flavorings that are not an ingredient with a nutritional content, are not made from animal products, and have not been connected to health hazards. The **Food and Drug Administration** currently has no definition for "natural" and often discourages the use of "natural" on labels because it is notoriously difficult to define.

The current USDA definition remains ambiguous. The use of "natural" typically implies that the food is superior, fresher, safer, and more healthful than its counterparts. Arsenic is natural, but it is far from safe for consumption. Even safe, natural substances at certain levels can prove unsafe. Vitamins A and D can be toxic at high levels. With the use of the "natural" term, consumers make many inferences that stretch beyond what the label actually denotes. According to philosopher Peter Singer, "Animals can be confined to bare concrete all their lives and fed chicken litter, antibiotics, and hormones, but the U.S. government says you can call their meat 'natural' as long as you don't add anything artificial to the meat itself." Moreover, it is questionable whether it is natural to add any substance to a product, whether that substance is itself "natural" or not. Some theorists believe the popularity of this label among consumers is due to a reaction to processed, industrialized foods, a tendency toward a "back to the land" approach to food. Throughout history, human beings have gradually given up much control over food they once had as farmers, hunters, and cooks. The "natural" label offers a primordial comfort, allowing consumers to believe that they are asserting control over what items they put into their bodies, how those items are grown or raised, and how they are cooked. The presence of the label can remind consumers how far from basic food they have come, essentially taking consumers' peace of mind and reselling it to them for the price of the product.

The overuse of this label can cause "label fatigue" among consumers. Some food producers have argued for stricter regulations to decrease the use of the label and gain a marketing advantage. In 2006, Hormel and Sanderson Farms Company asked the USDA for a stricter definition of "natural." Meat processors commonly inject chicken with natural **additives**, such as saline solution, arguably not fundamentally altering the raw product. These two companies wanted a stricter definition so that consumers could see a distinction between their product and the products treated with salt and other additives. Regardless of the ambiguity in the definition, food manufacturers and advertisers use this term while consumers undeniably buy products that carry this label.

See also: Additives and Preservatives; Appendix 12: Excerpts from 21 United States Code Sections 341 and Others.

Stephanie Jane Carter

NEIGHBORHOOD COVENANTS

Neighborhood covenants are property restrictions written into property deeds and titles that restrict the use of the property. This restriction refers to the use of the land in ways beyond zoning. It can include the manner in which is building is situated on a site and its orientation to the street, the size of a building in relation to the lot, the colors used, and the style of building, to name just a few of the possible restrictions. These rules can apply to commercial properties, such as restaurants and grocery stores, as well as residential properties.

Neighborhood covenants are often created when a subdivision or development is created under the auspices of one developer or development group. These rules are adopted while the developer owns the land and then follow the land as each subsequent owner buys and sells the property. These covenants are thought to create a unified look in a development thereby protecting property values.

Covenants are not the same as zoning rules or ordinances. Zoning represents a plan of development, growth, or land use that is adopted and enforced by government. Covenants, on the hand, are voluntary restrictions adopted by the community through deeds to ensure that the neighborhood retains its value and that property will be maintained. Some covenants contain provisions that allow neighborhood associations to assess fines and issue voluntary citations for violations as a form of enforcement. Usually the specific details of covenants are filed with country land offices and are referenced in deeds.

Covenants can affect parking, types of businesses allowed in a subdivision, signage, landscaping, and changes in the property. Besides compliance with zoning rules, businesses subject to neighborhood covenants must also comply with the covenants. Starting a business can be a difficult issue when it must be done in compliance with covenants. This can affect where trash can be stored, visibility of parking, and inability to use certain alternative energy sources when they are visible from the street.

An analogous business-driven neighborhood organization is called business improvement districts (BIDs). In addition to zoning, BIDs are defined areas that voluntarily allow for the collection of fees from those properties located within the district. In return, the district receives special services such as special patrolling, cleaning, landscaping, or even marketing. These services are not in lieu of governmentally provided services, but in addition to governmental services. The unified planning restrictions of covenants are usually not adopted by BIDs because the districts are already established and not created by one developer. However, in business park developments, covenants or a combination of covenant and BID can ensure that the business park maintains a uniform look and that property values are protected. The BIDS are a form of public/private partnership. They require enabling legislation to function.

Food businesses, whether a restaurant, grocery, or other business, have to consider the location and the particular rules and regulations applicable there.

Further Reading Nestle, Marion. *Food Politics: How the Food Industry Influences Nutrition and Health.* Berkeley: University of California Press, 2007

Elizabeth M. Williams

NESTLE, MARION (1936–)

Marion Nestle, influential and award-winning nutritionist, author, scholar, and teacher, is a leading independent voice in the food politics arena. Since the 2002 publication of her seminal book *Food Politics: How the Food Industry Influences Nutrition and Health*, Nestle has been at the forefront of the food social movement, raising awareness and shaping the debate around the often insidious interplay of food, nutrition, and politics in the United States. Through her research, writing, and lectures, Nestle has profoundly impacted Americans' understanding of the relationship between their food choices and consumption patterns on the one hand and the food industry's marketing and lobbying efforts that drive those choices on the other.

Her own recognition of that intrinsic relationship between consumer choice and food industry lobbying was forged in 1986 to 1988 during her brief stint in government as senior nutrition policy advisor in the **Department of Health and Human Services** (HHS) and managing editor of the 1988 *Surgeon General's Report on Nutrition and Health*. Nestle observed firsthand "that everything is political, especially when it comes to dietary advice." Her real "lightning bolt moment," as Nestle describes it, came in the early 1990s during a National Cancer Institute meeting on behavioral approaches to cancer prevention, when a fellow presenter pulled back the curtain on the cigarette industry's strategy of marketing to youngsters. Immediately making the connection to child-directed marketing by food companies, Nestle began compiling research and writing articles on the subject, out of which the highly influential and controversial *Food Politics* was born, inciting a new food-focused dialogue across the country.

Nestle originally tackled food industry marketing toward children, but gradually her policy reform target expanded to include aspects of both production and consumption while she explored the raging obesity epidemic debilitating Americans. In part, Nestle attributes rising obesity rates to the Reagan administration's deregulating industry and lessening agricultural controls, which indirectly encouraged American farmers to produce more food. As the daily available per capita caloric supply increased to 3,900, Americans consumed more food, making obesity commonplace. On Wall Street, far from the agricultural production venues, the "shareholder value movement" had stockholders demanding that food manufacturing companies create higher yields by increasing revenues in already excessive caloric foods and food categories. The American three-meal-a-day norm, practiced for decades, quickly gave way to between-meal snacks, increased and excessive portion sizes, packaged convenience foods, and frequent meals consumed outside the home. Americans grew accustomed to and expected lower food prices, ease of access, and "super-sized" portions. Nestle exposed and argued that the food industry and their lobbying groups effectively created a new platform for U.S. food consumption and with that a platform for obesity and related health risks.

As the food industry grew and refocused its attention on high caloric, high fat, low nutrient, and high profit food, it attempted publicity spins by aligning itself with nonprofit organizations, health-related publications, sponsored journals and research—all attempting to promote positive health images to products. The result is increasingly tainted scientific claims and a more confused public, unsure of whom to believe. Nestle argues that suspect nutrition labeling, such as "low-fat," "heart healthy," "anti-oxidant," and "organic," functional foods, and supplements promulgated by the food industry further confuse the general public. Nestle has become a vocal watchdog and inquisitor of the food industry.

Following the success of *Food Politics*, Nestle's scope broadened to include food safety (*Safe Food: The Politics of Food Safety*, 2003, updated edition 2010); public guidance on healthy food choices in the face of often intentionally misleading dietary messages and advertising claims (*What to Eat*, 2006); practices and perils of the pet food industry (*Pet Food Politics: The Chihuahua in the Coal Mine*, 2008, and *Feed Your Pet Right*, 2010, with co-author Malden Nesheim); front-of-package food labeling; and, in a forthcoming book, the myths and science surrounding calories. Throughout all of Nestle's publications and international speaking engagements runs the common thread of the role of politics—both governmental and big business—in shaping policy and behavior, often in spite of the science and to the detriment of the consumer.

In addition to writing books and articles, Nestle influences and directs nutrition and food policy dialogues through ongoing public health nutrition research and advisory work. She has served on a wide array of government, professional, and community advisory committees and boards, among them the Food and Drug Administration Food Advisory Committee and Science Board; the **US. Department of Agriculture**/DHHS Dietary Guidelines Advisory Committee; the Commission on Federal Leadership in U.S. Health and Medicine at the Center for the Study of the Presidency and Congress; the Harvard Business School and John F. Kennedy School of Government's Private and Public, Scientific, Academic and Consumer Food Policy Committee; and the *Journal of Public Health Policy*. Her research interests have continued to evolve throughout her eclectic academic career, centering on the development and analysis of food policy and dietary guidelines; social and political drivers of food choice; the politics of food safety; and the impact of corporate food advertising on children's eating habits and health.

Nestle has a Ph.D. in molecular biology and an M.P.H. in public health nutrition from the University of California, Berkeley. She has taught at Brandeis University and the University of California–San Francisco School of Medicine. From 1988 until 2003, Nestle chaired New York University's Department of Nutrition, Food Studies, and Public Health, in 1996 launched the pioneering graduate program in Food Studies, and laid the ground work for a food movement and today's food revolution sweeping the nation. She teaches courses in Food Policy, Ethical Perspectives in the Food Supply, Food Sociology, and Nutrition in Public Health. She is Paulette Goddard Professor in the Department of Nutrition, Food Studies, and Public Health at New York University and Professor of Sociology at New York University and Visiting Professor of Nutritional Sciences at Cornell University.

Although sometimes derided in a sexist manner by pro-industry groups as "hysterical," Nestle's style tends on the contrary to be characterized by reasonableness and common sense, her outrage generally tempered by amusement and grounded in scientific fact. Her impact on policy and regulations, while largely indirect, has been substantial.

See also: Pollan, Michael.

Further Reading Nestle, Marion. *Food Politics: How the Food Industry Influences Nutrition and Health.* Rev. ed. Berkeley: University of California Press, 2007; Nestle, Marion. *Food Politics* blog. http://www.foodpolitics.com/; Nestle, Marion. *Safe Food.* Berkeley: University of California Press, 2004.

Meryl Rosofsky and Jennifer Berg

NORTH AMERICAN COLD STORAGE CO. v. CHICAGO

The case of *North American Cold Storage Co. v. Chicago* (1908) came to the United States Supreme Court from the Circuit Court of the United States for the Northern District of Illinois. This case discusses several constitutional issues regarding the relationship between city and state law and the U.S. Constitution, as well as due process, and property rights.

The city of Chicago had adopted regulations (Section 1161 of the Revised Municipal Code of the City of Chicago for 1905) that allowed city inspectors to enter cold storage facilities to inspect stored products for health and safety reasons. If the food was found to be tainted, the inspectors were authorized to destroy it. In this case, the inspectors found what they claimed to be spoiled chicken. They ordered the plaintiff to destroy the product, and the plaintiff refused. Instead of complying, the plaintiff sought an injunction to prevent the destruction of the product.

The basis for the injunction and the subsequent lawsuit was the issue of due process of law. The question posed was, did the regulations of the city of Chicago violate the plaintiff's rights to due process by allowing for the destruction of tainted or unwholesome food without a hearing or notice, and without an opportunity for the plaintiff to present its position.

Because the city ordinance is considered a law of the state of Illinois, the Fourteenth Amendment to the U.S. Constitution makes the Constitutional right of due process applicable to the city ordinance. The Fourteenth Amendment makes the Constitution applicable to the states. Thus, the plaintiff argued that it was entitled to notice and a chance to present its side before the action of destroying the chicken. The plaintiff argued that it could have sold or used the chicken for other purposes than for human consumption, for example, animal feed, had it not been destroyed. This action by the city inspectors deprived the plaintiff of money that could have been recouped by repurposing the tainted chicken.

The U.S. Supreme Court argued that the basis for the city regulations was the constitutional recognition of police powers to government, one of which is to protect the health and safety of the citizens within the particular jurisdiction. In this case, the destruction of tainted food that was designated for human consumption was within the legitimate police powers of the city of Chicago. The Court found that just because it could have been sold for some other purpose, such as animal feed, does not mean that the plaintiff was planning to so use the product.

The original petition claimed that the plaintiff, North American Cold Storage Company, received the shipment in question in October 1906. The shipment was made up of 47 barrels of chicken. The dealer who shipped the poultry to the plaintiff intended for it to be stored until the dealer ordered it removed. It was in good condition at the time it was received by the plaintiff. The poultry could have remained wholesome for up to three months if it had remained in cold-storage.

The same day that the shipment arrived the health inspectors demanded to see the shipment in question. The inspectors alleged that the chicken was spoiled and had to be destroyed. The plaintiff refused to tender the chicken stating that the due process rights were being violated by the seizure and destruction order. The plaintiff was being deprived of property without due process of law. In response to the plaintiff's position, the inspectors refused to allow the plaintiff to continue to conduct business, threatening to arrest anyone who acted to deliver or remove goods from the facility.

The U.S. Supreme Court found that the individuals sued, the Director of the City Health Department, the individual inspectors, and other officials were acting in their official capacity and that they were immune from personal suit in this matter. The inspectors and others were acting within the police powers granted to the state of Illinois and delegated by the state of Illinois to the city of Chicago. But the lower court dismissed the claim for lack of jurisdiction. It was this decision by the lower court that formed the basis for the decision of the Supreme Court.

The lower court stated that the claim of the plaintiffs was based on the U.S. Constitution principle of due process. Because the matter was a state and local matter, the Constitution principle did not form a basis for jurisdiction. The Supreme Court said that the lower court erred in this decision, finding that the plaintiff claimed the due process rights through the Fourteenth Amendment. The Supreme Court had found that the Fourteenth Amendment to the Constitution makes the protections such as due process afforded by the Constitution applicable to the states, thus the state must comply with due process requirements. Because the plaintiff claimed the rights under the Fourteenth Amendment there was jurisdiction.

But in addition to the jurisdictional claim, the Supreme Court also reviewed the merits of the case. It was their determination that the police powers of the state did allow the immediate destruction of the putrid food. However, the Court did say that a hearing to determine the correctness of the destruction could protect the due process rights of the plaintiff. If it were found that the actions of the inspectors were unwarranted, the plaintiff could pursue monetary remedies. The threat to public health requires the ability of inspectors to take immediate action. The ability to recoup some value in putrid food is not a sufficient interest to protect when balanced against the possible health risk of having the food reach consumers. The decision made by the lower court finding that the destruction of the food was a valid police power was upheld by the Supreme Court.

This case is often cited to illustrate the legal principle that loss of property can be remedied by the payment of damages; thus, swift action that is taken prior to a hearing can be sanctioned when done for a reason greater than mere due process. Public health is one such reason.

See also: Court System; Appendix 5: *North American Cold Storage Co. v. City of Chicago.*

Further Reading North American Cold Storage Co. v. Chicago, 211 U. S. 306 (1908).

Elizabeth M. Williams

NUTRACEUTICALS

Physician Stephen DeFelice is credited with coining the term "nutraceutical" in 1989. It is formed by combining the words, "nutrition" and "pharmaceutical." The American Association of Nutraceuticals calls nutraceuticals "functional foods," citing their potential in preventing disease and encouraging health. The American Dietetic Association defines functional foods as "products whose nutritional value is enhanced by the addition of natural ingredients." Essentially, nutraceuticals are foods that have been altered in a way that adds **dietary supplements** or subtracts undesireable components to offer health benefits beyond the nutritive value of the foods themselves. Nutraceuticals are an outgrowth of the Dietary Supplement and Health Education Act (DSHEA) of 1994, which relaxed the restrictions on claims of health properties allowed on dietary supplements. Specifically, the DSHEA restricted the enforcement powers of the **Food and Drug Administration** (FDA) by loosening the restrictions on the claims that dietary supplements could make about their products. The supplement industry experienced enormous growth with the new labeling rules. Adding dietary supplements to their products allowed the food industry to take advantage of the dietary supplements' labeling rules. Nutraceuticals are also known as designer foods, functional foods, and techno-foods. They are regulated by the FDA under the authority of the Food, Drug, and Cosmetic Act, even though they are not specifically defined by law. Nutraceuticals are highly marketable.

The first nutraceuticals were fortified or enriched. Originally, foods were enriched or fortified to correct deficiencies. In 1924, it became common to add iodine to salt to prevent goiter. Vitamin D was added to milk starting in 1931. In 1942, the FDA established a standard of identity for enriched flour. A standard of identity establishes criteria that must be met before a product can be labeled a certain way. Standards of identity for other products followed. Over the years, the food industry found that foods that make health claims are highly marketable. Once they were able to make health claims for foods, the food industry introduced a wide array of nutraceuticals. Some of these seem helpful to the public. Others, such as foods made with Olestra, a fat-substitute, encourage the public to eat more "junk foods," rather than changing dietary patterns. Examples of nutraceuticals include vitamin-enhanced water, vitamin-supplemented Gummi-Bears, Benecol spreads that claim to lower cholesterol, and vitamin-supplemented cereals.

Many regulations that pertain to nutraceuticals and health claims on foods are directly tied to the history of regulation of **dietary supplements**. This paved the road for relaxed standards of health claims. The DSHEA of 1994 defined a dietary supplement as "a product taken by mouth that contains a dietary ingredient intended to supplement the diet." A "dietary ingredient" is, or is a combination of, "a vitamin, mineral, herb, or botanical, amino acid, dietary substance used to increase the total dietary intake, or concentrate, metabolite, constituent, or extract." The FDA is required to apply a different set of standards to its regulation of dietary supplements than it applies to "conventional" food products and drugs. The FDA considers dietary supplements to be different from prescription and over-the-counter drugs, and different from food.

In 1976, Congress introduced the Proxmire Amendment to the Food, Drug, and Cosmetic Act. The Proxmire Amendment stated that the FDA may not set limits on the amounts of vitamins or minerals allowed in a supplement, classify the supplement as a drug if its dose exceeds what the FDA considers nutritionally rational, or restrict the combinations of vitamins and minerals in a supplement. This was a major step forward for the dietary supplement industry. If supplements had been classified as drugs, they would be subject to much more regulation. Later that year, the FDA proposed that supplements be treated as over-the-counter drugs and carry a label that stated that they should only be used when their need has been determined by a doctor. The FDA withdrew this proposal, but maintained that if dietary supplements claimed that they treated, cured, mitigated, or prevented any diseases, then they were marketing themselves as drugs, and they would be treated as drugs by the FDA.

The next set of landmarks in dietary supplement regulation came in the 1990s. The Nutrition Labeling Act of 1990 (NLEA) forced the FDA to start authorizing health claims for foods and supplements. Before this, health claims were forbidden. However, there were very difficult standards to get these claims approved. The claims had to be substantiated by significant scientific evidence. The FDA also had to develop separate authorization process for supplement health claims and had to decide whether to authorize 10 specific health claims. A major controversy in the supplement regulation debate was whether they should be regulated as food or as drugs. The supplement industry preferred to be considered food so they would be subject to less regulation.

Senator Orrin Hatch (Rep-Utah) introduced the Health Freedom Act of 1992, which was to block the FDA from using health claims as an excuse to regulate dietary supplements as drugs. Hatch was reportedly concerned that the FDA could put anyone out of business through over-regulation. The act did not pass, but Congress did pass the Dietary Supplement Act of 1992, which barred the FDA from applying the forthcoming food labeling rules to dietary supplements for a year, giving the dietary supplement industry time to organize an opposition. This led to a major advance for the supplement industry, the DSHEA.

The DSHEA broadened the definition of supplements to vitamins, minerals, amino acids, botanicals, metabolites, and diet products. It makes the FDA responsible for proving that a product is harmful, rather than making the manufacturer prove it is safe. Given the budget constraints in the FDA, this charge proved difficult. The DSHEA ended the FDA's authority to remove harmful products from market. It allowed for products to remain on the market even while court proceedings against them are under way or while approvals are obtained. It also authorized the structure/function claims when a disclaimer is included that states that "the statement has not been evaluated by the FDA and that the product is not intended to diagnose, treat, cure, or prevent any disease." It allowed supplements a place in the food category, but not identical to foods. Under DSHEA, it is the burden of the manufacturer of a dietary supplement to ensure the safety of the supplement prior to reaching the marketplace. In most instances it is not necessary for the manufacturers to register dietary supplements with the FDA or get approval from the FDA before introducing the supplements into the marketplace. It is also the manufacturers' responsibility, not the FDA's, to ensure that the labeling information of the product is truthful and not misleading. The DSHEA provided that foods could be advertised as dietary supplements, changing the regulations to which they were subject. In 1997, The **Food and Drug Modernization Act** of 1997 (FDAMA) required the FDA to permit nutrient content and health claims for conventional foods when the claims are substantiated by published, authoritative statements by the federal public health agencies or the National Academy of Sciences. These criteria apply to supplements as well. In 1998, *Pearson v. Shalala* took more regulatory authority away from the FDA. The FDA was authorized by Congress in NLEA to pre-approve health claims about foods, but the FDA created a difficult standard to approve such claims. After 10 years, only 10 claims had been approved. Durk Pearson and Sandy Shaw were supplement manufacturers who thought that they had the evidence to make four health claims on their packages, claims that were substantiated by scientific data. The scientific data were also widely accepted and commonly repeated in mainstream media. The FDA withheld approval of these claims, causing Pearson and Shaw to sue. The D.C. Court of Appeals ruled that dietary supplement labels may contain health claims when they also contain a disclaimer that such claims have not been approved by the FDA. The Grocery Manufacturers of America told the FDA that this decision meant that the standards that govern dietary supplements also apply to foods. In 2001, the FDA warned the food industry that botanicals could not be assumed to be approved food additives or generally recognized as safe (**GRAS**). However, the food industry responded against that warning.

In May 2009, the FDA warned General Mills about cholesterol-lowering claims the company made for its Cheerios cereal. The press gave the warning more coverage than it may have in the past, signaling that the FDA and the public may consider a stricter treatment of this industry.

There are several issues with nutraceuticals. Firstly, they occupy a middle ground between food and drugs, which arguably blurs the distinction between these categories. This may cause more confusion among a public that is already confused about proper nutrition. Since nutraceuticals are so marketable, it is very common to create these kinds of foods. As a result, some nutritionists question whether it may be too much of a beneficial food. They further wonder what the effects of too much of these supplements may be. Another way of looking at it is they give people an excuse to eat more "junk foods." Once a junk food can make a health claim, it seems to look less bad. However, the foods are still not healthy. As a result, many consumers do not change their diets when they need to eat better. Instead, they choose the healthier versions of the junk foods they were previously eating.

See also: Advertising of Food; Diet Foods; Federal Trade Commission; Lite Labeling.

Stephanie Jane Carter

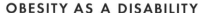

OBESITY AS A DISABILITY

Obesity, defined by the National Institutes of Health as a person whose body mass index is over 30, has been described as a disability under the **Americans with Disabilities Act** (ADA). When the person's obesity is such that it is a physical impairment that prevents or interferes with performance of major life activities, the cause of the impairment is a disability. Although obesity is not specifically listed as a disability in the act, the nature of the disease is such that it can result in a disability. When a person with an obesity-related disability applies for a job, the restaurant or other food service industry employer must make reasonable accommodations to allow the potential employee to work at the place of employment when that person is the best qualified candidate. The employer must be alert to obesity as a disability under the ADA.

Other forms of obesity-related disability may manifest themselves in the Social Security system, which provides for disability payments to the qualified disabled. Prior to 1999 obesity was considered an impairment, that is, a person who met certain height-weight guidelines was considered automatically impaired. This meant that meeting the criteria allowed a person to avoid a hearing, but many people were disabled and did not necessarily meet the set of height-weight guidelines. Under current regulations of the Social Security Administration (SSA) the obesity is considered a disability after confirmation by a physician and when the condition makes the obese person unable to perform the basic activities for work. The degree of disability is determined on a case-by-case basis.

In some cases where the problem caused by the obesity, for example, musculoskeletal deterioration, is the cause for disability, the SSA may say that the obesity is equivalent to musculoskeletal deterioration. This allows the determination to be made on the basis of something other than obesity.

In 2009, the American Medical Association voted to not support the principle that obesity is a disability. Some doctors argue that patients can be offended by a suggestion that they lose weight and that physicians may wait until the person has a treatable related condition, like high blood pressure, before discussing weight. Insurance companies also will generally not cover obesity treatments, but only related conditions.

Case law under both the ADA and the SSA clearly do not automatically link the condition of obesity with disability. The law clearly states that obesity can be a cause of a disability, but obesity is not automatically considered a disability. The person who claims the disability must show that the condition causes the person to be disabled. A mere showing of obesity is not enough to meet the legal standard.

The **Centers for Disease Control and Prevention** have listed a number of consequences of obesity such as high blood pressure (hypertension), increased risk of Type 2 diabetes, coronary heart disease, increased risk for certain cancers, osteoarthritis, and sleep apnea. The Centers for Disease Control and Prevention has stated that in the United States about 30 percent of the adult population is obese. These conditions may cause symptoms such as fatigue, shortness of breath, and joint problems, any of which may be deemed a disability—interfering with a person's ability to perform a job or requiring some reasonable accommodation so as to perform the job.

In addition to being a potential legal disability, obesity can also be considered a social disability. The need to sit in a special seat in a theater, because a person is too large to fit in a regular seat, or the need to purchase a second seat in an airplane, takes a social and emotional toll. This is true even when the obese person is totally mobile and not otherwise disabled. The social stigma of obesity may include embarrassment caused by body odor, the inability to find or afford appropriate clothing, and the inability to ride in a car or bus, as well as myriad other daily indignities. There is a need to find a way to deal with the social problem of obesity. The problem, however, is quite complex, and the law is only just beginning to address its impact.

See also: Americans with Disabilities Act and Restaurants; Obesity Lawsuits.

Elizabeth M. Williams

OBESITY LAWSUITS

A series of private law suits that attempt to both rectify what could be considered the damage wrought by fast-food companies and to duplicate the success of the smoking lawsuits against tobacco companies are collectively referred to as the obesity lawsuits. John F. Banzhaf III, a public interest lawyer and professor at George Washington University Law School in Washington, D.C., is an architect of the plan that features the use of the courts to, if not actually collect damages, at least provoke changes in corporate behavior. The first suit was filed against McDonald's, Burger King, KFC, and Wendy's on behalf of a middle-aged obese man in 2002. This suit was withdrawn.

These lawsuits seem to be tools in the arsenal of lawyers with an agenda. The cause of action and controversy generally required by the **court system** are not clearly based on conventional causes of actions and conventional duties. The arguments that have been made by the lawyers have been novel. They do bring attention to the matters of concern to the lawyers, but they do not seem to actually bring matters to resolution through the court system.

The theory of these cases is that fast food is so full of fat, salt, and sugar that it is almost addictive. In addition the portions are too large to be healthful, and the fast-food companies encourage patrons to eat even larger portions by making larger portions better bargains. By making this food available at inexpensive prices, patrons cannot resist the food. They eat too much and they become obese and unhealthy. The plaintiffs argue that they are unable to resist eating this food, and thus they have no responsibility in the matter of overeating and becoming obese.

As lawsuits have matured in their techniques and strategies, they now not only attack directly the question of growing obesity, but they also indirectly attack situations that activists see as contributors to obesity, particularly childhood obesity. By zeroing in on childhood obesity, the cases can avoid the question of personal choice that may overcome the "fault" of the product. For example, cases have been brought against Kraft because it failed to disclose that Oreo cookies contained trans fat and against Big Daddy's Diet Ice Cream for labeling inaccuracies affecting its diet status. Cases trying to ban the serving of soft drinks in schools, because soft drinks are linked to obesity, also fit into the category of obesity lawsuits.

These lawsuits do not address any of the other factors that might have contributed to obesity. That means that the failure to exercise, the trend in schools to limit physical education courses, the increased watching of television and use of computers and video games, for example, are not addressed in the lawsuits. All of the responsibility for obesity falls on fast-food and prepared food corporations.

These lawsuits may also claim that corporations and food manufacturers have a duty to the public to disclose ingredients and other nutritional information beyond what is actually required by labeling laws. The question has been raised as to whether the nutritional concerns expressed by the plaintiffs in these lawsuits are based on solid science.

In addition to Banzhaf, the **Center for Science in the Public Interest** (CSPI) has used the public relations technique to cause change as well as legal actions. Often the lawsuits that are brought are class actions, which will increase damages, if awarded, and will discourage the behavior that forms the basis for the suit. Here, the lawyers look for a suitable plaintiff instead of a plaintiff feeling wronged and deciding to hire an attorney. The suits are lawyer-driven and designed primarily to garner maximum publicity and change corporate behavior rather than resolve a dispute.

A counter balance to these lawsuits is an organization supported by restaurants, food manufacturers, as well as the public, the **Center for Consumer Freedom**. This organization counters the actions of the trial lawyers and represents the positions of restaurants and food manufacturers. It is the position of the Center for Consumer Freedom that adults should be allowed to choose what they eat. Restaurants and manufacturers should not be penalized for creating food that tastes good.

The CSPI took a strong stand against butter and in favor of the use of margarine. Now that scientists are watching trans fats for health problems, the CSPI is advocating against margarine and in favor of butter. It seems that the opinion of scientists may still be theoretical when the CSPI begins to try to influence eating and behavior.

Several states have enacted laws that do not allow the prosecution of obesity lawsuits. The National Restaurant Association and other food industry groups and restaurant associations have been supporters of these bans. The House of Representatives also passed a bill in 2004 and again in 2005 that would prohibit the pursuit of obesity lawsuits against restaurants and food manufacturers, but it was never enacted into law. The bill became known as "the Cheeseburger Bill."

Taxing Sugar-Sweetened Soft Drinks

There have been studies that correlate the drinking of sugar-sweetened soft drinks with obesity according to the April 2007 issue of the *American Journal of Public Health*. The beverage industry argues that no single food can be the cause of obesity. The reviewers in the article suggest that those who drink these beverages actually eat more and do not compensate for the extra calories by eating less. In addition, the article cites a correlation with an increase in Type 2 diabetes. One reaction has been a move to increase taxation of soft drinks to discourage consumers, especially youth, from drinking sweetened drinks. The Senate Finance Committee considered such a tax in 2009 as a source of income to fund a national health care program, citing the link between obesity and health costs. The proposal has not been adopted, but in 2010 President Obama said that he considers the tax worth exploration.

Critics of the bill argued that since the courts had generally found that the cases could not be supported, as they failed to state a claim or had no merit because the parties chose to eat, that there was no need for the bill.

These lawsuits have not generally been successful in actually awarding damages to plaintiffs who have become obese. In fact, the predicted unleashing of obesity lawsuits has never materialized in part because the suits have been dismissed as failing to state a claim that can be resolved by the courts. Because there is more recognition of the many factors that contribute to obesity, it is becoming harder to sustain the original basis for these suits. However, the use of the courts to bring attention to a matter and to force changes in either government positions or in consumer or corporate behavior continues.

See also: Labeling, Nutrition; Labeling, Quantity; Lite Labeling; Appendix 3A: *Pelman, et al. v. McDonald's Corporation*; Appendix 3B: *Pelman, et al. v. McDonald's Corporation*, Amended Complaint; Appendix 3C: *Pelman, et al. v. McDonald's Corporation*.

Elizabeth M. Williams

OCCUPATIONAL SAFETY AND HEALTH ADMINISTRATION AND SLAUGHTERHOUSES SAFETY

Slaughterhouses and meat processing are big business in the United States. It takes approximately 10 billion animals annually to feed the meat-eating needs of the country. It is estimated that 28.1 billion pounds of beef were eaten by people in the United States in 2007. There are many potential problems that arise when animals are killed in such significant numbers. The amount of meat consumed continues to rise. Working in a slaughterhouse is a physically difficult and demanding job. Slaughterhouses face many environmental problems.

In 1970 the Occupational Safety and Hazard Act was adopted with the purpose of protecting the safety of workers. By promulgating regulations for workplace health and safety standards, the Occupational Safety and Health Administration (OSHA) can reduce work-related accidents, occupational illnesses, and deaths. There are myriad regulations that set different standards based on the type of workplace and the special conditions of that workplace. Yet, general regulations apply to all facilities. First aid, for example, would apply to most workplaces, including slaughterhouses. OSHA uses workers as informal inspectors, assuming that they know best the conditions of the workplace; thus, workers have the opportunity to report unsafe conditions, bring lawsuits against the employer, and call for inspections all without retaliation.

OSHA has a big job, regulating and monitoring workplaces around the country. There are over 200 OSHA offices around the country. There are regular inspectors throughout the United States in addition to many other types of employees and technical personnel who together support the agency. Physicians, engineers, and others write the standards for each type of workplace. It is the job of OSHA to promulgate its standards after they are adopted. In addition, it is responsible for enforcement and for education of both employers and employees in the technical aspects of OSHA compliance.

OSHA places certain requirements on the workplace. The primary requirement is to maintain a workplace that is free from known safety and health hazards that have the potential to cause death or serious bodily harm. If workers are working with or are exposed to hazardous materials, they must be so informed by their employer. When necessary, employers must provide special training necessary to properly and safely perform workplace duties. Employers must maintain records of those incidences that reflect work-related injury and death and also exposure of employees to hazardous materials or toxins.

Employees may bring lawsuits directly against the employer asking the court to rectify conditions that are not in compliance with OSHA standards. States have worker compensation laws that provide for compensation to employees when there is a workplace injury or illness. When those conditions are related to a substandard workplace caused by a violation of OSHA or state standards, the employee may be able to receive more than the normal amount of compensation. If OSHA finds a dangerous condition to exist, it has a number of remedies at its disposal. It may require that all employees to be evacuated from an unsafe area. It may issue an order to employers to repair equipment that is dangerous or unsafe. It can require that the employer clean an area or remove scattered materials that could cause a hazard. It can require an employer to adopt and implement cleaning and storage standards to maintain safety.

Retaliation against workers for reporting unsafe workplace conditions or other safety violations is prohibited, but it still might occur. When a worker considers actions taken by an employer to be retaliatory, the worker may report this occurrence to OSHA. OSHA regulations set a window of 30 days from the time of the retaliation in which a worker must report retaliation to OSHA and to the Department of Labor. This complaint triggers an investigation. Should the investigation find that the action is retaliatory (this would often be as severe as a termination of the worker or a disciplinary action), OSHA can order the employer to rectify the action by restoring the worker to the pre-retaliation position. Findings and subsequent action by OSHA is only one remedy available to the worker. The employee may also have the additional remedy of bringing a legal action against the employer.

The rate of injury at slaughterhouses is several times higher than at other factories. Work at these facilities is still extremely dangerous. The work is partially automated, which makes it impossible for workers to control speed. They must conform to the speed of the line. It requires use of sharp objects like knives and saws. The work is quick, messy, repetitive, and dangerous. One typical injury is being cut by a knife. This may occur because of the speed of the line. The speed and pressure coupled with the repeated killing and carcass-filled environment may cause psychological stress and other psychological disorders.

The disassembly line is the single most dangerous area of the slaughterhouse, usually where the most injuries occur. The speed of the line and the number of injuries are directly correlated. The speed at which animal slaughtering has taken place has increased dramatically. In the early 20th century, the stockyard facilities in Chicago, subject of the early muckraking novel *The Jungle* (1906), by **Upton Sinclair**, killed about 50 heads of cattle an hour. Improvements in technology over the years more than tripled that number by the 1980s. It is now reported that some facilities reach up to eight times that number. Keeping up with the line can result in repetitive injuries such as tendonitis, locked joints, and carpal tunnel syndrome. Slipping knives can cause different levels of abrasions and lacerations. Workers report back problems and physical and psychological stress disorders. The meat inspectors from the Food Safety Inspection Service (FSIS) do not police the work safety issues, but merely the food safety issues. OSHA inspectors may respond to complaints from workers, but do not inspect for food safety.

Because psychological stress disorders can develop as workers cope with the relentless pressure in their attempt to keep up with the speed of the production lines, workers have developed coping mechanisms that may be unhealthy. The high-pressure environments have given rise to a drug subculture in the meatpacking industry; employees sometimes develop dependencies on "speed" and other drugs like methamphetamines. Worker turnover in slaughterhouses is high.

See also: Appendix 9: Twenty-Eight Hour Law of 1873 as Amended in 1994.

Further Reading U.S. Department of Labor, Occupational Safety and Health Administration, http://www.osha.gov.

William C. Smith and Elizabeth M. Williams

ORGANIC FOODS PRODUCTION ACT

The Organic Foods Production Act (OFPA) was adopted by Congress in 1990. It is the enabling legislation for the National Organics Program (NOP). Through this law and the NOP regulations, promulgating the list of acceptable production inputs, known as the National List, and all of the regulations that inform farming practices for organic food are authorized. The act places the regulatory authority under the **U.S. Department of Agriculture** (USDA). In addition it establishes the **National Organic Standards Board** (NOSB).

This legislation got off to a rocky start. The regulations were not ready by the 1993 goal, partly because funds were not appropriated to develop them. The OFPA states that the cost of maintaining the program will be self-generated from the fees paid by those applying for organic certification. However, the program was delayed in its early implementation because funding was slow in the initial states.

The NOSB makes recommendations for organic standards to the USDA. The Secretary of Agriculture and staff promulgate the proposed rules. Initially, the rule promulgated under the OFPA received such extensive comments that the time for commenting was extended. This also meant that additional time was needed to consider the comments before the final regulations could be published.

The law was a result of lobbying by various groups, including the American Farm Bureau and the National Association of State Departments of Agriculture, which wanted to have one national standard instead of having to deal with standards set in various states. Compliance with multiple standards, plus the cost of applying for certification in each state, made organic farming in interstate commerce expensive and uncertain. In addition, the lobbying groups considered differing standards a point of confusion for consumers who would not know what was "organic" from state to state.

The law also applies to foods that are multi-ingredient. To qualify as organic, the components of multi-ingredient products must conform to the NOP. But before the NOP, it was difficult for these products to comply with the organic standards of the various states, plus the various state labeling laws. These products also supported a national standard. Before the adoption of national standards, meat and seafood could not be labeled organic. Organics were a growing international market that could not be exploited without a national standard. Importing of products labeled organic also requires a national organic standard.

Currently, products that meet the standards set by the NOP may display the "USDA Organic" seal on the package. Although organic farms represent a small fraction of the total land being farmed in the United States, the field is growing. It is believed that the added value represented by the ability to display the seal is worth the cost of compliance with regulation. In addition, the idea of eating healthily is being identified with eating organic, so the consumer is looking for organic products.

The NOP sets regulations for handling and production. The rule requires that 50 percent by weight of ingredients must be organic for the product to be labeled organic. If less than 50 percent by weight of ingredients are organic, the "organic" descriptor can be used in the regular ingredient list. The law includes the National List, which is a list of substances that have been pre-approved for use in organic products. The law provides for a protocol for applying for inclusion in the National List. The program has a certification program for food and for farms.

Because the need for certification is more extensive than can be handled by the USDA alone, there is a project (part of the NOP) that accredits the certifiers. The regulations include considerations and minimum standards for importation. They also cover labeling.

Organic standards and their application are still controversial. Farmers complain that the language is vague and nonspecific. They also complain that the cost of certification and re-certification is not worth it. Some farmers who qualify for the organic label have opted out of the system and merely rely on loyal customers who know their methods to pay organic prices for noncertified products. Other farmers complain that certification can be obtained by simply complying with the standards on the days of inspection and not necessarily complying on other days. The enforcement provisions are contained in the NOP, but since the program is supposed to be self-supporting, the number of inspectors and enforcement personnel is inconsistent.

Many organic consumer groups such as the Organic Farmers Marketing Association object to the NOP, claiming that standards are not truly organic. They argue that allowing as much as 20 percent of animal feed to be nonorganic cannot produce an organic animal. The farmers argue that some nutrients necessary for the health of the animals are not available organically. Farm animals may also be treated with antibiotics for health reasons, although not to encourage growth. Organic consumer groups do not approve of this practice. Irradiation is allowed, which some consider a nonorganic practice. **Genetic engineering** is also allowed, which is objected to by many organic practitioners.

Organic consumer groups have objected to the language in the statute that purports to describe a holistic method of tending the soil, farming, and processing. In particular, such phrases as "where possible" and "without use of extraneous synthetic additives or processing" are considered objectionable because they create a toehold for those who wish to circumvent the organics standard when it is difficult. Although any NOP must be reduced to specific definable standards, organic consumer groups claim that current standards do not reflect a concern for sustainability in practice that true adherence to organic standards represent. The conflict between organic consumers and the government standards seems to be a difference between those who consider organic farming a lifestyle and those like organic agribusinesses that consider it a business. Businesses can comply with the organic standards without having embraced the philosophy and world view. They merely comply with the standards. Organic consumer groups worry that by merely complying with standards that agribusinesses will also look for legal loop holes, because they are merely businesses without a moral commitment to an organic life.

See also: Milk, Organic.

Elizabeth M. Williams

P

PACKERS AND STOCKYARDS ACT

The Packers and Stockyards Act (PSA) was adopted by Congress in 1921 in response to an investigation by the **Federal Trade Commission** (FTC), which was looking for ways to keep the cost of food down. Food prices—especially meat prices—were rising at a rate that alarmed consumers and the federal government during World War I; one response to this price increase was the search for economies in production and packing. In addition, the FTC began to look for cooperative efforts in the food chain that kept prices high. Today, the law not only covers stockyards and meat packers, but poultry dealers and pig dealers.

The result of the FTC investigation was an initial recommendation that the government take over the stockyards, because of their corruption. The FTC found that the stockyards and meat packers were generally cheating the meat producers and cattlemen, manipulating the markets to increase prices, and cheating consumers. Rather than nationalizing the stockyards, Congress decided to authorize the regulation of the stockyards and related activities. At the same time that Congress was debating regulation of the industry, the Justice Department was considering taking action under the Sherman Antitrust Act. This threat was an attempt to get the meat packers out of every aspect of the industry and limit them to meat packing. This would mean disentangling the meat packers from the stockyards, retail and wholesale sales of meat, as well as storage of product. The industry was controlled by five companies known as the "Big Five." These companies were Armour, Wilson, Swift, Cudahy, and Morris. They finally reached a settlement agreement with the Justice Department about limiting their activities to meat packing in 1920.

Although the power and influence of the meatpackers were greatly limited by the settlement, Congress passed the PSA with the intention of regulating international and national commerce in meat, poultry, eggs, and dairy products. For good measure, the act prohibited antitrust activities as well as unfair and deceptive practices in the industry. Although the law did not nationalize the stockyards, meat packers and their employees were required to register with the government. Most importantly meat packers could not sell or broker the meat that came through their yards. This was a significant limitation on free trade.

The limitations and restrictions on commerce were challenged by the industry as restraint of trade in violation of the **interstate commerce** clause in the case of *Stafford v. Wallace*. The case was resolved by the U.S. Supreme Court in 1922. The court upheld the law as constitutional, stating that regulation was constitutional and that it was not unreasonable.

The **U.S. Department of Agriculture** (USDA) was given regulatory jurisdiction under the PSA. That jurisdiction was expanded from stockyards and meat-packing facilities to auction markets through amendments to the PSA. The PSA has been expanded over the years through amendments. Today, the USDA has the ability to assess civil penalties, through the Grain Inspection, Packers and Stockyard Administration, overseas regulations that include bonding of packers and protection of producers from nonpayment by packers, and regulation of the entire meat-packing and distribution chain. This authority covers beef and pork industries.

See also: Appendix 5: *North American Cold Storage Co. v. City of Chicago*; Appendix 9: Twenty-Eight Hour Law of 1873 as Amended in 1994.

Elizabeth M. Williams

PELMAN, ET AL. V. MCDONALD'S CORPORATION

The *Pelman, et al. v. McDonald's Corporation* lawsuit made the fast food industry concerned about the possibility of further **obesity lawsuits**. The case also triggered the introduction of **legislation** into Congress and in some states, for example, Georgia and Illinois, that would limit the ability to sue a restaurant for personal obesity. The bill passed in the House of Representatives but not in the Senate; thus, it never became law.

The case was originally brought in the U.S. District Court for the District of New York in 2002. The basis of federal jurisdiction is diversity. The plaintiffs were a mother, Roberta Pelman, on behalf of her minor daughter, Ashley, by Roberta on her own behalf, and by Israel Bradley, on behalf of his minor daughter, Jazlen, and by Israel in his own right. The lawsuit also sought to have certified a class of people similarly situated, making the suit a class action. The suit raised several issues against McDonald's Corporation, including deceptive practices under the New York Consumer Protection Statute in that McDonald's fraudulently advertised that consumption of its food—chicken nuggets, hamburgers, and other products—could form part of a balanced diet and that they were nutritionally beneficial. The complaint further stated that purchasers of the food sold by the defendant's restaurants relied on general definitions of potato, chicken, beef, and other foods when assuming what they were choosing at the restaurants. The complaint stated that the defendant was negligent in that it sold harmful products without warning its patrons, and further alleged that the defendant's products were psychologically addictive, the sale of which was also negligent.

The plaintiffs claimed that the foods were not nutritious and that McDonald's France, a part of the defendant's international corporation, had warned that the food was not nutritious. According to the complaint, the complainants acted on the belief that the food was nutritious and the plaintiffs ate the food regularly and often. The plaintiffs were obese and this obesity was blamed directly on the regular consumption of the unhealthy food that the defendant wrongfully sold at its restaurants.

The lawsuit has been seen as an abandonment of personal responsibility. However, there has been some concern that the defendant did inject its products with certain additives without informing its patrons, calling the additives flavoring.

Some of these actions resulted in foods that were not reflective of the nutritional content of those foods without additives, and there is a question raised about the duty to warn patrons of these alterations. The complainant did not let patrons know that the "flavorings" were altering the nutritional content of the foods. Some of these issues have been mooted by restaurant nutritional disclosure regulations and the defendant's ultimate conformance with these regulations.

The district court held that the lawsuit did not adequately allege facts that constituted deceptive practices as defined by the New York statutes. It went on to state that the complaint failed to establish a connection between the alleged harm and the deceptive practices. The action in tort or negligence failed to establish that the negligence was the proximate cause of the injury. However, the court allowed the plaintiffs leave to replead, which they did.

The court's first opinion was rendered in January 2003. The second opinion, after the repleading, was rendered in September 2003. The court once again stated that the complainants had failed to establish that they had relied on McDonald's advertisements and had failed to establish probable cause. In addition, all of the claims made by the adults were barred by the statute of limitations.

The court in dicta was critical of the defendant, because the defendant had—if not been deceptive—at least relied on people's common understanding of food in making choices about the healthfulness of the products. But the judge did not find that there were deceptive practices or sufficient connection to cause harm.

The complainants appealed to the Second Circuit Court of Appeals. The appellate court determined that the trial court had erred in its dismissal vis à vis deceptive practices, the standard being met. The appellate court said that questions raised by the trial court could be addressed in discovery. Thus, the court remanded the case to the trial court in 2005. In 2006, the trial court required the complainant to reply to the second amended complaint.

The trial judge ultimately stated that there was a failure in the complainants' establishment of causation between the consumption of the food sold by McDonald's Corporation and the obesity suffered by the plaintiffs. The judge considered that there could be many factors contributing the obesity of the plaintiffs including family history, other foods eaten by the plaintiffs, the amount of exercise engaged in by the plaintiffs, and other factors. The judge also discussed the difficulty of establishing a single string of causation when there were several plaintiffs who may have different life styles and family histories. Causation might be easier to establish with an individual plaintiff. The trial judge opened the way for pretrial discovery.

The lawsuit or the threat of a lawsuit is said to have made fast-food restaurants rethink elements of their menus in favor of healthier choices such as salads, yogurt, and fruit. The restaurants deny any relationship between these changes and the pressures brought by the lawsuit, stating that the changes were already under consideration based on changes in consumer demands.

The settlement of a lawsuit may resolve things that are at issue in a particular lawsuit, but not the global issues of the case that might be decided by a court judgment. Often large corporate defendants will settle a case so as to keep the case from reaching judgment, and several other cases involving issues of food have been settled.

See also: Additives and Preservatives; Court System; Liability; Torts; Appendix 3A: *Pelman, et al. v. McDonald's Corporation;* Appendix 3B: *Pelman, et al. v. McDonald's Corporation,* Amended Complaint; Appendix 3C: *Pelman, et al. v. McDonald's Corporation.*

Further Reading Frank, Theodore H. "Taxonomy of Obesity Litigation." *University of Arkansas at Little Rock Law Review* 28, no. 3 (2006): 427–41.

Elizabeth M. Williams

PERISHABLE AGRICULTURAL COMMODITIES ACT

The Perishable Agricultural Commodities Act (PACA) is a federal law that prohibits unfair trading practices by buyers and sellers in the fruit and vegetable industry. Because fruits and vegetables are perishable goods that lose their value in a short period of time, traders in these goods can be exposed to a great amount of risk if there are problems with shipments and payments. The PACA establishes standards for fruit and vegetable trading practices and provides for enforcement by the PACA Branch within the Agricultural Marketing Service of the **U.S. Department of Agriculture** (USDA). The act also creates a dispute resolution process to handle PACA contractual disputes more expeditiously and at lower cost by keeping them outside of the civil **court system**.

Congress approved PACA during the economic troubles of the Great Depression in 1930 and created the standards of fair trade practices to protect the often smaller growers and fruit and vegetable supplies from the large dealer and grocery merchant buyers. Congress amended PACA in 1984 following a period of complaints by suppliers that dealers were delaying and withholding payments from suppliers. Among other changes, refinements, and expansions, the amendments to PACA created a trust system whereby unpaid fruit and vegetable suppliers maintain a statutory trust claim on the buyer, when the buyer failed to pay for the produce and/or entered bankruptcy.

The PACA defines perishable agricultural commodities as all fresh fruits and vegetables, whether frozen, packed in ice, or otherwise. Courts and USDA regulations interpret this definition as continuing to apply to fruits and vegetables that have been minimally processed as well, including sliced or pitted produce. The test is whether the produce retains its essential nature, or changes to a different kind or character of food. For example, raw potatoes that have been coated with oil in preparation for frying are still considered perishable agricultural commodities.

The PACA applies to three categories of people, including dealers, that is, buyers or sellers of fruits or vegetables. The act also applies to commission merchants, that is, those who buy or sell on behalf of another party. A third category, brokers—persons negotiating interstate commercial fruit and vegetable sales—also falls under PACA. In addition, anyone who is not required to obtain a dealer may voluntarily apply for a dealer license. To deal in fresh fruits and vegetables, these commercial interstate buyers and sellers must obtain a PACA license from

USDA by filling out an application available on USDA's Web site. The USDA also maintains a database of current PACA licensees.

Dealers, brokers, and commission merchants who sell more than 2,000 pounds of perishable agricultural commodities must register with USDA for a PACA license to track and enforce compliance. The PACA licensees may use different trade names under one license without requiring new licenses, but the USDA may disapprove of trade names that would be deceptive, misleading, or confusing. Retailers are exempt from the license requirement until their purchases of fresh and frozen fruits and vegetables exceed $230,000. There is also a limited exemption for brokers who deal only in frozen products on behalf of the vendor if the value of the contracts is less than $230,000 per year. Finally, growers who sell only their own products are not required to register under PACA.

Annual PACA fees are $550 for a single business and $200 per branch location for the tenth branch location and additional branches with an annual cap of $4,000 per business. As allowed by amendments to the act in 1995, the USDA proposed to increase the fees by regulation for the first time to $995 per business, $600 for every branch location, and an annual cap of $8,000 with the effective date of October 2010. The PACA program is supported by user fees, and the USDA has authority to increase them when operating reserves fall below 25 percent of projected annual costs. The 1995 act also created a one-time fee for new retailers and grocery wholesalers that are dealers, and gradually eliminated annual fees for existing retailers and wholesalers that would otherwise need to pay fees as dealers.

Failure to maintain a license is punishable by a fine of up to $1,000 per offense and up to $250 each day a firm continues to do so. The USDA can file actions in a civil proceeding to recover the fines, or it may seek an injunction in an appropriate court. If any license violations are the result of inadvertence, a person may instead pay the license fee and up to a $250 penalty. The USDA will also refuse licenses to applicants that have had revoked licenses or other serious PACA violations within the previous two years or were declared bankrupt within three years. After that two-year period, the applicant may receive a license if they post a surety bond in an appropriate amount with the USDA. The USDA may further withhold a license pending an investigation.

The PACA prohibits the use of unfair, discriminatory, or deceptive practices in the weighing, counting, or quantity determination of perishable agricultural commodities in all commerce and also prohibits false or misleading statements in any transaction. The act also prohibits any dealer from rejecting delivery or failing to deliver according to the terms of a perishable agricultural commodity contract. The act further prohibits commission merchants from discarding, dumping, or destroying perishable commodities without reasonable cause.

Any person involved in a perishable agricultural commodity transaction must correctly account for and make full payment promptly within 10 days in a fruit or vegetable transaction and fulfill any other duty arising from the transaction, barring reasonable cause for failing to do so. The act also specifically makes it unlawful to misrepresent by any word or marking the character, kind, grade, quality, quantity, size, pack, weight, condition, maturity, or geographical place of origin of any perishable agricultural commodity. The act also prohibits tampering with any quality or grade certificate from a federal or state inspector about a perishable commodity or to substitute goods after an inspection, unless it is for re-sorting and discarding inferior produce.

In the 1984 amendments to PACA, Congress created a statutory trust provision for fruit and vegetable suppliers. Prior to the trust, sellers of fruits and vegetables with unpaid bills were treated as other business creditors in **bankruptcy** proceedings, recovering from the bankruptcy estate only after secured creditors such as banks. With dealers, merchants, and large retailers often financed by banks, the options for fruit and vegetable sellers for recovering from a bankrupt buyer were often reduced. The PACA trust, on the other hand, provides produce sellers with superior claims in bankruptcy.

A trust is a legal obligation where one party, the trustee, holds property, the trust assets, for the benefit of another, the trust beneficiary for a trust purpose. Under PACA, buyers are the trustees; sellers are the beneficiaries; the trust assets are the buyer's inventory of produce, processed products, or cash proceeds from sale; and the purpose is to protect unpaid fruit and vegetable suppliers. To be a beneficiary of the PACA statutory trust, sellers must notify the buyer that they intend to preserve trust benefits. Today, this may be accomplished by a standard clause on an invoice or bill; previously, a separate written notice was required. The notice has to be provided within 30 days of the expiration of the parties' contract terms.

Buyers of PACA-covered produce must maintain sufficient assets to pay PACA trust claims. The enforcement of the terms of the PACA trust operates under existing general trust law. Sellers may enforce the terms of the trust through injunctions from a court, which can freeze assets and seek trust assets through personal **liability**, protection in bankruptcy proceedings, and recovery of assets transferred to third parties. Overall, the terms of PACA provide produce industry sellers with significant and unique protection from unpaid bills unusual in other areas of business law.

In addition to the trust claim option, when a party to a fruit or vegetable transaction believes that another party has failed to pay or violated the act, that party may file a PACA complaint with a $100 filing fee either via letter or electronic mail to a USDA PACA Branch office. The complaint has to be filed within nine months of the alleged violation and must briefly state the facts and provide supporting documentation. State offers and agencies may also file PACA complaints. If the USDA determines the complaint warrants an action, it forwards it to the defending party who must answer the complaint in writing or satisfy the claim. The PACA Branch of USDA is headquartered in Washington, D.C., with regional offices in Tucson, Arizona; Fort Worth, Texas; and Manassas, Virginia.

If the USDA finds that a PACA-licensed firm has failed to pay, its license is suspended and it is prohibited from operating until the order is paid to satisfaction. For other violations of PACA, the USDA may suspend or revoke a firm's license depending on its discretion based on the severity of the violation. For violations of false inspection markings, the USDA may suspend a license for up to 90 days or revoke the license for repeated or flagrant violations. While a license is suspended, the firm's officers are prohibited from affiliation with any other PACA licensed firm as well. The USDA may also revoke the license of any applicant who obtained the license through false or misleading statements. Instead of suspension or revocation, the USDA may instead seek civil penalties of up to $2,000 per transaction or day of violation. If not paid, the USDA must take civil penalties for enforcement to the U.S. Attorney General, who can pursue them in a U.S. district court.

If there are reasonable grounds for a complaint, the USDA may investigate and expand the investigation to include any other additional PACA violations that are found. If it finds sufficient evidence, the USDA may bring a complaint against a person who has an opportunity for a hearing before an administrative law judge for cases where the amount claimed is more than $30,000 in damages. For lesser amounts, the complaint and answering may be conducted by deposition or other verified statements of fact.

If the USDA administrative law judge finds that a complaint is valid or the accused party fails to answer the complaint, then the judge will determine the amount of damages owed to the complainant and order the offending party to pay reparation. The judge will also order that the losing party to the dispute pay the prevailing party's reasonable fees and expenses incurred in the hearing. If a losing party fails to pay by the date required in the administrative law judge's order, the prevailing party may bring a suit in federal district court within three years for the dispute. The USDA's judge's order is considered prima facie factual evidence, and the party bringing the suit may recover reasonable attorney's fees. If a party fails to pay a reparation order or appeal, the USDA suspends its PACA license.

Either party adversely affected by an order for reparation by USDA administrative law judge may appeal it by way of a lawsuit in U.S. district court within 30 days of the order. The appealing party must post bond with the clerk of the district court in an amount double the amount of reparations. In the district court, the appeal is a trial de novo, meaning that the final decision of the USDA judge does not hold weight in the decision, but the facts in the USDA order are considered prima facie evidence of such.

To facilitate compliance and enforcement, PACA requires that dealers, brokers, and commission merchants keep accounts and records of their produce transactions. They must also disclose these transactions and the true ownership and stockholding in PACA-regulated businesses. Failure to keep proper records may result in a license suspension of up to 90 days.

See also: Code of Federal Regulations; Interstate Commerce.

Andrew G. Wallace

PESTICIDES

A pesticide can be a single material or combination of materials used for the control of pests. This generic term may be applied to preventive substances as well as those that kill pests. Repellants or substances that minimize pests are also included in the term. The word "pesticide" does not only refer to insecticides, which control insects. Herbicides, used to control weeds and other unwanted growth, and fungicides, used to control fungi, are included. A pesticide can be synthetic or natural. For example, botanicals such as tobacco, chrysanthemum, and pyrethrum have been used as the foundations for pesticides. The **Environmental Protection Agency** (EPA) monitors and controls pesticides and their use in the United States.

Pesticides first gained national attention in the early 1960s with the publication of *Silent Spring* by biologist **Rachel Carson**. The book called attention to the results of the use dichlorodiphenyltrichloroethane (DDT) on the environment and suggested that it was carcinogenic. Carson questioned the logic of spraying chemicals into the environment without adequate research on the chemicals' effects on the environment, wildlife, and human health. As the U.S. public became outraged at the use of pesticides, nongovernmental organizations found an audience. The common 1960s' view on pesticides was summarized on the International Union for Conservation on Nature's (IUCN) Commission on Ecology's statements on policy published in 1966. The expressed views are still common. The statements recognized that pesticides may be necessary on some level. They stated that food production and the elimination of vectors of diseases makes pesticide use necessary. However, some aspects of pesticide use must be taken into account, such as the broader ecological consequences; that unnecessarily clean farming and monoculture carry inherent risks; that biological control methods can present alternative and long-term strategies; that chemicals should be applied in the minimum amount necessary to be effective; that more specific pesticides are needed; and that in some circumstances, some pesticides may be dangerous to wildlife and others. Although these points were not new, the publication of and response to *Silent Spring* meant more people were willing to listen. The 1970s saw an argument for the gradual development of alternatives and the spread of integrated pest management thinking.

Organic foods began to become popular in the 1970s. Beginning in the 1970s and increasing radically after that, organic foods were no longer relegated to specialty stores. They were commonly available in most markets in the United States. Organic foods are now purchased by people of all ethnic backgrounds and of all economic classes. By the 1990s, U.S. consumers wanted to be sure that the food they were buying was actually produced in an organic matter if the label claimed that it was. In 1990, the U.S. Congress authorized the **U.S. Department of Agriculture** (USDA) to establish a standards and certification scheme so that consumers could purchase organic foods with confidence. They called these criteria "USDA Organic." The **Organic Foods Production Act** (OFPA) was contained in Title 21 of the 1990 **Farm Bill**. The OFPA authorized the promulgation of regulations describing food production and handling standards that would allow food that was produced in compliance with the regulations to be called organic. The act was the basis for the USDA National Organic Program (NOP), which established minimum standards for agricultural products, outlining standards for processing, growing, and handling of the products. The NOP has the job of monitoring the mandatory certification program of the producing of organics. If a producer is in compliance with the standards promulgated by the NOP, that producer's products may be labeled "USDA Certified Organic." In addition, the 1990 Farm Bill created the **National Organic Standards Board** (NOSB), which makes recommendations to the Secretary of Agriculture regarding the standards for the NOP. Among the regulations for a product to adhere to so as to qualify as organic is that organic products must eliminate synthetic pesticides. Also, it allows that a pesticide made with all organic products can be labeled "organic." The standards took over 10 years to develop. This allows the consumer to have some control over the pesticides they are using and also the ones they are eating.

According to ethicist Peter Singer and Jim Mason, authors of *The Way We Eat and Why Our Food Choices Matter* (2006), organic foods have significantly fewer pesticides than conventionally produced foods. In a 2002 study, a Consumers Union research team found that, in 94,000 samples of food, 73 percent of the conventionally grown foods had pesticide residue on them. This figure was much higher for certain foods, such as strawberries. Only 23 percent of the organic foods had pesticide residue and when they did, it was at much lower levels than the amount of residue on conventionally grown foods.

There are many issues with the use of pesticides. Although pesticides increase crop production, they also entail negative consequences. Sometimes pesticides affect more than they were intended to affect. Many people believe the ban on DDT allowed the bald eagle to survive in the United States. In 1980, New York honey production was negatively affected by the use of pesticides meant to target the gypsy moth and protect sweet corn. Pesticides can pollute the environment and farmers and farm laborers working with them can have health problems. Long-term effects have not been well documented, but some theorists believe that farmers who use pesticides have a greater risk for developing certain types of cancer and Lou Gehrig's disease. Consumers have reported problems such as nausea, lung and eye irritation, and temporary nerve damage as a result of pesticide exposure. Children may be at a greater risk than adults in their exposure to pesticides. Children eat more fruits than adults. They also eat more of the kinds of fruits that have heavy amounts of pesticides.

On the other hand, pesticides have some benefits. They arguably can help people in developing countries to feed themselves. Also, even natural pesticides can still be toxic. Another issue is that food that is produced without pesticides can have a higher price tag at the supermarket. Without using pesticides to farm, farmers cannot use modern conservation tillage techniques that have been enormously successful in reducing soil erosion. Since the issue of using pesticides is often grouped with organics and organic farmers tend to use fewer pesticides, it makes sense to mention the effects of organic farming on the environment. Organic farming takes up much more space than nonorganic farming, meaning that organic farming on a large scale could mean the loss of forests.

See also: Children and Food; Labeling Definitions; Pricing; Soil, Organic; Sustainability.

Further Reading Brian P. Baker, Charles Benbrook, and Edward Groth III. "Pesticide Residues in Conventional, IPM-Grown and Organic Foods: Insights from Three U.S. Data Sets," *Food Additives and Contaminants.* Pp 427–446. 2002; Boardman, Robert. *Pesticides in World Agriculture.* Houndmills, Basingstoke, Hampshire: Macmillan, 1986; Goldstein, Myrna Chandler, and Mark A. Goldstein. *Controversies in Food and Nutrition.* Westport, CT:

Greenwood Press, 2002; Singer, Peter, and Jim Mason. *The Way We Eat and Why Our Food Choices Matter*. New York: Rodale, 2006.

Stephanie Jane Carter

PET FOODS, ORGANIC

The **U.S. Department of Agriculture** (USDA) has not adopted organic standards for pet foods. Federal organic rules are found in the **Organic Foods Production Act** (OFPA), which was part of the 1990 **Farm Bill**. The bill authorized the National Organic Program (NOP) under the USDA to promulgate regulations defining what is organic in all areas. As yet organic standards with regard to some foods for human consumption are still under development. With no specific standards for pet foods, in order for pet food to be certified organic, it must follow those organic standards set up for food for human consumption. This delay in establishing standards for organic pet foods mirrors the delay in establishing organic standards for food for human consumption.

It is currently possible for producers of pet food to comply with already published organic standards. By using products that are already certified as organic in the manufacturing process the manufacturers of pet food can at least become compliant in anticipation of standards being adopted. In light of the recent scare over imported pet foods that were mislabeled and contained melamine and that caused harm to pets, there is a greater push to establish these standards.

Currently the use of the word "organic" is permissible on pet food labeling if all of the ingredients are certified organic. The standards for manufacturing processes have not been established specifically for the pet food industry. However, there are currently rules that allow the use of certain incidental products in the manufacture of food. There is an approved list of these products, and pet food manufacturers must use products on the list in order to be "organic." Because there are currently no standards, certification is optional. However, certification does mean that an outside party has reviewed the practices of the manufacturer.

Some pet food standards proponents are particularly vehement in their support because they believe that pet food standards in general are too low, and that the adoption of organic standards for pet food will inform all consumers of the gap between high quality pet food and pet food with what they consider unacceptable additives.

Elizabeth M. Williams

POLLAN, MICHAEL (1955–)

Michael Pollan is an award-winning author who focuses on the problems with food production in the United States and the rest of the world. Born in 1955, Pollan grew up on Long Island, New York, to a family of plant-growing enthusiasts. His father very rarely mowed their front lawn, which caused a commotion in their meticulously pruned suburb. Pollan also remembers his grandfather's enormous vegetable gardens in which he planted grocery-store varieties of fruits and vegetables, savoring the knowledge that he was saving money on his fresh produce. Pollan relates stories of trying to create his own little gardens in his suburban backyards, squeezing them between the hedge and the fence and creating an oasis of food next to the foundation of his house.

This intimate relationship with food and nature's bounty at an early age seems to have eventually led Pollan to the stories he writes today. He attended Bennington College, Oxford University, and Columbia University and earned a master's degree in English. He served for several years as the executive editor of *Harper's Magazine*, and in 1987 he began writing articles for the *New York Times Magazine*. Most of these articles focused on home gardening, and the battles between nature and human needs for neat lawns and perfect vegetable gardens. "Gardening Means War," "A Gardener's Guide to Sex, Politics, and Class," and "This Bud's for You" all concentrated on the larger implications of gardening as Pollan chronicled his struggles in his own backyard to make sense of the natural world. He wrote his first book, *Second Nature* (1991), drawing these topics together in an exploration of society's perceptions of nature and how to control it in a garden.

After several years of this approach, Pollan discovered the world of feed lots and commercial animal farms during a trip through California. While driving down Route 5 he passed a feed lot and found what he described in a PBS interview with program host Bill Moyers as "this nightmare landscape where there were mountains of manure the size of pyramids, and mountains of corn the size of pyramids, and cows, black cows as far as you could see. . . ." This experience motivated him to delve into the world of commercial meat production, following the food chain through politics and lobbyists, corn subsidies, and oil prices. His books and articles follow those connections and have introduced the public to many of the more troubling aspects of the commercial food industry. He has also written about genetically modified vegetables, the actual costs of food, and the government's role in food and meat production. In Pollan's 2001 book, *The Botany of Desire: A Plant's Eye-View of the World*, he connected his earlier writing on gardens and plants with worldwide food production, showing the evolution and impact of four important plants in human society: the apple, potato, tulip, and marijuana. This book brought a new concept of plants and the co-evolution of other species with people.

Pollan's next book, *The Omnivore's Dilemma: A Natural History of Four Meals* (2006), continued in this unique approach to food and eating, this time exploring the intricate food chains that make up simple, everyday foods like a McDonald's chicken nugget. He revealed the American dependence on corn and corn products that make up a great deal of modern day food and the related dependence on oil and petroleum. The next book from Pollan, *In Defense of Food: An Eater's Manifesto* (2009), breaks down what he found in *The Omnivore's Dilemma*, encouraging his readers to eat food that is "real," or unprocessed and local, and to rely less on the ubiquitous nutritional information. His latest book, *Food Rules: An Eater's Manual* (2010), lays out simple rules to eating well. The mantra: "Eat food. Not too much. Mostly Plants." sums up Pollan's approach to healthy eating. He continues to write about the dangers of the typical modern American diet, targeting additives and corn syrup most frequently.

Although Pollan's writing and advocacy have yet to bring tangible results, his books and articles have drawn attention to American production and marketing of food. Pollan's 1998 article "Playing God in the Garden," which discussed genetically modified plants, caught the attention of some members of Congress. His work has also brought responses from the agri-business giants, causing them to print statements dismissing Pollan's positions, and letters from companies such as Whole Foods, which thought that he misrepresented them. Pollan sees this as a sign of a more healthy way to address the issue, as it becomes a matter of public debate instead of closeted political decisions.

Pollan has won numerous awards for his writing and there was even some pressure for him to be nominated to President Barack Obama's cabinet in 2009 as Secretary of Agriculture. Although Pollan emphasized that his place was in media, it was a sign that at least some of the American public was ready for serious change in the way agri-business was handled. Today, Pollan is Knight Professor of Science and Environmental Journalism at University of California, Berkeley, and he continues to live by many of his food rules.

Further Reading Pollan, Michael. *The Omnivore's Dilemma: A Natural History of Four Meals.* New York: Penguin, 2006.

Kelsey Parris

PORTION SIZES

The **U.S. Department of Agriculture** (USDA) defines portion size in its 1980 *Dietary Guidelines* as "the amount of food consumed on one eating occasion." There are several resources for determining appropriate portion sizes. The USDA publishes a *Food Guide Pyramid* and *Dietary Guidelines*. The emphasis of the current *Food Guide Pyramid* is that one size does not fit all, meaning that portion sizes should vary among individuals depending on their dietary needs, activity levels, and genetic make-up. For this reason, there are no prescribed portion sizes on the pyramid. Instead, individuals are encouraged to enter their own data into a Web site to discover what portion sizes suit them. The USDA now refers to the *Food Guide Pyramid* as *My Pyramid* to emphasize the importance of tailoring nutrition needs and portion sizes to the individual. Based on a daily consumption of 2,000 calories, the *Food Guide Pyramid* would prescribe 2.5 cups of vegetables, 2 cups of fruit, 6 ounces of grain, 5.5 ounces from the milk and beans group, and 6 teaspoons of oil. The Harvard School of Public Health and the University of Michigan also offer food guides.

Many consumers have found it difficult to visualize what a portion size should be, based on how much it should weigh. For example, a serving of meat is defined as two or three ounces. Two to three ounces of meat looks similar in size to a deck of cards. An appropriate serving of pasta is half a cup and would look similar to a woman's fist. Portion sizes have grown partly because consumers enjoy what they perceive to be a good value: getting more food for a lower price. For this reason, the increase in portion sizes has been partly consumer-driven. In 1980, 7-Eleven convenience stores introduced the Big Gulp, which, at 32 ounces, was the largest single portion of a beverage many people had seen. Now they sell the Super Big Gulp, which contains 64 ounces of liquid. A standard bag of chips has at least doubled in size over the last 20 years. Nutritionists believe that another contributor to the increase in the portions Americans feed themselves is the amount of **diet foods** on the market. Instead of cutting down on portion sizes, many Americans buy "diet foods" and eat more. They also end up gaining more weight on a diet of less appetizing food.

One criticism of past *Food Guide Pyramids* was that they allowed less nutritious foods to qualify as part of a food group. For example, cake could qualify as a grain. In fact, under the Reagan Administration, there was a push to include ketchup as a vegetable. For this reason, the USDA was blamed for promoting poor eating habits. In the current pyramid, the USDA does make some qualifications regarding what foods fit into each food group. For example, the USDA recommends that half of one's grain intake be whole grains. According to the USDA, a serving of meat is two or three ounces. A serving of bread is equal to half a cup of pasta or one ounce of cereal. The dietary guidelines seek to promote health and reduce the risk of chronic diseases through diet and exercise. The dietary guidelines recognize that weight issues are a major health factor in the United States.

Many theorists believe that portion sizes were driven up by the simple economic idea of supply and demand. Portion size gained national attention with the 2004 documentary, *Super Size Me* by filmmaker Morgan Spurlock. In the film, Spurlock ate McDonald's, and nothing else, for breakfast, lunch, and dinner for a month. Spurlock gained weight, increased his cholesterol, and experienced other negative side effects such as liver problems and loss of sex drive. The film generated enormous negative publicity for the fast-food industry. McDonald's stopped selling portions called "Super-Size." Wendy's stopped selling portions called "Biggie." However, the restaurants continue to sell large portion sizes. More importantly, consumers continue to eat them, and demand them. Wendy's started calling the portion of beverage formerly known as "Biggie" medium. It added a size large that is bigger than "Biggie." Advertisements for food often use the size as a selling point because it works to sell the product. Denny's offers a Grand Slam Breakfast, and Ruby Tuesday's, which found that customers were outraged when they decreased portion sizes, offers the Ultimate Colossal Burger. While consumers were appalled by what they saw in *Super Size Me*, they still demand more food at value prices.

See also: Advertising of Food; Children and Food; Labeling, Nutrition; Trans Fat; Appendix 3A: *Pelman, et al. v. McDonald's Corporation*; Appendix 3B: *Pelman, et al. v. McDonald's Corporation*, Amended Complaint; Appendix 3C: *Pelman, et al. v. McDonald's Corporation*.

Further Reading My Pyramid Web site. http://www.mypyramid.gov/; Nestle, Marion. *Food Politics: How the Food Industry Influences Nutrition and Health*. Berkeley: University of California Press, 2007; Schlosser, Eric. *Fast Food Nation: The Dark Side of the All-American Meal*. Boston: Houghton Mifflin, 2001.

Stephanie Jane Carter

POULTRY PRODUCTS INSPECTION ACT

The Poultry Products Inspection Act (PPIA) of 1957 is applicable to those facilities that process and slaughter poultry and operate in foreign **interstate commerce**. The act mandates federal inspection at these facilities. The PPIA parallels the meat inspection requirements in that inspection takes place while the poultry is alive, at the carcass stage, and then again before the poultry is processed. Imported poultry must be inspected at entry points before being allowed into the country.

The PPIA also required that plant facilities be sanitary, that slaughtering and processing plants be inspected, and that labeling of products be accurate and truthful. Regulation of poultry was not included in other acts regarding meat or meat products. In 1968 Congress amended the PPIA, again mirroring the laws applicable to meat inspection, but making the inspection and inspection standards applicable to all in-state facilities killing or processing poultry, if the state's laws and standards did not meet the federal standards. The amendments also apply to poultry and poultry products that are distributed out of interstate commerce, totally within that state.

This amendment means that federal minimum standards for poultry slaughter and processing now apply to all facilities whether they operate fully and wholly within the boundaries of a state or operate freely over state lines. The inspections may be made by state inspectors, but the federal standards will apply. There are certain exceptions to the provisions of this law. When a facility killing and processing poultry is exempt under this law, it does not have to submit to daily inspections on a bird-by-bird basis from federal inspectors and it does not need to be operated under the aegis of a federal certification. Those facilities inspected by state inspectors may not be distributed outside of the state.

The most obvious exemption to the need for inspection applies to poultry slaughtered for personal use and also when the killing and processing are customized. It is thought that the consumers in the custom slaughter will be more able to make their own inspection. Additional exemptions are based on the size of production. Operations that raise fewer than 1,000 birds annually to up to 20,000 birds are exempt under the law. There are other exemptions.

The exemption only exempts a slaughterhouse from the requirements of the presence of federal bird-by-bird inspection. It does not exempt facilities from upholding the protections of the law for consumers. These smaller facilities must still comply with minimum standards set by the law. This means in particular that the poultry processed and produced by any facility that is intended for human consumption must not be misbranded and adulterated.

More than half of the states support state-based meat and poultry inspection programs. These state programs support approximate 2,000 small slaughtering and processing facilities. These facilities may not sell in interstate commerce, operating as they do, without federal inspection. Other food products that are subject to state inspection in compliance with federal standards are restricted to sales within the state.

Congress passed the PPIA because the market for poultry that was processed and ready for cooking grew quickly and the industry was seen as taking shortcuts that could adversely affect consumers. During World War II, demand for poultry increased sharply because of its availability and low cost. The U.S. military, concerned about the health and safety of the food that it fed to its troops, set its own standards and would only purchase poultry that was processed and complied with its standards. The **U.S. Department of Agriculture** agents regularly inspected poultry plants to determine whether operators were compliant with its regulations.

Further Reading U.S. Department of Agriculture. http://www.fda.gov/RegulatoryInformation/Legislation/ucm148721.htm.

William C. Smith and Elizabeth M. Williams

PREPARED FOODS, TAXES ON

Taxes on prepared foods are a sales tax imposed by state or municipal governments on food products meant to be consumed in the same location where they were purchased. Taxes on prepared foods are a tax on an item rather than an individual, so they are considered indirect taxes. Groceries are typically defined and taxed differently from prepared foods. Although definitions of groceries and prepared foods vary from state to state, there are some common, general definitions. Groceries are generally foods meant to be consumed in a location other than the location of purchase. A prepared food, in contrast, is typically defined as a food prepared for immediate consumption at the place of purchase. A prepared food can be considered a grocery item if it is a cold, prepared food meant to be reheated at home for home consumption. For states that tax these items differently, a grocery store with a dining area may have to charge sales tax on the items meant to be consumed there and no sales tax on the typical grocery items. Taxes on prepared foods vary by state and local government.

In 1921, West Virginia became the first state to impose a sales tax. By 1940, 30 states had a sales tax. By 2009, 45 states and the District of Columbia imposed a sales tax. Thirty-one states and the District of Columbia exempt grocery items from the sales tax. Although a state may exempt a grocery food item, it may not exempt prepared food items from the sales tax. Arkansas, Mississippi, Tennessee, Utah, Virginia, and West Virginia tax groceries at a lower rate than other products. The five states with no sales tax, and therefore no prepared food tax, are Alaska, Delaware, Montana, New Hampshire, and Oregon.

States differ in their definition and treatment of prepared food items. Texas requires that sales tax must be paid on individually packaged foods that are sold at the same register as prepared foods meant to be eaten on the premises if the store has a dining area. The idea is that the consumer also intends to eat these on the premises. In Texas and many states, a bakery item is not taxable until it is sold with a plate or eating utensils. Texas requires that sales tax be charged on all food kept hot and food sold with plates or eating utensils. Texas charges sales tax on food mixed from at least two ingredients and sold by weight or volume. Salad bar items are an example. Frozen sandwiches are exempt from sales tax in Texas, while other sandwiches are not. If food is expected to be reheated at home before consumption, Texas does not charge sales tax. Items that would qualify are the prepared food dinner items stored in a cold case. Those items are meant to be reheated and consumed at home. If food has simply been cut, pasteurized, or repackaged, it is not subject to sales tax and is still viewed as a simple grocery item in Texas.

A growing number of states impose what is known as a Streamlined Sales Tax. The Streamlined Sales and Use Tax Agreement (SSUTA) is an agreement between member states to streamline or simplify the different state sales tax laws. The Streamlined Sales Tax Governing Board is an organization that assists states in creating a more uniform sales tax system. States become members once they adopt and are in compliance with the board's guidelines. Rhode Island adopted the streamlined sales tax in 2007, changing its definition of prepared foods from one meant for "immediate consumption" to a definition recommended by the Streamlined Sales Tax Governing Board. Other states that are full members of the Streamlined Sales Tax are Arkansas, Iowa, Kentucky, Minnesota, Nevada, North Carolina, Oklahoma, South Dakota, Washington, Wisconsin, Indiana, Kansas, Michigan, Nebraska, New Jersey, North Dakota, Vermont, West Virginia, and Wyoming. Ohio, Utah, and Tennessee are scheduled to become full members by 2011.

Although not all states adopt the Streamlined Sales Tax, their definitions of prepared foods and groceries are similar to those described by the Streamlined Sales Tax Governing Board. The Streamlined Sales Tax Governing Board defines "prepared food" as a food that the seller serves or sells in a heated state. When two or more items are combined and sold as one item, that item is considered a prepared food. If these combined items are sold in an unheated state, they are not considered to be prepared foods if sold without a utensil or plate. Bakery items are not considered prepared foods until they are sold with utensils or on a plate.

Stephanie Jane Carter

PRICING

The price of food is determined by many factors. Traditionally, these factors have consisted of basic items needed to get products from the farm or manufacturer to the consumer. These basic items include cost to raise crops; land cultivation, and fertilizers; cost to feed animals; and slaughter and transport to customers. Pricing of food can be affected by bad weather, such as droughts or freezes. Food prices generally have remained steady since World War II with low rates of inflation and steady rates of economic growth.

In recent years, however, the price of food has been more turbulent. In 2007, for example, food prices rose by 4 percent, the highest rate since 1990. Higher prices of oil have affected food production, and many farmers in the Midwest are growing crops such as corn more for fuel than for consumption. Also, food reserves worldwide have decreased to meet consumer demand. Overseas, many countries have implemented price controls to avert food crises. The cost to produce food for human consumption has become much more complicated as the global economy has grown.

Contributors to rising prices of food and crops include soil and productivity losses from idled farmland that has been set aside as part of agricultural subsidies, and financial speculation that has eroded investment in food commodities. Other factors that affect pricing are as follows:

- *Cost of Fertilizer:* The price of oil and gas has increased in recent years, and because oil and natural gas are used in the manufacture of fertilizer, the cost of fertilizer has increased dramatically, in some cases doubling in cost. This increase in costs of fertilizer increases the farmer's costs and thus the cost of food.

- *Smaller Food Stockpiles:* In years past, many nations created economic policies that called for sizable food stockpiles. In recent years, stockpiles have been allowed to become smaller. Therefore, when events happen that affect the availability of a nation's food supply, countries have no ability to provide additional food to their citizens. Thus with decreased supply in general and increased demand, prices rise.

- *Additional Resources Needed:* In developing nations where food production has increased and more meat is being eaten, more resources are required to produce food. For example, the production of beef to keep up with new demand requires additional land, water, and grain. The additional resources cost more money which creates a rise in food prices.

- *Crops Grown for Biofuel:* Recently, farmers have cultivated crops for the purposes of fuel instead of food. An estimated 100 million tons of grain—primarily corn—have been grown for biofuel. The farm acreage formerly dedicated to raising crops has been taken out of circulation. The result is less food produced for consumption, especially in developing nations. This reduces supply and increases cost.

- *Rise in Consumption:* Consumption has risen in numerous countries, notably India and China. The rise of the middle class and a change to a more Western diet has created a demand for greater variety of foods and the eating of more food, that forces prices upward.

- *Protective Measures:* Some nations have imposed tariffs or blocked exports of food or crops to ensure they remain available for domestic consumption and to combat inflation. These protective measures add cost to the price and drive prices higher for nations that seek to import goods, and they isolate nations that try to protect internal markets.

See also: Appendix 7: *In the Matter of McCormick & Company, Inc.*

William C. Smith

PRISON FOOD

Prison food law differs greatly from the food law that applies to free citizens. Governed by the **Food and Drug Administration** (FDA), the **U.S. Department of**

Agriculture (USDA), **legislation** such as the **Federal Meat Inspection Act of 1906** and the **Pure Food and Drug Act of 1906**, numerous state and local agencies that regularly inspect food establishments for sanitation and safety, and others, the general public benefits from a complex network of what can collectively be termed "food law." However, these food laws are rarely applied to prison food. Prison food is overseen by the **court system** through decisions based on constitutional law and by voluntary self-regulation. There are some nonprofit accreditation organizations that provide oversight of the prisons that choose to participate in them.

Reasons for Differences between Food Law and Prison Food Law

There are several reasons for the differences between prison food law and food law for the general public. Theorists believe that the difference between the protection afforded the general public and the protection afforded prisoners stems from the punitive nature of prisons. Prisons are purposefully unpleasant. Other theorists question the role food plays in punishment. It is questioned whether inflicting obesity and food-borne illness is part of the punishment of inmates.

General food law is typically a product of consumers demanding legislatures to act. An obvious example is the actions after **Upton Sinclair** published his 1906 muckraking novel, *The Jungle*. The public was outraged and worried about the conditions in the meat industry. Congress quickly passed the Meat Inspection Act of 1906. As prisoners are a small percentage of the population, it is difficult for them to affect such change. Moreover, 48 states do not allow prisoners to vote. Similarly, inmates live controlled lives while the general public constantly makes choices in a highly competitive food market.

Although it can be argued that a system composed of rules created piecemeal through the courts may not be the best system, it can also be argued that the FDA is not suited for the task. Many methods the FDA employs to govern the food industry could not work in prisons. For example, the FDA recalls food found inappropriate for consumption. This only works in the marketplace. Press releases and recalls create bad publicity, making it in the company's best financial interest to improve or close its doors. Prisoners, unlike free citizens, cannot choose to eat or buy something else. As discussed, fines could only work if they were imposed on a private company running the food program in prisons. Otherwise, fines would simply move money between government agencies. The FDA tries to educate consumers to help them make better food choices. Again, inmates have few choices.

History of Prison Food Law

Prison food law is an outshoot of prison law, and it is difficult to discuss them as separate entities. Until recently, prisons were not used as a form of punishment in themselves, but as holding cells until the actual punishment could be administered. For 3rd-century Roman jurist Ulpian, prisons were for custody. This rule was restated in the 13th century by a British jurist known as Ralegh-Bratton. Colonial America continued to use prisons as a holding area. The French royal prisons in the 14th century were the only prisons known to have any regulation. The jailer was responsible for providing some food. The French prisons were also reported to have been inspected periodically. The punishments that the prisoners were waiting on usually involved shaming or execution. The Enlightenment changed some of the thinking about prisons and several writers questioned the use of execution for crimes that did not seem grave enough to warrant it. In the United States, William Bradford wrote a piece in 1793 entitled, "An Enquiry How Far the Punishment of Death Is Necessary in Pennsylvania, with Notes and Illustrations." During the 1800s, there were few attempts at prison reform, although several proposals were made in response to reports of overcrowding, filth, and not enough food. Prisons were governed exclusively by prison wardens. However, the courts began accepting claims in the 1960s under the idea that the prisons may be violating the Eighth Amendment, which prohibits cruel and unusual punishment. At the beginning, the courts heard only claims that involved prison discipline because that practice fell clearly within the lines of punishment. With that, the courts began creating some sort of prison law and prison food law. In the 1970s, the courts began hearing a wider range of prison practices, opening the gates to a flood of lawsuits. However, the Prison Litigation Reform Act (PLRA) was passed by Congress in 1996. Congress believed that the prisoners were filing frivolous lawsuits, tying up the courts' time, resources, and taxpayer money. They also thought that in some cases the courts overstepped their boundaries. The PLRA restricted prison litigation in what remedies could be had. Injunctions or consent decrees had to be strictly based on a federal right and had to be the "least intrusive" correction to the violation of a federal right. The PLRA also created a requirement that inmates pay a filing fee to file a claim. Moreover, a limit was placed on the attorneys' fees prisoners can claim if they succeed in their claims. The PLRA only allows inmates to file certain types of claims. A "physical injury" must have occurred for the inmate to file a suit. Also, there must be no other administrative remedy available before the suit can be filed. The PLRA had the effect of cutting back on court oversight and reducing the number of lawsuits brought by prisoners before the courts. If inmates can establish the denial of a federal right, they can file suit under 42 U.S.C. Section 1983.

As a result of this history, prison food law is litigated on the basis of the Constitution. Without mechanisms available in general food law such as fines, penalties, and laws, the courts offer an opportunity to enforce minimum standards in prisons. Many lawsuits stem from the Eighth Amendment prohibition of cruel and unusual punishment, yet many stem from the First Amendment rights to free speech, freedom of religion, and due process, and the Sixth Amendment right to counsel as part of the right to a fair trial. Suits have also been litigated on the basis of the Fifteenth Amendment right to refuse medical treatment. For sanitation and nutrition to be considered cruel and unusual, they would have to be objectively cruel and violate "contemporary standards of decency." Since contemporary standards of decency are constantly evolving, there is no static test for this. They would also have to meet the requirements of punishment. Prison officials would have to know about the conditions. Interestingly, the Eighth Amendment requires a minimum of adequate food. There has been criticism that protection awarded by courts is difficult for prisoners to obtain without proper knowledge of food safety. Others also note that this style of enforcement forces judges to become involved to a greater extent than they are equipped.

Today, prison food law is governed in three ways. First, the courts assume the role that the FDA plays in free society. Through litigation, the courts create some enforceable body of rules regarding prison food. Second, some prisons self-regulate by setting standards and complying with them voluntarily. There are several non-profits that publish standards to aid in this self-regulation. For example, the American Public Health Association requires an onsite dietitian to supervise the planning of nutritionally adequate menus. Third, accreditation is available. Accreditation organizations inspect the prisons to ensure that they are complying with their standards. At least 80 percent of state departments of corrections are involved. Some theorists believe that accreditation benefits the prisoners by providing regular inspections of prison facilities. Other theorists point to one of the stated goals of the accreditation organizations, that accreditation provides a defense against lawsuits by demonstrating a good faith effort to improve the conditions, and wonder whether the accreditation organizations are actually designed to benefit the prisoners.

Special Diets

Because prison food issues must be litigated in the constitutional realm, religious diets receive a large amount of protection through the first amendment right to freedom of religion. Special medical diets are also litigated under constitutional law. The American Diabetes Association notes that most diabetes cases are litigated under the Eighth Amendment prohibition of cruel and unusual punishment. In *Johnson v. Harris* (1979), the court ruled that it was cruel and unusual punishment when the prison failed to provide Paul Johnson with proper meals for a diabetic. The provided meals caused harm to Johnson, manifested in the amputation of a leg infected with gangrene. In some cases, for example, *Mullins v. Cranston*, courts have held that prisoners with special dietary needs must choose the correct foods on their own, rather than having a special tray prepared for them. In *Johnson v. Harris,* Johnson claimed that he would have to choose between eating harmful foods or not eating at all.

Hunger Strikes

The decision to not eat is also an issue in prisons. Hunger strikes are a form of protest by which the prisoner refuses to eat. If the hunger strike receives publicity, it can be a very effective tool of protest. The prison will receive negative publicity if a hunger striker dies. Hunger strikes have been ended by forced feeding of inmates. Although Guantanamo Bay in Cuba is not an example of a regular prison, hunger strikes by so-called enemy combatants garnered national attention in 2005. By September 11, 2005, 131 prisoners were reportedly on hunger strikes. The *New York Times* reported on February 9, 2005, that the strikers were restrained and force-fed. The military commander confirmed this report.

Hunger strikes are both a legal and ethical issue in prisons. A major issue has been whether physicians should force-feed hunger strikers. Although it may seem to be a question of preserving life or allowing suicide, many theorists believe this question approaches the subject in the wrong way. Most hunger strikers do not want to die. They are striking so that they may obtain a change.

In 2010, a Connecticut state judge ruled in favor of force-feeding an inmate who had been striking for over two years. In response, law professors filed an amicus brief claiming that forced feeding could violate constitutional and international law. The World Medical Association (WMA) Declaration of Malta states in Article 21 that force-feeding is inhumane and degrading. It further states that "forced feeding contrary to an informed and voluntary refusal is . . . never ethically acceptable . . . [and] feeding accompanied by threats, coercion, force, or use of physical restraints is a form of inhuman and degrading treatment." The American Medical Association is a member of the WMA but is not bound by it.

The constitutional issues can be found in the First Amendment right to free speech, which includes the right to protest. By force-feeding the prisoners, it effectively ends the protest, to which they have a right. Other parts of the Constitution seem to endorse force-feeding. The Eighth Amendment prohibition against cruel and unusual punishment obligates prisons to keep prisoners alive and not to demonstrate deliberate indifference if there is a substantial risk of serious harm. The **Code of Federal Regulations** states that the health and welfare of each inmate must be monitored and preserved. It would follow that forced feeding is allowable if this action is needed to preserve the prisoner's health and welfare.

What these guidelines and law seem to say is that if there is no medical need to force-feed strikers, then the strikers should not be force-fed. A medical need arises when there is cognitive decline and significant weight loss. Some theorists believe that the use of a restraining chair during forced feeding demonstrates that the prisoner is still strong enough. However, other theorists argue that cognitive decline can create the type of behavior that may warrant a restraining chair.

Nutraloaf

Nutraloaf, also known as food loaf, is a full meal in loaf form served to prisoners who have misbehaved. It is served without utensils on a piece of paper and is not part of the regular prison menu. Nutraloaf recipes vary by state. Illinois' nutraloaf is made from canned spinach, baked beans, tomato paste, margarine, applesauce, breadcrumbs, and garlic powder, whereas California's version is made with meat and fresh, natural ingredients. Vermont's nutraloaf comprises whole wheat bread, nondairy cheese, spinach, seedless raisins, beans, vegetable oil, tomato paste, powdered milk, and dehydrated potato flakes. Some prisoners have argued that nutraloaf is so unappetizing that it should be considered cruel and unusual punishment. They have also claimed that being served nutraloaf as punishment violates their due process rights. In *LeMaire v. Maass*, Samuel LeMaire's claim was denied because "the Eighth Amendment requires only that prisoners receive food that is adequate to maintain health; it need not be tasty or aesthetically pleasing." The cruel and unusual punishment claims are generally denied, but there is usually a restriction placed on how many consecutive days a prisoner can be subjected to the nutraloaf diet. The limit on how many days nutraloaf can be served and the recipe for nutraloaf vary by state. For example, Vermont limits the nutraloaf diet to one week. Other relevant court cases include a 1978 ruling by the Supreme Court that said a concoction similar to nutraloaf known as "gruel," may be cruel if served for weeks or months, but a few days is fine. In 1988, a federal judge ruled that the nutraloaf served by the Michigan Department of Corrections was punishment and that prisoners must go through a disciplinary process landing them in segregation before it can be served. A 2008 case in Vermont claimed nutraloaf violated due process rights. The Vermont Supreme Court also held that nutraloaf is served as punishment and that intention obligates the state to allow the inmate due process protections. Another restriction courts have placed on nutraloaf is that this punishment should only be used if the offence was related to food. Possible offences could be throwing food, using eating utensils to throw feces, or injuring an inmate or officer with eating utensils.

Last Meals

There is no legal requirement that special last meals be given before execution. However, it is customary in prisons to provide inmates a last meal of their choice before execution. The rules regarding the meals vary by state. Virginia limits the inmate to one of the meals in the 28-day cycle of meals the prison provides. The prison in Huntsville, Texas, tries to accommodate any request, making changes where necessary. One Huntsville inmate asked for 24 tacos, but only received four. Florida requires that the last meal must be purchased locally and that it must cost no more than $40.

The tradition of last meals demonstrates the importance society places on food. Last meals are of such interest to the public that the Texas Department of Criminal Justice posted the last meals on its Web site until people complained that it was offensive. The last meal it posted was in 2004. It is also common for a prison spokesperson to announce the last meal to the public. However, it is usually respected when a prisoner asks that his or her last meal not be announced.

Private Contracts with Prisons

Funding has been a consistent problem in the history of prisons. It has also been widely accepted that food in prisons can often be unsanitary and unhealthful. Many theorists point to the issue of funding as a cause of those problems. In fact, a 2003 article in the *Seattle Times* reported that there was a trend in legislatures pressuring prisons to reduce prison food expenses. Private companies that contract with the state to provide food in prisons often reduce costs in the prison system.

There are two general views on the private contracts. Private companies are profit-driven, so they are more motivated to save money. This motivation is often good news for under-funded prisons and for taxpayers. However, others point out that the very drive for profit may result in worse prison food conditions as the companies strive to cut costs. Aramark was a recent contractor in the Kentucky prison system. In 2009, a bill was proposed to cancel Aramark's contract with Kentucky prisons. Advocates of the bill point to inmate riots partially caused by the state of the food at the facility. Among complaints were grub worms found in the food. A prison official claimed that one grub worm was found and that it was promptly removed. Courts have constantly ruled that occasional foreign objects in food at prisons do not constitute cruel and unusual punishment. Those who criticized the bill pointed out that Aramark saved Kentucky at least $4 million dollars a year. A decision regarding House Bill 33 was expected in 2010, but it has stalled in the House Budget Committee. If the bill passed, it would limit food service to inmates, volunteers, and government employees.

Still, many believe that the elements of competition and the drive for profits may improve the food situation in prisons. After all, the contract could always be cancelled in the case of a sufficient breech. The kitchen would simply be taken over by another company. A problem many see with the government-run system is that fines levied in the marketplace in the case of a breech cannot be applied to government-run prison food programs because money would just move between government agencies.

See also: Diet Foods, Special; Kosher and Halal Labels; Litigation; Appendix 4: *Arnett, et al. v. Snyder.*

Further Reading American Diabetes Association. "Claims Related to Medical Care for Prisoners with Diabetes." http://www.diabetes.org/assets/pdfs/know-your-rights/for-lawyers/correctional-institutions/atty-prison-cases-memo1-11-10.pdf (Retrieved April 25, 2010); Greenwood, Alin. *Taste-Testing Nutraloaf.* Slate.com, June 24, 2008. http://www.slate.com/id/2193538; Howe, Patrick, *Cash-Hungry States Cutting Prison Fare.* The Seattle Times, May, 14, 2003 *Johnson v. Harris.* 479 F. Supp. at 335; *Lemaire v. Maass.* 1992 12F3d 1444; *Mullins v. Cranston* U.S. App. LEXIS 32580 (6th Cir. Dec. 9, 1999); Naim, Cyrus. "Prison Food Law." *LEDA at Harvard Law School* (2005.) http://leda.law.harvard.edu/leda/data/733/Naim05.html (Retrieved March 10, 2010); World Medical Association. *Declaration of Malta.* http://www.wma.net/en/30publications/10policies/h31/index.html.

Stephanie Jane Carter

PROBIOTICS

A "probiotic" is an expansive term referring to bacteria and other microorganisms that can be found in a number of food products and have generally been considered to be beneficial to human health. Knowledge of the functions of probiotics goes back several hundreds of years, as people used them to create and preserve foods such as dairy products, meats, and baked goods. In the early 1900s, more scrutiny was directed at the microbes in human bodies. Researchers determined that benign and helpful microbes could be introduced into the body through eating. They worked with the research of Bulgarian scientist Stamen Grigorov, which indicated that Bulgarian yogurt was fermented with the help of the starter culture *Bacillus bulgaricus.* They determined that the bacteria found in that particular yogurt and sour milk were not to be found naturally in the human intestinal tract. Researchers also observed that there were an extraordinary number of Bulgarians who were over 100 years old compared with people in other countries studied. They concluded that the consumption of the yogurt, with its special bacterial composition, was linked to the longevity of Bulgarians. The microbe was renamed *Lactobacillus bulgaricus.*

Fellow Institute scientist Henry Tissier was studying the presence of bacteria in children at the same time, and his research indicated that those children who were breast fed by their mothers had higher levels of the bacteria *Bifidobacterium bifidum* than children who were not breast fed. When he also discovered that sick children's stool contained fewer numbers of the *Bifidobacterium* than healthy children's, he suggested that treatment start with the administration of these bacteria. The work of these scientists indicated that specific microbes could be digested to improve the health of the intestines. It soon became apparent that it was almost commercially impossible at the time to create an ingestible bacteria formula that would help cure intestinal problems. Research continued through animals and occasionally people, but it did not take off particularly well until renewed studies in the United States indicated their benefits.

Nutritionist Werner Kollath seems to have coined the word "probiotic" in 1953 as he discussed the benefits of foods that contained helpful bacteria as opposed to harmful antibiotics. After that, the definition has been debated and hashed out, resulting in medical, pharmaceutical, and alimentary probiotics. Alimentary probiotics are used in food production and fermentation. The two strains first promoted by Metchnikoff and Tissier, *Lactobaccillus* and *Bifidobacterium*, have been most used to produce food and supplements that are probiotic.

There are many health claims for probiotic supplements and foods—from helping inflammatory bowel disease to diarrhea, eczema symptoms, bad breath, and respiratory problems. However, the lack of regulation in the claims of these products is beginning to become a problem as illness caused by food-borne microorganisms become more common. The World Health Organization and the **Food and Agriculture Organization of the United Nations** convened in 2001 to examine the health claims of probiotic foods and to determine what was accurate and appropriate for mass consumption. Following the study, the organizations determined that there should be a standard to judge and evaluate any product that claims to have beneficial probiotics. The groups formed a set of guidelines that addressed the basic problems. Basically, the probiotic had to be specifically identified, tested thoroughly, and labeled with information such as proper storage, minimum bacteria count left at the expiration date, and exactly what they claimed it would do. Even with these guidelines, there is no legal regulation regarding the labeling of probiotics in the United States.

Health officials are addressing the lack of regulation, and organizations are meeting to craft **Food and Drug Administration** (FDA) requirements for proper labeling, description, and evaluation of health claims. The number of ways that probiotics can be consumed means that the FDA will have to consider each possibility in a different category: food, drugs, and supplements. They introduced a regulation for "Dietary Supplement Current Good Manufacturing Practices and Interim Final Rule" in 2007 that required dietary supplements to be produced in a clean and consistent manner to maintain proper quality of the supplement. Probiotics have shown that they have promise to help with a variety of human health complaints, but further research and regulation seem to be necessary to monitor their quality and effects.

Further Reading FAO/World Heath Organization. "Probiotics in Food." ftp://ftp.fao.org/docrep/fao/009/a0512e/a0512e00.pdf; Rusch, Volker. "Probiotics and Definitions: A Short Overview." http://www.old-herborn-university.de/literature/books/OHUni_book_15 _article_1.pdf; Sonal, Sekhar P. "Probiotics: Friendly Microbes for Better Health." http://www.ispub.com/journal/the_internet_journal_of_nutrition_and_wellness/volume_6 _number_2_10/article_printable/probiotics_friendly_microbes_for_better_health.html.

Kelsey Parris

PURE FOOD AND DRUG ACT OF 1906

The Pure Food and Drug Act of 1906 (PFDA) was a product of its time. It was passed in tandem with the Meat Inspection Act of 1906 during the presidency of Theodore Roosevelt. The laws were a response to widespread lack of regulation that allowed the sale of products like patent medicines, which could be poisonous; allowed the sale of tainted and adulterated food; and allowed for mislabeling and unsanitary processing conditions. With more and more people living in cities and purchasing processed foods that could not be checked by simple inspection, the political climate was ripe for government regulation.

The law was applicable to both food and drugs, observing the thin line that may exist between them. It was a major expansion of the foreign and **interstate commerce** clause, banning adulteration and mislabeling in sale, production, and transportation. Notably the law provided for enforcement of the law in the form of seizure and destruction of products. It also provided for fines and jail sentences. This law led the way for consumer protection laws that followed and expanded through the 20th century.

The new act adopted the *U.S. Pharmacopoeia* (USP) and *National Formulary's* standards as the standard of the United States. This was significant because these standards were produced by private concerns and not created by a government agency. These books had respected standards of quality and were constantly being updated. These books set dosage standards and standards of purity. In addition these books set standard tests to verify the standards through product testing. For example, the 1906 law used the USP as the benchmark in defining an adulterated drug. That is, if it was found in the USP, but did not meet USP standards, the drug was adulterated. An exception was made for a drug that was labeled as not being in accordance with USP specifications.

This law was the first one that alluded to misbranding. Misbranding is labeling that fails to list certain addictive or dangerous drugs. This list included alcohol, found in many patent medicines; and various opiates like morphine and opium, found in "sedatives" and cocaine and "pick-me-up" patent medicines. A product was considered misbranded if any of the aforementioned substances, or others mentioned in the act, were contained in the products but the label did not list them or their amounts. It is significant that the law only applied to labeling and not to advertising of the product. Advertising regulations were to come later.

In the beginning, the enforcement of the law was tame by today's standards. The products that were previously sold as cure-alls, making "false and misleading" claims on their labels, were seized and destroyed. The sellers and manufacturers were generally fined. Claims that these products could cure many maladies, ranging from baldness to cancer, were rampant.

This law and the enforcement agency were the precursors to the **Food and Drug Administration** (FDA). Today, the FDA regulates food, drugs, biologics, medical and radiologic devices, diagnostic agents, and cosmetics. Its consumer protection role is massive and a critical part of the health of the citizenry.

The effort to enact the Pure Food and Drug Act was led by Harvey W. Wiley, who was the leader of the Bureau of Chemistry in the **U.S. Department of Agriculture**. He was concerned that there were unscientific claims made about the safety of certain preservatives. He wanted to find the effects of preservatives and know what quantities were safe. He created the "poison squad" in 1902. This was a group of volunteers who agreed to eat measured doses of preservatives in use at the time, such as formaldehyde and boric acid. They ate large doses of these and other preservatives and substances used to color food. The squad became ill from these experiments. Wiley became known as "the Crusader" because of these extreme experiments. The squad and Wiley were immortalized in song, and his experiments and the sacrifices of the squad had the intended effect. Manufacturers could not continue to make claims about the safety of the additives in food when clearly the poison squad had been made sick by ingesting them.

The Jungle by **Upton Sinclair** was published in 1906. The novel uncovered the dirty secrets about deplorable and unsanitary conditions of the meat-packing plants and slaughterhouses in Chicago. The book was graphic and direct, especially for its time, and its revelations made it a bestseller. Another result was that people stopped eating as much meat out of disgust and a fear of the unsanitary conditions. Readers were sickened by the descriptions of the conditions in the facilities—tubercular workers who spit on the floors and the casual disregard of the rot of meat all around. The fear of the contents of sausages was fueled by this book. The cries for reform became too much for Congress to ignore.

Critics charged that regulation was needed not only in the meat–packing industry, but also in other areas of consumer purchases. After the Civil War the sale of patent medicines became rampant. People took these medicines as a cure for many ills. It was an easy solution to many problems. These drugs were called "patent" because their formulas or recipes were secret, known only by the manufacturer. The reference to patent did not mean that the chemical formula had been patented. In fact the secret and proprietary nature of the formula was the justification for not labeling the package with the ingredients, thus those who used these products had no knowledge of their contents. The patent medicine industry was highly competitive, and this led to some of the most widespread national advertising campaigns. The advertising became important to the press, which also affected their reluctance to expose dangerous products. This factor slowed the spread of knowledge of the potential danger of these products.

Wiley created alliances with legitimate food producers and drug companies, the American Medical Association, the General Federation of Women's Clubs, and other consumer groups. The opponents of reform were those meat-packing facilities known as the "Beef Trust," the congressmen of the southern states who were concerned about federal erosion of states' rights, and the patent medicine manufacturers.

Although the act was difficult to enforce, had limited remedies, and was thwarted by industry, it was the beginning. Enforcement was made difficult by the high standard of proof required in court to have a product declared harmful. There was little money appropriated to monitor the entire country. One important victory was the elimination of what was known as the "dead horse racket." This term described the practice of the meat industry, which would send trucks around a town, pick up horses that were lying dead in the streets, return the dead horses to the butchering facility, and then sell the meat as beef. Wiley was unsuccessful in eliminating the sale of products containing caffeine, saccharine, and sodium benzoate, all of which he considered unsafe or addictive. Wiley is credited with eliminating cocaine from drinks known collectively as coca beverages. These included Coca-Cola. Caffeine was then substituted in those products so the drinker could continue to get the desired rush of energy.

The 1906 law was strengthened by the Food, Drug, and Cosmetic Act of 1938, which is now considered the most important legislation regarding food in the United States. The law is applicable to manufacturers of food, drugs, and vaccines for human beings and animals; medical devices; and cosmetics that are engaged in interstate commerce. After its passage facilities manufacturing these products were inspected. All aspects of the manufacturing process were covered. Each step in the process from raw materials, through manufacture and the final product, was subject to review for sanitary conditions and safe ingredient compliance. Enforcement expanded so that impoundment, fines, prosecution for intentional violations and fraud, and cease and desist injunctions became part of the arsenal.

As pharmacological advances were made, it became necessary in 1951 to amend the law further. This amendment made it illegal to sell drugs without a prescription when those drugs required medical supervision to be properly used. In 1958 another amendment provided for the burden to shift to manufacturers to prove to the FDA the safety of an additive before it could be legally used in a food or drug product. Consumer laws continued to be passed. In 1960 the law was amended again to provide for the safety of colorants used in food, drugs, and cosmetics. This began the controversial automatic congressionally mandated ban on products that were shown to cause cancer in animals. In 1962, the law was amended to require that drug companies prove not only the safety of their products, but also the effectiveness of the products. This caused the burgeoning of trials to prove effectiveness. Drugs, such as antidepressants and hallucinogens, which were subject to potential abuse, became subject to strict control and regulation through another set of amendments in 1965.

See also: Interstate Sales.

William C. Smith and Elizabeth M. Williams